A Casebook of Cognitive Therapy for Psychosis

This book is a unique volume in which leading clinicians and researchers in the field of cognitive therapy for psychosis illustrate their individual approaches to the understanding of the difficulties faced by people with psychosis and how this informs intervention.

Chapters include therapies focused on schizophrenia and individual psychotic symptoms such as hallucinations and delusions (including paranoia). Beck's original case study of cognitive therapy for psychosis from 1952 is reprinted, accompanied by his 50-year retrospective analysis. Also outlined are treatments for:

- bipolar disorder
- dual diagnosis
- schema-focused approaches
- early intervention to prevent psychosis
- adherence to medication.

This book will be useful to clinicians and researchers alike, and will be an invaluable resource to mental health practitioners working with individuals experiencing psychosis.

Anthony P. Morrison is Senior Lecturer in Clinical Psychology at the University of Manchester and coordinator of a specialist programme of care for people with early psychosis.

Contributors: Christine Barrowclough, Aaron T. Beck, Andy Benn, Richard P. Bentall, Max Birchwood, Alison Brabban, Jennifer Day, Hazel Dunn, Daniel Freeman, Paul French, Philippa A. Garety, Paul Gilbert, Gillian Haddock, David Healy, Peter Kinderman, Alice Knight, Shôn Lewis, Alan Meaden, Jan Moring, Fiona Randall, Julia Renton, Anne Rogers, Jan Scott, Nicholas Tarrier, Peter Trower, Douglas Turkington, Lara Walford, Steven Williams, and Pam Wood.

A Casebook of Cognitive Therapy for Psychosis

Edited by Anthony P. Morrison

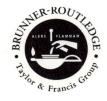

First published 2002 by Brunner-Routledge
27 Church Road, Hove, East Sussex BN3 2FA

Simultaneously published in the USA and Canada
by Taylor & Francis Inc.
29 West 35th Street
New York, NY 10001

Brunner-Routledge is an imprint of the Taylor & Francis Group

Typeset in Great Britain by RefineCatch Limited, Bungay, Suffolk
Printed and bound in Great Britain by Biddles Limited,
Guildford and King's Lynn

British Library Cataloguing in Publication Data
A catalogue record for this book is available from the British Library

Library of Congress Cataloging-in-Publication Data
A casebook of cognitive therapy for psychosis/edited by Tony
Morrison
        p. cm.
Includes bibliographical references and index.
ISBN 1–58391–205–3 (hbk)
1. Psychoses—Treatment. 2. Cognitive therapy. 3. Psychoses—
Treatment—Case studies. 4. Cognitive therapy—Case studies.
I. Morrison, Tony, 1969–.
   RC512.C367 2001
   616.89'142—dc21

                                        2001035706

ISBN 1–58391–205–3

Contents

List of figures and tables	viii
List of contributors	x
Preface by Anthony P. Morrison	xiii

PART I
Cognitive therapy basics   1

1 Successful outpatient psychotherapy of a chronic
   schizophrenic with a delusion based on borrowed guilt:
   A 1952 case study   3
   AARON T. BECK

2 Successful outpatient psychotherapy of a chronic
   schizophrenic with a delusion based on borrowed guilt:
   A 50-year retrospective   15
   AARON T. BECK

3 Cognitive therapy for paranoia   19
   JULIA RENTON

4 Cognitive therapy for psychosis: Emphasising engagement   37
   HAZEL DUNN

5 The search for meaning: Detecting congruence between life
   events, underlying schema and psychotic symptoms   59
   ALISON BRABBAN AND DOUGLAS TURKINGTON

PART II
Specific cognitive therapies for psychotic symptoms   77

6   The use of coping strategies and self-regulation in the
    treatment of psychosis   79
    NICHOLAS TARRIER

7   Shame, humiliation, and entrapment in psychosis: A social
    rank theory approach to cognitive intervention with voices and
    delusions   108
    MAX BIRCHWOOD, ALAN MEADEN, PETER TROWER,
    AND PAUL GILBERT

8   Cognitive therapy for drug-resistant auditory hallucinations: A
    case example   132
    ANTHONY P. MORRISON

9   Anxiety, associated physiological sensations, and *delusional*
    catastrophic misinterpretation: Variations on a theme?   148
    STEVEN WILLIAMS

10   Cognitive therapy for an individual with a long-standing
    persecutory delusion: Incorporating emotional processes into a
    multi-factorial perspective on delusional beliefs   173
    DANIEL FREEMAN AND PHILIPPA A. GARETY

11   Attributional therapy: A case of paranoia and hallucinations   197
    PETER KINDERMAN AND ANDY BENN

PART III
New developments in cognitive therapies
for psychoses   217

12   Cognitive therapy for preventing transition to psychosis in
    high-risk individuals: A single case study   219
    PAUL FRENCH, ANTHONY P. MORRISON, LARA WALFORD,
    ALICE KNIGHT, AND RICHARD P. BENTALL

13   Cognitive therapy for clients with bipolar disorder   236
    JAN SCOTT

14 Cognitive behaviour therapy for patients with co-existing psychosis and substance use problems 265

GILLIAN HADDOCK, CHRISTINE BARROWCLOUGH, JAN MORING, NICHOLAS TARRIER, AND SHÔN LEWIS

15 Enhancing appropriate adherence with neuroleptic medication: Two contrasting approaches 281

FIONA RANDALL, PAM WOOD, JENNIFER DAY, RICHARD BENTALL, ANNE ROGERS, AND DAVID HEALY

Index 299

Figures and tables

Figures

3.1 The generalised model of information processing changes
     following mood change   26
3.2 The personalised model of information processing changes
     following mood change   27
3.3 Adapted automatic thoughts records used in therapy   29
3.4 Adapted pie chart sheets used in therapy   31
3.5 Developmental formulation based on Beck's model of
     emotional disorders   34
3.6 Behavioural experiment form   35
4.1 Initial formulation maintenance cycles   47
4.2 Final formulation examples   56
5.1 A classical cognitive formulation of Helen's problems   70
5.2 The bucket-filling analogy describing the stress
     vulnerability model   71
6.1 Heuristic model of the determinants of positive psychotic
     symptoms   81
6.2 Factors that maintain negative self-schema in sufferers of
     severe mental illness   99
6.3 Problem and intervention sequences indicating coping
     methods and belief maintenance   101
7.1 Karen's delusional beliefs: Formulation   116
7.2 Harjinder: Formulation   120
8.1 Steven's PSYRATS delusions scores   138
8.2 Formulation for voices   143
8.3 Steven's PSYRATS hallucinations scores   145
9.1 Symptom level formulation   168
9.2 Longitudinal formulation   169
10.1 A multi-factorial model of the belief maintenance factors   183
10.2 Percentage ratings of delusional conviction   189
10.3 Personal questionnaire ratings of dimensions of the delusion   190

10.4   Depression and anxiety scores   191
11.1   A diagrammatic representation of the attributional model
        of paranoia   198
12.1   Model of development of early psychotic symptoms   224
12.2   John's PANSS scores   227
12.3   Initial formulation   229
12.4   Idiosyncratic model of emergence of psychotic symptoms   231
13.1   Beck's Integrative Model: Activation of the mode   238
13.2   Basic conceptualisation of bipolar disorder   240
13.3   A more detailed conceptualisation of bipolar disorder   242
15.1   Distress caused by BC's unusual experiences   291
15.2   Frequency of BC's unusual experiences   292

Tables

4.1   Early warning signs of relapse and strategies to be implemented   54
4.2   Pre- and post-treatment data   55
7.1   The ABC model   113
8.1   Steven's PANSS and PSYRATS scores pre- and post-treatment   135
8.2   Maintenance formulation for delusions   136
8.3   Maintenance formulation for voices   138
8.4   Evidential analysis for interpretations of voices   141
9.1   June's ratings for weeks one, two, and three   156
9.2   June's PSYRATS delusions scores   166
11.1   Formal symptomatic assessment using the PANSS and
       PSYRATS   203
11.2   Psychological assessments   204
12.1   John's prioritised problems and goals   230

Contributors

Dr Christine Barrowclough, Reader in Clinical Psychology, University of Manchester, Academic Department of Clinical Psychology, Tameside General Hospital, Ashton-u-Lyne OL6 9RW.

Aaron T. Beck, University Professor of Psychiatry, University of Pennsylvania, Department of Psychiatry, Room 754 Science Center, 3600 Market Street, Philadelphia, PA 19104–2648, USA.

Andy Benn, Principal Clinical Psychologist, Rampton Hospital, Woodbeck, Retford, Nottinghamshire DN22 0PD.

Professor Richard P. Bentall, Department of Psychology, University of Manchester, Oxford Road, Manchester M13 9PL.

Professor Max Birchwood, Director, Early Intervention Service, Harry Watton House, 97 Church Lane, Aston, Birmingham B6 5UG and University of Birmingham, Department of Clinical Psychology.

Alison Brabban, Consultant Clinical Psychologist, Maiden Law Hospital, Lanchester, County Durham DH7 0NQ.

Dr Jennifer Day, Department of Psychology, University of Manchester, Oxford Road, Manchester M13 9PL.

Hazel Dunn, Principal Cognitive Therapist, Psychology Services, Mental Health Services of Salford, Prestwich Hospital, Bury New Road, Manchester M25 3BL.

Dr Daniel Freeman, Department of Psychology, Institute of Psychiatry, King's College London, University of London, Denmark Hill, London SE5 8AF.

Paul French, Cognitive Nurse Therapist, Psychology Services, Mental Health Services of Salford, Prestwich Hospital, Bury New Road, Manchester M25 3BL.

Professor Philippa A. Garety, Department of Academic Clinical Psychology,

GKT School of Medicine, King's College London, University of London, Saint Thomas' Hospital, London SE1 7EH.

Professor Paul Gilbert, Mental Health Research Unit, University of Derby, Kingsway Hospital, Derby DE22 3LZ.

Dr Gillian Haddock, Senior Lecturer in Clinical Psychology, University of Manchester, Academic Department of Clinical Psychology, Tameside General Hospital, Ashton-u-Lyne OL6 9RW.

Dr David Healy, Reader in Psychological Medicine, University of Wales College of Medicine, Heath Park, Cardiff CF14 4XN.

Dr Peter Kinderman, Reader in Clinical Psychology, Department of Clinical Psychology, University of Liverpool, Whelan Building, Quadrangle, Brownlow Hill, Liverpool L69 3GB.

Alice Knight, Assistant Research Clinical Psychologist, Psychology Services, Mental Health Services of Salford, Prestwich Hospital, Bury New Road, Manchester M25 3BL.

Professor Shôn Lewis, School of Psychiatry and Behavioural Sciences, University of Manchester, Withington Hospital, Manchester M20 8LR.

Dr Alan Meaden, Department of Psychology, South Birmingham Mental Health Trust, Queen Elizabeth Psychiatric Hospital, Birmingham B15 2QZ.

Jan Moring, Clinical Psychologist, Psychology Services, Mental Health Services of Salford, Prestwich Hospital, Bury New Road, Manchester M25 3BL, and University of Manchester, Department of Clinical Psychology.

Dr Anthony P. Morrison, Senior Lecturer in Experimental Clinical Psychology, Department of Psychology, University of Manchester, Oxford Road, Manchester M13 9PL.

Fiona Randall, Department of Psychology, University of Manchester, Oxford Road, Manchester M13 9PL.

Dr Julia Renton, Clinical Psychologist, Psychology Services, Mental Health Services of Salford, Prestwich Hospital, Bury New Road, Manchester M25 3BL.

Professor Anne Rogers, Professor of the Sociology of Healthcare, National Primary Care Research and Development Centre, University of Manchester, Williamson Building, Oxford Road, Manchester M13 9PL.

Professor Jan Scott, University Department of Psychological Medicine, Gartnavel Royal Hospital, Glasgow G12 0XH.

Professor Nicholas Tarrier, Department of Clinical Psychology, School of Psychiatry and Behavioural Sciences, University of Manchester, Withington Hospital, Manchester M20 8LR.

Dr Peter Trower, School of Psychology, University of Birmingham, Birmingham B15 2TT.

Dr Douglas Turkington, Senior Lecturer and Consultant Psychiatrist, Department of Psychiatry, Royal Victoria Infirmary, Leazes Wing, Queen Victoria Road, Newcastle-upon-Tyne NE1 41P.

Lara Walford, Assistant Research Clinical Psychologist, Psychology Services, Mental Health Services of Salford, Prestwich Hospital, Bury New Road, Manchester M25 3BL.

Steven Williams, Cognitive Nurse Therapist, Psychology Services, Mental Health Services of Salford, Prestwich Hospital, Bury New Road, Manchester M25 3BL.

Pam Wood, Department of Psychology, University of Manchester, Oxford Road, Manchester M13 9PL.

Preface

This book is intended to illustrate the practice of cognitive behaviour therapy for psychosis in a clinician-friendly manner. It is a unique volume in which leading clinicians and researchers in the field of cognitive therapy for psychosis illustrate their individual approaches to the understanding of the difficulties faced by people with psychosis and how this informs intervention.

Each chapter contains an introduction to the theory concerned and has detailed clinical information regarding how this translates into therapeutic practice. Each chapter also contains information regarding assessment, formulation, and intervention components with reference to specific case material.

Chapters include therapies focused on individual psychotic symptoms such as hallucinations and delusions, as well as treatments at the cutting edge of current research for bipolar disorder, dual diagnosis, schema-focused approaches, and adherence to medication. The book begins with a re-examination of Beck's original (1952) case study (reprinted in full, with the permission of Guilford Press, New York), which was the inspiration for the other approaches outlined, with (in Chapter 2) his commentary on how he might approach the case now, almost 50 years later. Also in Part I are several chapters that illustrate many of the basic techniques and theoretical aspects of cognitive therapy. Renton's chapter illustrates how Beck's (1976) generic theory is applicable to working with psychotic patients, and Dunn's chapter focuses on the requirement of a sound therapeutic relationship. The chapter by Brabban and Turkington shows how Beck's schema theory is applicable to understanding psychosis and highlights the clinical implications of this.

Part II includes chapters that focus on the application of symptom specific theories. Many of the chapters show commonalities of approach as well as some interesting differences. Several of the chapters appear to be applying conceptualisations of psychosis that are derived from existing models of emotional disorders. Tarrier's chapter provides a theoretical basis for coping strategy enhancement that is rooted in the stress, appraisal, and coping literature, and goes on to show how this translates into practice. Birchwood and colleagues' chapter illustrates their application of Paul Gilbert's social rank theory of depression to the understanding and treatment of voices and paranoia. The chapters by Morrison and Williams show how specific cognitive models such as Clark's (1986) cognitive model of panic is applicable (with modifications) to formulating the development and maintenance of hallucinations and delusions and intervening accordingly. The chapter by Kinderman and Benn applies attribution theory, which has long been used in explanations of depression, to the theory and treatment of persecutory delusions, and Freeman and Garety incorporate factors related to both anxiety and depression in their attempt to provide a comprehensive framework for the same kind of difficulties.

The final part includes chapters that demonstrate how cognitive behavioural therapy is being applied to other difficulties faced by people with a psychotic diagnosis. The chapter by Randall and colleagues shows how cognitive behavioural principles can be used to enhance adherence to medication in a way that empowers patients. Haddock and colleagues' chapter shows how a combination of cognitive behaviour therapy, family intervention, and motivational interviewing can be a successful treatment for people with psychosis who also abuse substances. Scott illustrates how the generic cognitive model can be applied to understanding and treating bipolar disorder, and French and colleagues demonstrate how cognitive therapy can be used with people at high risk of becoming psychotic for the first time.

This book is intended to demonstrate the transition from theory to therapy in a way that will be useful to clinicians and researchers alike, and it should be an invaluable resource to mental health practitioners working with individuals with psychosis. It is hoped that it will encourage clinical psychologists, nurses, social workers, psychiatrists and occupational therapists to understand people with psychosis from a psychological perspective and help to inform the delivery of their interventions, whether psychological, social, or biological.

The contributors to this book represent the majority of the different groups of clinicians and researchers that have pioneered these treatments and the development of models for understanding the problems faced by people with psychosis. There have now been several randomised controlled trials of such approaches that have found very promising results and it is to be hoped that these treatments will be available to all people with a psychotic diagnosis in the near future. However, the current situation appears to be that it is only a select few who have access to such evidence-based psychological therapies, usually by virtue of geography, where there is a research trial being conducted or a critical mass of local expertise (Birmingham, London, Manchester, Newcastle and Southampton probably have a disproportionate amount of services for these reasons). Initiatives to ensure the implementation of these approaches do exist (the Thorn/COPE courses and Birchwood and colleagues' Initiative to Reduce the Impact of Schizophrenia, IRIS); however, much higher priority needs to be given to such implementation nationally. It is hoped that this book will make a contribution to ensuring such access for all.

Anthony P. Morrison
June 2001

Part I

Cognitive therapy basics

Successful outpatient psychotherapy of a chronic schizophrenic with a delusion based on borrowed guilt

A 1952 case study[1]

Aaron T. Beck

The increasing number of case reports of successful psychotherapy of patients with chronic schizophrenia has attested to the validity of this approach and has done much to dispel the former pessimism and skepticism (Arnow, 1951; Betz, 1946; Kellerman, 1949; Knight, 1946; Lafourge, 1936; Lindsay, 1948; Rosen, 1947; Sechehaye, 1951). Most of the papers, however, have dealt with hospitalized patients; relatively little has been written on the treatment of schizophrenia on an ambulatory basis.

This report of the outpatient psychotherapy of a chronic schizophrenic with paranoid delusions is presented because of three noteworthy features. First, although patients as acutely disturbed as this man would generally have been referred to a mental hospital, he was treated (for reasons to be described below) in a mental hygiene clinic where he was seen only once a week for a total of 30 interviews. With this arrangement, and without being removed from the setting in which his delusion was anchored, he experienced an almost immediate improvement in his general condition and level of functioning. Second, despite the fact that his delusional ideas were of seven years' duration, they proved to be amenable to interpretation and, as the patient gained insight into them, they faded away. Thirdly, a prominent mechanism in the formation of the delusion was found to be the phenomenon of "borrowed guilt", which has found scant attention in the literature (Lampl, 1927).

This report will include a discussion of the reasons for the favorable outcomes of the therapeutic venture, of the techniques that were employed, and of the dynamics of the delusional formation.

PRESENTING ILLNESS

A 28-year-old World War II veteran was first seen in February 1951 on a referral from his family physician who felt he needed immediate attention. At that time he reported his chief complaint as follows:

Fifty men, many of whom were in my outfit overseas, are now being employed by the FBI to investigate me. They appear one at a time in the store where I work and secretly observe my speech and behavior. They have concealed, somewhere in the store, an elaborate system of microphones that can pick up anything I say and, possibly, can even record my thoughts. They are trying to build up some case against me, the substance of which is unknown to me.

This idea first began to take form when he was overseas in 1944. It was preceded by obsessional thoughts that he had syphilis, that he looked like a "queer", and that he might stab somebody. Also, he experienced compulsions to use "blasphemous language" and to gouge his eyes out. Shortly afterwards he began to believe that 50 men in his medical outfit, whom he thought were actually encephalographic technicians, had been given the special assignment of looking after him and checking his movements. After he returned to the United States in 1946 and started to work in his father's small retail store, he spotted some of these men posing as customers. There also appeared, so he thought, to be a number of recent additions to the group. Although he assumed at first that their function was to protect him and look out for his interests, he felt a good deal of annoyance that they were going about it in this way, and that they would not admit what they were up to. When one of these men would enter the store, he would react in one of several ways. He would either put up his guard so as to prevent the man from detecting his real reactions, or he would try to imitate him—that is, he would respond to a smile with a smile, to a stare with a stare, and so on. He finally came to the conclusion that these men were actually FBI agents, and, a few months before starting therapy, he began to suspect that they were trying to convict him of something and were probably out to harm him.

Concomitantly, he began to experience severe episodes of anxiety, fears of going out of control, repeated nightmares, bizarre physical symptoms, and feelings of unreality. As his condition deteriorated he found himself unable to work, and, on the advice of his family doctor and his frantic parents, he sought help at the clinic.

BACKGROUND

The patient is the oldest of three children of foreign-born parents. His two married sisters show no gross evidence of emotional disturbance. The patient's father had encephalitis while serving overseas during World War I, and a few years later began to develop post-encephalitic Parkinsonism. This was slowly progressive until two years ago, since which time it has been fairly well controlled with drugs; his chief symptoms have been weakness of the right arm and leg, spasmodic blinking of the eyes, facial tics, and a constant state of drowsiness. The father is an outgoing person and is fairly well liked, but has shown signs of "weak character" at times by cheating in business, lying, and carrying on clandestine extramarital flirtations. The patient feels a good deal of shame about this and also suspects that his father may have associated with prostitutes in the past.

His mother is a highly moralistic, overprotective, fearful woman who has constantly reminded the children of all the sacrifices she has made for them and has placed great emphasis on integrity, duty, and achievement. She has never tired of demonstrating to them that she has exceptional judgement and foresight. The patient always felt that his mother knew what was best for him and that all of her predictions would inevitably come true. He came to believe that he didn't have a mind of his own. He was extremely attached to her and considered himself "tied to my mother's apron strings".

> In the course of therapy the patient gained some understanding of his strong need to idealize his mother and to assume a completely passive puppet-like role in the relationship with her. However, these feelings appeared to be too deeply buried to be accessible to scrutiny. On the other hand, his resentments towards his father were relatively close to the surface and could be mobilized and ventilated. Evidently the hostility towards his mother was of a more primitive and violent character and therefore had to be more vigorously defended against. Successful attempts to break through the repressions might have aroused a dangerously high level of anxiety and led to a further disintegration.

On the surface, the father and mother had a happy marital relationship, with the mother maintaining the dominant position and indulging the father's various needs in a maternal way. At times, however, she betrayed a contemptuous attitude towards her husband for his lack of success in business and his great dependence on her.

The patient was a sad, lonely, withdrawn child to the extent that contemporaries nicknamed him "Blue Boy". On his mother's caution he avoided contact sports and any other activity that might have exposed him to injury. He was not expected to perform any chores around the house; he recalls ruefully that his mother made his father, instead of him, take care of the garbage. He had at times almost overwhelming feelings of weaknesses, inferiority, and inadequacy. One of his most vivid memories is of being chased by a gang of rough boys in the neighborhood. Nevertheless, he got good grades in school and gradually developed a few close friendships.

The age of 13 stands out in his mind as a turning point in his life. At that time class work began to slip. He started to feel increasingly self-conscious, and he suspected from time to time, when called on for a recitation, that his teachers could detect his reactions, such as embarrassment, resentment, and competitiveness. He would then try to foil them by acting contrary to the way he was feeling. Despite his difficulties, he succeeded in getting through school without anybody suspecting that there was anything wrong with him. After graduating from high school he went to college for two years. He was drafted at about the time he felt he was developing self-confidence and forming rewarding friendships with other students. He served three years in the armed forces overseas and was discharged on the point system in 1946.

COURSE IN THERAPY

When first seen in the mental hygiene clinic, the patient appeared anxious and tense and in some distress over his paranoid obsessional ideas. He showed facial grimacing and verbal peculiarities. He spoke of feeling that he was falling apart, of being a Jekyll–Hyde personality, and of spells in which his mind was completely blank. Although he seemed to be very precariously balanced, the staff felt that it was worth taking the risk of treating him on an outpatient basis rather than recommending hospitalization. On the positive side he showed a fairly good preservation of intellectual functioning, a strong motivation for therapy, and a capacity to view his symptoms and experiences with some objectivity. Although there was some inappropriateness of affect, he was in general responsive and sensitive and revealed a fairly free play of emotional expression. The initial diagnostic impression was chronic schizophrenia, and this diagnosis was later supported by a battery of psychological tests, which showed numerous signs of chronicity and paranoid thinking.

The patient was seen for a total of 30 interviews over a period of 8 months. At the very beginning I felt a good deal of interest in and empathy for him. In the earlier interviews I was quite active in discussing his current problems with him, counselling him about his relations with other people, and recommending recreational activities. My role in this phase was predominantly supportive and educative. At the same time I was relatively non-directive in allowing him to bring up whatever he felt was important. He expressed a wish to go over his war experiences with me, and experienced a profound catharsis in bringing out his resentments toward the other members of his outfit who had belittled and humiliated him. He reported an almost immediate relief from his anxiety, feelings of depersonalization, and nightmares. After the third interview, he remarked that he felt that the FBI men would soon feel they had accumulated all the evidence they wanted, would decide that he wasn't guilty, and would "close the case".

The patient then expressed a strong inclination to understand the various elements in the development of his illness and began to survey his past experiences with a good deal of thoughtfulness and reflection. At the outset of an appointment that proved to be probably the most dramatic one, he stated that he wanted to tell me about a family secret that had tormented him for a long time and that he had never before confided to anyone. This had to do with disability compensation (for the sequelae of his encephalitis) that his father had begun to receive when the patient was 13 years old. He stated that when his father had first filed for the disability benefit he had made a false or misleading statement in the application. Each month thereafter when the check arrived, his parents acted in a very furtive manner, as though they were afraid that the circumstances of his father's dishonest act might leak out. The patient himself was under almost constant dread that a Federal investigator would be summoned to look into the case and would expose his father's misrepresentation. He recalled having experienced intense guilt over this, just as though he himself had committed perjury.

In presenting this material the patient spoke with a great deal of emotion. While describing his present feelings about his father's misdeed, he remarked that he now felt as bad about it as he ever did. He stated that he had been feeling worse ever since "the FBI men moved in and started checking on my father in the store". He went on to say that "they are coming in posing as customers and have planted microphones in the store to gather evidence against my father". He described his reactions to them as follows:

> When one of them comes in I cover up and make out I don't know what he's up to or else if he smiles, I smile back. If he stares, I stare back at him. . . . I wish they would leave him [his father] alone. He's such a good guy. Sometimes I suppose they know what a good guy he is and won't do anything to him. Maybe they're really looking out for him.

It was quite striking that this account was couched in practically the same language the patient had used previously in referring to the men who were supposedly assigned to investigate him. I promptly pointed this out to the patient. He appeared to be dazed for a moment and then with an expression of surprise he blurted out that somehow he had himself all mixed up with his father. As he tried to straighten this out he arrived at the conclusion that basically he must have thought the men were checking on his father, but in order to protect his father he had concealed this idea from himself by assuming himself to be the victim. We discussed at length how he had put himself into his father's shoes, had taken over the guilt for his father's dishonest act, and had expected punishment for it. At the end of this hour the patient declared that he felt he had really accomplished a great deal during the appointment.

Following this interview he discussed the disability insurance with his father and, for the first time, scolded him for always complicating things unnecessarily. His father reacted in a sheepish way, and the patient felt relieved that he had talked it out with him. This interview was, in retrospect, a turning point in the therapy. From that time on the patient found it increasingly easy to reject his irrational ideas. In the next few interviews he brought out a good deal of important historical material, which filled in many of the gaps in the original history and paved the way to further formulations and interpretations (described later).

It was easily recognized that one of the most critical periods in his life had occurred in his thirteenth year. It was at that time that he felt the full impact of the fact that his father was a sick man. Up until then the patient had been able to write off his father's tendency to doze off during the day as being due to "laziness", which was the explanation his mother had given. As his father's symptoms became worse, however, both the patient and his mother realized that his lethargy was due to his illness. In describing this, the patient remarked that as far back as he could remember he was always "revolted" at the sight of anyone who was physically handicapped, with the single exception of his father. It was also at that time that his father started to receive disability benefits, and the patient, learning of his father's misrepresentations, began to worry about exposure of this. He felt increasingly self-conscious in school, and he began to suspect that the teachers could perceive his feelings. Then he committed the first dishonest act in his life. Following the lead of a large group of other students, he cheated on an examination, and was caught. Because he was the only one who was caught, the principal decided to make an example of him and suspended him from school for a short period.

At about the same time he developed a fascination for mystery movies and experienced particular relish when the hero was falsely accused of some crime but was, in the end, vindicated. Finally, in the same year, he developed occasional involuntary blinking of his eyes. Although his father had had the same symptom for many years previously, the patient had not been consciously aware of it; in fact, it was only two or three years before the time of his therapy that the patient first recognized this symptom in his father. Sometime after the acquisition of this first symptom, the patient began to show grimaces that closely paralleled his father's facial tics. The patient's two years in college were characterized by a desperate and partially successful attempt to become a "real person" and to gain a sense of belonging. He showed a strong tendency to "ape" the other men in his fraternity house and to adopt their mannerisms, their style of speaking and joking, and their values. In looking back at this year in college, the patient stated reminiscently: "I was really well liked, I had 50 good friends then".

The patient made a fairly good adjustment in basic training in the army, but after he was shipped to the European theater he started running into difficulties. The men in his medical unit had backgrounds that were completely different from his, and they impressed him as being rugged, crude, and almost barbaric in their values and behavior. His old feelings of not belonging, not being wanted, and being different were reactivated. He felt threatened by these men and at times was alarmed at the thought that they might attack him while he was asleep and "make me sterile". He was also haunted by the idea that he had syphilis (although he had never had any sexual experiences), and he made weekly visits to the medical officer for a physical examination and a blood test. At about this time he was also distressed to learn that his father had lost his job for an alleged theft and was being employed as an elevator boy at a wage of $18 a week.

The patient felt somewhat better when he was temporarily detached to a small station where he worked with only two other men. He made a strong effort to neutralize his fears of being a "queer" by plunging into intense heterosexual activity. He selected a German woman many years older than himself and began to have sexual relations with her every night. One night, however, her face seemed to take on the form of his mother's. He was startled by this, became impotent, and immediately began to be plagued with two sets of "vile thoughts". The first was that he should gouge his eyes out, and the other thoughts, which he labeled as "blasphemous", consisted of a constant repetition of an Italian expression meaning "God is swine", which he had learned from some other man in his outfit. Later, when he was reassigned to another medical unit that was about to return to the United States, he began to experience almost constant anxiety and intense feelings of loneliness. At this time he started to feel that the other men considered him a "queer". His feeling gradually expanded into the conviction that the men were watching him.

In the patient's presentation of this material it appeared that several of his autistic ideas were closely linked. His obsession that he had syphilis had occurred after he had seen the routine army movies on venereal disease. The part of the movie that had impressed him the most dealt with central-nervous-system syphilis. In discussing this he recalled having had a vague thought that syphilis of the nervous system was the same thing as encephalitis, although he knew from his scientific training that this was not so. Then, in describing a group of technicians who he had felt were watching him, he first referred to them as "encepha-something". The word encephalographer was suggested, and he responded that that was what he was thinking of. Once, in referring to them, he made a slip of the tongue that sounded like "ensyphilitics". He felt that their function as encephalographers was to treat people with diseases of the brain by means of electric shocks.

As certain prominent themes became clear, I pointed them out to the patient and later developed them more fully. One of the central interpretations was that he had identified himself with the weak side of his father and had adopted many of his father's physical and emotional characteristics—for example, his involuntary eye-blinking, his physical weakness, and his feelings of helplessness. I also suggested that as he himself began to feel more and more helpless he must have longed for somebody strong to bolster him up and to look after him. He supported this by citing a few examples of his need to turn to strong figures for support. I then suggested that when his need for protection became intensified in the service, he turned desperately to the idea that a group of men were looking out for him. He accepted this formulation tentatively, taking the attitude that it sounded logical but he wasn't sure about it. In subsequent discussions, however, he indicated that this explanation was beginning to feel more real and convincing to him.

The persecutory aspect of his delusions was discussed, first in terms of the borrowed guilt—his need to assume the responsibility for his father's misdemeanors—and then as an expression of his own feeling that he should be punished for his own weakness. His borrowed guilt extended also to his father's qualities, such as his father's general slyness and his extramarital flirtations. In discussing this he was able to release some resentment toward his father.

During the period when the content of the delusion was discussed and interpreted, the patient only rarely experienced the feeling of being watched. On the occasions when he would start to suspect that one of his customers was an agent, "I would reason myself out of it". He reported that he was able to narrow down the original group of 50 to 2 or 3 possibilities and that he felt he would soon be able to eliminate them completely. In the 10 months following termination of therapy, he did not have any recurrence of his delusional ideas.

In one of his last appointments he expressed considerable optimism about the future and was in the process of evolving plans for obtaining some on-the-job training in writing advertising copy, for which he had a special talent. His outlook at that time was expressed in the following statements:

> Since I was 13 I have been completely arrested. I had one maladjustment after another. It was a lapse of time just like Rip Van Winkle's. Now I'm moving again and I'm making the right adjustments. I'm not feeling inferior or out of place any more. I've got my feet on the ground.

DISCUSSION

Several factors may be advanced to explain why this patient, with a chronic psychotic disorder and a recent acute decompensation, was able to respond favorably to outpatient psychotherapy at weekly intervals. First, his ability to relate to other people was sufficiently preserved to permit a working therapeutic relationship practically at the outset. He showed a fairly good measure of adaptiveness, spontaneity, and sensitivity, all of which favored emotional communication. Secondly, despite the strong disorganizing tendencies, he retained sufficient intellectual integration to take some distance from his autistic productions, to define his difficulties, and to examine meaningfully his life experiences. He was also able to identify and verbalize his feelings as well as to grasp the interconnection between external stresses, emotional responses, and symptoms. Thirdly, his delusional ideas had not substantially invaded his relations with his family and friends or severely damaged his reality situation. In addition, he had sufficient resources to resume his job, to expand his social life, and to take up new activities, all of which served as integrating forces and fulfilled important needs. Finally, his delusion had not completely "set"; it had a certain plastic quality that spoke for its reversibility. Although it is true that it had taken on a more malignant aspect as indicated by the persecutory overtones, this was of relatively recent occurrence.

The major force in the therapeutic process appears to have been the emotional experience between patient and therapist. Important components in the therapist's attitude were a strong liking for and interest in the patient. No fixed system of therapeutic techniques was employed other than an attempt to perceive the patient's needs and to deal with them in a flexible way. At first this took the form of reassurance and guidance with his environmental problems, and later of clarification and interpretation of his distorted and conflicting attitudes toward himself and others. As the level of the patient's tensions and anxieties was reduced, he was able to relax his pathological defenses, to discriminate more sharply between fantasy and reality, and to discard many of his autistic attitudes. It appears that his insight into his delusional ideas played a major role in their disappearance.

Despite the relative paucity of childhood material, it is possible to reconstruct the development of the patient's illness from the time of his adolescent crisis. He entered adolescence as a somewhat withdrawn, passively oriented, timid boy. His mother, with her numerous methods of control, had prevented him from developing any sense of autonomy and had instilled in him a rigid set of moral values. His father, who served as the chief model for identification, was broken by physical illness and showed many traits that were in conflict with the patient's own strict standards. His identification with his father was not a completely stable one and as late as his college years he was still struggling to find a mold to fit himself into. In addition, in place of having a strong father whose strength he could draw on, he was expected to provide the emotional support for his father. In the army, his old feelings of loneliness and lack of sense of identity were revived. Furthermore, he had to cope with particularly intense aggressive and homoerotic impulses that were stimulated by his role as a soldier and by his close proximity to other men. In this setting his delusion developed.

The delusion itself can be analyzed like a dream, in terms of the imagery, the latent content, and the dynamic processes employed. Although not all of its aspects can be traced back to their origins, the patient provided enough clues to explain many of its elements. In elucidating the significance of the *encephalographers*, one finds the following pertinent material: (a) the close linkage of *syphilis*, *encephalitis*, and *encephalographer* (as connoted by the condensation "ensyphilitics"); (b) the conception that syphilis causes encephalitis, and the underlying theme that promiscuity is punished by disease (as affirmed in the movie on venereal disease); and (c) the association to encephalographers, that "They treat brain disease with electric shock".

With this data we can construct the following sequence. As he became aware of his father's infidelities the patient deduced that his father's encephalitis had resulted from a syphilitic infection that he must have acquired from an extramarital contact while overseas in World War I. According to his characteristic mode of assuming the responsibility for his father's deeds, he assigned the guilt for this "sin" to himself. When the patient was placed in a similar situation in World War II, his impersonation of his father was consolidated and became manifest in his fantasy that *he* had syphilis: he, then, was the guilty one. The encephalographers entered the picture to determine whether he was really guilty and, if he was, to punish him with electric shock. The latent thought, thus, is: "I am assuming the responsibility for father's sin and these men will observe me to decide whether I shall be punished".

The transition of the group of encephalographers into FBI agents is a continuation of the same theme. As I have previously pointed out, the choice of FBI agents was conditioned by his long-standing fear that the government would prosecute his father for his dishonesty. The patient's feeling of guilt, however, was probably abstracted not from a single "immoral" act by his father, but from the latter's sporadic unscrupulousness and infidelities. The selection of the number 50 in the delusion can be linked to the *50 close friends* he fantasized he had in college. This association gives the delusion a somewhat different twist. It is as though the patient is trying to reassure himself: "These men in the group are my friends. They are here to help me not to harm me". This element thus served as a check against the persecutory aspect of the delusion.

From the standpoint of the dynamic mechanisms involved, the delusion may be regarded as a composite picture arising from a fusion of the following elements: first, the projection of certain feelings that were consciously repudiated and repressed (including his rage and homoerotic impulses); secondly, the fantasized wish fulfilment of his strong longings to be cared for and be protected; and thirdly, the fantasized punishment for fantasized crimes, which embodies the mechanism of borrowed guilt.

The phenomenon of borrowed guilt has been seldom described. In one case reported by Lampl (1927), a patient developed his guilty feelings because his father's affair with a mistress represented the satisfaction of his own unconscious wishes. He thus acquired, by means of identification, his father's guilt and his life from then on was dominated by an immense need for punishment. The dynamics appear to be more complicated in this case. On the one hand, the pressure from his overbearing and punitive superego pushed him to repudiate or condemn any moral frailties in his father, as well as in himself. This was particularly disturbing because the idea of censuring or resenting his father was intolerable to him. On the other hand, it appears that he found gratification of his own repressed impulses by participating vicariously in his father's conniving tactics and sexual escapades. His solution to this dilemma was to take over completely the responsibility for his father's act and to assign the guilt and need for punishment for himself. The delusion in this instance served the dual role of providing a means of expiating his borrowed guilt and a method of concealing his critical attitudes and hostile feelings towards his father by projecting these feelings onto others and then making himself the victim. The formulation was confirmed by the patient's almost immediate emotional response to the interpretation that he had identified himself with his father and assumed his father's guilt. With this insight he was able to drop this defense and, for the first time, to express some resentment towards his father.

SUMMARY

A case of chronic schizophrenia with a delusion of seven years' duration is presented as an example of the favorable outcome that can be obtained when selected patients, such as this one, are treated in an outpatient clinic on a one-visit-a-week basis. Despite the long-standing nature of the delusion it proved to be interpretable to the patient. The factors contributing to the favorable outcome, the course in therapy, and the dynamics of the personality disorder and the delusion have been discussed. The mechanism of borrowed guilt, which assumed an important role in the delusion formation, has been described as the central core of the illness. The good outcome in this case suggests that careful appraisal of even chronic schizophrenics may permit the selection of treatable cases, and that the presence of chronicity and delusion formation is not invariably ominous for the prognosis.

REFERENCES

Arnow, E.J. (1951). The Influence of an intense transference on a schizophrenic patient. *Bulletin of the Menninger Clinic*, *15*, 100–106.

Betz, B.J. (1946). Experiences in the psychotherapy of obsessive-schizophrenic personalities. *Southern Medical Journal*, *39*, 249–257.

Kellerman, E.A. (1949). Psychotherapy with favorable outcome in a chronic schizophrenic. *Psychiatric Quarterly*, *23*, 96–107.

Knight, R.P. (1946). Psychotherapy of an adolescent catatonic schizophrenia with mutism: a study in empathy and establishing contact. *Psychiatry*, *9*, 323–339.

Lafourge, R. (1936). A contribution to the study of schizophrenia. *International Journal of Psychoanalysis*, *17*, 147–162.

Lampl, H. (1927). A case of borrowed sense of guilt. *International Journal of Psychoanalysis*, *8*, 143–158.

Lindsay, D.S. (1948). Psychotherapy in schizophrenia. *Canadian Medical Association Journal*, *59*, 142–144.

Rosen, J.N. (1947). The treatment of schizophrenic psychosis by direct analytic therapy. *Psychiatric Quarterly, 21*, 3–37.

Sechehaye, M.A. (1951). *Symbolic realization: A new method of psychotherapy applied to a case of schizoprenia.* New York: International University Press.

NOTES

1   This paper was reprinted, with permission, from Beck (1952). Successful out-patient psychotherapy of a chronic schizophrenic with a delusion based on borrowed guilt. *Psychiatry, 15*, 305–312.

Chapter 2

Successful outpatient psychotherapy of a chronic schizophrenic with a delusion based on borrowed guilt

A 50-year retrospective

Aaron T. Beck

Although 50 years have passed since I treated this patient (see Chapter 1), I am surprised to note how close my thinking about the nature of psychotic symptoms was then to what it is today. If I were treating this patient today, I would develop the conceptualization of the case as a framework for the therapy much earlier in the treatment process. In the actual treatment, my conceptualization unfolded as the therapy progressed and, as I shall explain, served as a major component in promoting the improvement. My current approach would be to draw initially on the presenting phenomenology and then attempt to fit it into the generic cognitive model. I would, for example, extract the data relevant to the patient's self-image and images of other people, particularly outsiders. I would then establish and define the interaction between his sense of vulnerability and his misperception of being under surveillance by others. I would also attempt to pinpoint the patient's beliefs (e.g. "I appear weak"), and specify how these beliefs made him hypersensitive to other people's expressed criticisms and negative attitudes. In conjunction with this, I would explore how these beliefs developed during adolescence, and later were applied erroneously to ambiguous situations he encountered as an adult (for example, customers entering the store).

The phenomenology of the patient's disorder can be readily recognized in the description of his life history, delusions, and behaviors. One can discern specific threads running through childhood, adolescence, and adulthood that are woven into the fabric of his delusions. In his early years he perceived himself, and was perceived by others, as different and apart from his peers. The label applied to him, "Blue Boy", helped to solidify this devalued self-image. Presumably, the relative social isolation not only deprived him of corrective feedback for his various misinterpretations but also failed to provide an opportunity for learning the interpersonal skills required for a more rewarding social adjustment. Consequently, the patient's own sense of self was unstable and poorly formed. In misguided attempts to compensate for this deficient sense of self, he was prone to extrapolate and incorporate specific characteristics of other people, particularly his father.

In terms of cognitive structure, he failed to develop stable representations (schemas) of other people that would enable him to read or interpret accurately their verbal and non-verbal behavior. It is likely that during his development he did not develop the skills necessary to read other people's intentions accurately. His appropriation of his father's weakness, physical problems, and moral failings was facilitated not only by his permeable self-image but also by its congruence with his own pre-existing self-image of weakness, deviance, and vulnerability. Consequently, under the stress of army life, he reverted to a pre-formed "theory of mind" that other people watched and demeaned him.

The instability of his self-image also led to his assuming characteristics of other people. The patient, for example, attempted to fortify his shaky self-image by imitating his peers. His experience of a sense of guilt over his father's failing was perhaps accentuated by his internalizing his mother's strong code of morality. In addition, the patient was highly imaginative, and, like many psychosis-prone individuals, lacked the skills to reality test his imaginary ideas. Thus, when he felt that the teachers could read his mind, he accepted this as a fact, without attempting to evaluate its validity. The sense of malleability of his mind was an aspect of his self-image of a puppet.

As the patient gradually developed psychotic features, his information processing became increasingly more egocentric. The interaction of his own sense of vulnerability with his mixed view of his fellow soldiers crystallized into the largely self-conscious belief that they were not only watching him, but were also watching *over* him. Although this benevolent view served for a while to compensate for his sense of powerlessness and vulnerability, it could not endure because of the background images of his peers as rejecting. The latter images became activated by noxious experiences with other soldiers and carried over into civilian life. Thus, the delusion that crystallized when he returned home contained elements of his fear of punishment for his father's presumed misdeeds as well as concern over the continued antagonism of his fellow soldiers.

Unfortunately, the published version of his case history does not include information regarding any specific precipitating event that led up to the patient's decompensation (fears, agitation) so it is not possible to present a formulation regarding this aspect of his breakdown.

In summary, the patient's self-schemas were so poorly defined that he expropriated the images of another person—his father. Similarly, his schema of outsiders was expanded into a broad image ("50 people watching me"). When this schema was energized, the specificity of other people as individuals was erased and superseded by a broad category, namely FBI men. The interaction of his self-image with that of the outsiders was expressed dramatically: he was powerless, exposed, and guilty, and the outsiders (the

"FBI men") were powerful, intrusive, and punitive. Perhaps, his identification with his father and the consequent fear of reprisal was activated by his continuous contact with his father in the store.

THE THERAPY

What was responsible for the improvement in this case? Because the patient was not taking antipsychotic medication (it had not yet been introduced), it is reasonable to assume that psychotherapeutic intervention played a decisive role. As I implied in the paper, my therapy with him had a soothing effect and the guidance not only provided practical benefits but also conveyed the notion that he was being looked after by a protective authority figure— something that he yearned for. The more specific interventions, namely interpreting his delusions in the context of his life history, provided a plausible *explanation* for the delusion: customers only seemed like FBI men because of his previous experience. Consequently he could accept the notion that he was misinterpreting the behavior of the customers.

The use of "alternative explanations" was made explicit in later writings (e.g. Beck, 1963). Also, although my interpretations of "borrowed guilt" prompted the patient to examine the perceived persecutors more closely, the strategy of focusing on delusions was not described until much later (Hole, Rush, & Beck, 1979).

In the light of my experience in recent decades, I would make the following changes in my therapeutic approach. First, I would follow the systematic structure of the interview as outlined in *Cognitive Therapy of Depression* (Beck, Rush, Shaw, & Emery, 1979). This structure, which has been generally used by cognitive therapists treating schizophrenia (including myself in the past year) consists, briefly, in setting an agenda, employing Socratic questioning, providing capsule summaries at intervals, eliciting feedback, and assigning homework. More specifically, I would encourage the patient to focus on the specific characteristics of the FBI men and attempt to define the features that differentiated them from other people.

In addition, I would stimulate his practicing making alternative explanations. What other motives could prompt the men to come to the store? What other reason could account for any one of them being out on the street? While attempting to sharpen his reality-testing in this way, I would also try to help him build up a more stable self-concept through a number of procedures. For example, I would engage him in completing a daily activity schedule in which he would rate his mastery experiences.

I would also have the patient focus on positive beliefs about himself, such as "I can control my own life", and look for evidence that helped support this belief. I might also employ imagery techniques, like having him imagine the way he perceives himself now (weak, helpless, vulnerable) and the way he would like to be (presumably, strong and self-reliant). Finally, I would conduct role-plays designed to empower him through assertive and social skills training.

Although I learned a great deal about this case through active questioning and guidance, I believe that the therapy could have been shortened if I had been able to apply some of the current approaches. A streamlined approach based on the cognitive model might also have provided a stronger foundation for a long-term recovery.

REFERENCES

Beck, A.T. (1963). Thinking and depression: Idiosyncratic content and cognitive distortions. *Archives of General Psychiatry, 9*, 324–333.

Beck, A.T., Rush, A.J., Shaw, B.F., & Emery, G. (1979). *Cognitive therapy of depression*. New York: Guilford Press. (Also published in Chichester: John Wiley & Sons, 1980.)

Hole, R.W., Rush, A.J., & Beck, A.T. (1979). A cognitive investigation of schizophrenic delusions. *Psychiatry, 42*, 312–319.

Chapter 3

Cognitive therapy for paranoia

Julia Renton

This chapter is dedicated to the client it refers to, who took his own life prior to publication. He had worked hard to utilise cognitive therapy and was excited when asked if his case could be written up in order to aid the learning of other professionals. His mother also wishes for the publication of this chapter in the hope that others who work with psychotic people might learn from the work completed and from the questions that his suicide raises.

THEORETICAL PERSPECTIVES

Cognitive therapy was devised by Aaron T. Beck in the early 1960s as a structured, short-term, problem and present-oriented psychotherapy for depression. It is described by Beck, Rush, Shaw, and Emery (1979) as "an active, directive, time-limited, structured approach used to treat a variety of psychiatric disorders (for example, depression, anxiety, phobias, pain problems, etc.)".

From observation of his patients, Beck hypothesised that irrationality could be understood in terms of inadequacies in organising and interpreting reality. In a paper in 1963, Beck writes that "the schizophrenic excels in his tendency to misconstrue the world that is presented . . .". While the validity of this statement has been supported by numerous clinical and experimental studies, it had not generally been acknowledged at that point that misconstructions of reality may also be a characteristic of other psychiatric disorders. Thus, based on his clinical experience, he expounded the view that psychological problems were not necessarily the product of "mysterious, impenetrable forces" but rather the result of faulty learning, making incorrect inferences on the basis of inadequate or incorrect information, and not distinguishing adequately between imagination and reality.

Thus, cognitive therapy is based on an underlying theoretical rationale that an individual's affect and behaviour are largely determined by the way in which they structure the world (Beck, 1976). Their cognitions (verbal or pictorial "events" in a person's stream of consciousness) are based on attitudes or assumptions (schemas), developed from previous experiences. Thus, Beck (1976) writes that "psychological processes can be mastered by sharpening discriminations, correcting misconceptions, and learning more adaptive attitudes". Thus, he commented, "since introspection, insight, reality-testing, and learning are basically cognitive processes, this approach to the neuroses has been labelled cognitive therapy".

However, it is important to note that, while the *means* of cognitive therapy is focusing on the patient's misinterpretations, self-defeating behaviour, and dysfunctional attitudes, the *goal* is the relief of emotional distress and other symptoms of emotional disorder. The therapeutic techniques of cognitive therapy are designed to identify, reality-test, and correct distorted conceptualisations and the dysfunctional beliefs underlying these cognitions. The patient learns to master problems and situations, which they previously considered insuperable by re-evaluating and correcting their thinking. The cognitive therapist helps the patient to think and act more realistically and adaptively about their psychological problems and thus reduces symptomatology.

Thus, in the broadest sense, cognitive therapy consists of all the approaches that alleviate psychological distress through the medium of correcting faulty conceptions and self-signals. As mentioned earlier, the emphasis on thinking should not obscure the importance of the emotional reactions, which are generally the immediate source of distress. It simply means that one can get to the person's emotions through their cognitions, and that by correcting erroneous beliefs one can dampen down or alter excessive, inappropriate emotional reactions (Beck, 1976). Beck (1976) continues that this can be done, first, via the "intellectual" approach, consisting of identifying the misconceptions, testing their validity, and substituting more appropriate concepts, and secondly, via the "experiential" approach, namely, exposing the patient to experiences that are in themselves powerful enough to change misconceptions.

Inherent within the practice of cognitive therapy are the main principles or features of this therapy that should enable practitioners to maximise their treatment efficacy and adherence to the model. Several authors—not least Beck himself (Beck, 1952)—have developed approaches to psychosis incorporating some or all of these principles (e.g. Chadwick, Birchwood, & Trower, 1996; Fowler, Garety, & Kuipers, 1995; Kingdon & Turkington, 1994; Morrison, 1998). A brief description of these principles follows.

Primarily, cognitive therapy is based on the cognitive model of emotional disorders and is thus theory and model-driven rather than a collection of techniques. Both the model and individual conceptualisations are explicitly shared with the patient throughout therapy.

Secondly, cognitive therapy is educational and collaborative. This means that the patient and the therapist agree on targets and then set out ways in which these can be achieved.

Thirdly, cognitive therapy aims to be time limited, the important feature being the explicit time limitation that is given to the patient with reviews being used to collaboratively decide on the need for further intervention. Within this time limited format, explicit and realistic targets or goals are collaboratively set, which are assessed by both parties to be appropriate for the decided number of sessions.

Fourthly, cognitive therapists primarily use the Socratic method (guided discovery). That is to say, that instead of providing answers to the patient's questions or problematic negative automatic thoughts, the therapist asks questions that help patients to provide their own answers. By utilising this therapeutic strategy, the patients will have an understanding of the process of therapy, rather than purely the results, and can therefore be active participants in their own recovery and relapse prevention.

Fifthly, a sound therapeutic relationship is a necessary condition of good cognitive therapy. A patient must be able to feel that she or he is able to trust the therapist and will be taken seriously by the therapist.

Finally, cognitive therapy is structured and problem-oriented. Each session starts with setting an agenda decided on by both the therapist and the patient, specifying which problems will be tackled within the session and any educational information that needs to be taught. The therapist will help the patient to identify the obstacles that hinder him or her in problem solving; either skill deficits or dysfunctional ideas that impede the use of previously acquired skills. Alongside this, "homework" is always given at the end of the session and should involve a task that is relevant to the present therapy task and decided on in collaboration. The homework should thus not only be relevant for the patient's progress in therapy, but also enable them to understand the process of therapy and therefore determine future directions for implementing their learned therapeutic techniques.

CASE EXAMPLE

Shaun, a 32-year-old man, was referred due to his persecutory beliefs that ruled much of his life. He believed that people were plotting against him and wished to "get into his mind to make him kill himself".

Pre-therapy assessment of psychotic symptoms

On his independent pre-therapy assessment, Shaun scored six on the delusions subscale of the PANSS and seven on the suspiciousness and persecution subscales, indicating a level of suspiciousness and persecution that impinged on his daily living and did not allow him to live independently. He did not, however, hear voices and was not thought disordered. On the delusions rating scale his conviction in his beliefs was 100%, and preoccupation with and duration of preoccupation was almost constant.

Reasons for referral

Shaun was referred to the service following his admission to the psychiatric hospital after he had taken an overdose. At this point his fears of conspiracy had become so widespread and his resultant anxiety so high that he had attempted to take his own life. He had gone by train to Wales, walked six hours into the hills and taken 100 paracetamol and 25 Melleril. He was only discovered because, following taking the tablets, Shaun had vomited and thus, thinking his overdose would be rendered ineffective, telephoned his mother and told her what had happened. His family were then able to notify the local police about his circumstances and whereabouts, who then found him.

Initial presentation

At the initial meeting, Shaun presented as highly anxious and agitated and, although not thought disordered, difficult to understand due to the incorporation of all events into his delusional belief. His description of his difficulties and present circumstances was littered with delusional explanations for everyday events. On route to the appointment, for example, the yellow car that had passed him meant that he was a coward and therefore the conspirators were going to continue until he had a heart attack. The letter that had been received earlier that week from the bank was also a warning. Shaun described how this new "blue" card was a reference to the fact that he had visited the home ground of his football team (blue strip) prior to going to Wales. Therefore, this advertising leaflet was not what it seemed; rather, it meant the conspirators were warning him to "leave the city now".

Shaun was mainly compliant with his medication regime but believed that the receptionists at his general medical practice were involved in the conspiracy and, therefore, found visiting the practice very difficult. Shaun's conviction in his delusional beliefs was 100% and had led to difficulties while on the wards. At this point, he believed that one of the nursing staff was involved in the conspiracy. He believed that her not saying hello on passing him in the corridor had meant she was trying to make him kill himself, and had led him to push her resulting in his transfer to a locked ward.

The development of a problem and goal lists

At the initial interview, the therapy began with the development of problem and goal lists to allow a collaborative and shared understanding of current difficulties and the desired outcome for these problems. The idea of this was sold to Shaun as a "map" for therapy to guide progress from current problems to a shared set of goals. Therefore, following an initial discussion of problems, these were then pulled together in session so that a shared problem list could be established.

Problem list

1   *His worries about conspiracy*: Thinking that everyone is plotting against him to cause him harm or to "get into his mind" so that he will harm himself. Believing that people follow him and that shopkeepers say things to him as a warning. Also, children playing in the street and taxi drivers are a warning to him to leave the city. Belief in both past and present theories 100%.
2   *Finding it difficult to go out*: Concerns and subsequent anxiety render it very difficult to leave the house.
3   *Not meeting people*: Finding it difficult to talk to other people due to his suspiciousness about their motives.
4   *Getting tongue-tied with friends and colleagues*: Again, this relates to his fear about the involvement of others in the plot to do him harm. However, Shaun told me that some of this related to levels of social anxiety that predated his delusional beliefs.

Goal list

His corresponding goals, again identified during the session, for each of the main identified problems were:

1   To find out more about what's going on and to be able to wake up and not feel watched.
2   To be able to socialise.
3   To do some voluntary work.
4   To have more confidence in himself.

Early experience

Shaun (35) was the eldest of two brothers born to Deirdre and Fred, who were still living together. He described having good childhood memories and enjoying primary school. He found making friends easy and made a best friend at secondary school. He recounted being big for his age and, therefore, never being threatened or bullied in any way.

Shaun described being "sensitive" and "a bit touchy" as long as he could remember although is unsure as to when this began. He described his mother as being similar and easily upset, although felt that this had not had any major effect on him. He told me that his mother believed Shaun to have a low opinion of himself, but was unsure as to whether this was true, although did describe always believing that people did not like him.

Shaun recounted that he attended secondary school regularly during the first three years, but on beginning the fourth year began to "play truant". He told me he would "hang out and chill" with his best friend in the country where they "dabbled" with magic mushrooms and speed. When questioned about his motives for missing school, he described being influenced by his friend who had since died through drug misuse. Shaun accounted that over the course of his final years at school, he attended for only half of the time, was put on report, and thus failed most of his CSEs. He described not being unduly upset at the time (although regrets this now) and told me that this did not cause any difficulties at home.

Shaun left home at 15 and began work with his father for a building firm. When he reached 16, the firm sent him on day-release to college as part of a youth opportunity scheme, but he told me that this reminded him of school and, therefore, he "wagged" it and was sacked. He then got another job and youth opportunity scheme place with a landscape gardener, which he enjoyed immensely and attended. However, after six months when he was about to graduate, he was made redundant because the company preferred to employ another trainee on a youth opportunity scheme rather than have a full-pay worker. Shaun described being devastated at this and, for the next four years, he entered numerous other training schemes and community programmes.

Onset of difficulties

During this period, Shaun described continuing with his recreational hallucinogen and amphetamine use at the weekends along with a group of friends. At age 21 Shaun began working with a building firm, which he very much enjoyed. Things continued smoothly until age 23 when he went on holiday to Morocco with a girlfriend. It was on this holiday that he began to smoke cannabis. He broke up with this girlfriend on returning to England but continued to smoke cannabis. He told me that pretty soon his life began to revolve around cannabis and he would smoke during the day and all evening: he began by smoking about one-eighth of an ounce a week, but this soon rose to about half an ounce. He withdrew from all social activity, stopped going out, and stopped seeing his old friends. Instead he associated only with others for whom smoking was their whole life.

At age 26 he was made redundant from work, although he believed this to be due to his personality change. He recounted becoming paranoid, very difficult and cheeky at work and told me that the quality of his work had suffered. Following this, Shaun was on the dole and doing bits of work that his friends found for him. Shaun recounted that each of these jobs ended in the same way with him becoming paranoid and leaving the job having fallen out with his boss and colleagues. He described the paranoia as "having taken over my whole life" at this point, and told me that every time he left the house he would have to carefully plan his route in advance.

At age 29 Shaun visited his GP who referred him to a psychiatrist. He was prescribed Melleril, which he felt (at the time) did not help, and thus stopped taking it. The following year, Shaun found a permanent job and began working as a driver. At this point he became paranoid about a conspiracy against him. Shaun recounts how five years earlier he had made a complaint against a chain of bookmakers following placing a bet. The horse he had backed won overseas, and, while the bookmakers had offered him odds of 20–1, he read in the papers that the odds overseas had been 100–1. Following this, he told me that he lodged a complaint with the bookmakers and, after an investigation, he believed a woman had been sacked directly as a result of his complaint. Shaun told me that following this incident he became convinced that this bookmaker, other bookmakers, his employer and colleagues, local shopkeepers, and residents had joined forces to punish him for the loss of this employee's job.

At this point, Shaun described thinking that everything he saw was related to him. He felt that the taxis driving past his house, cars, pedestrians and children playing were all there in order to give him a warning and a message. He left his job and again went to his GP. While waiting for an appointment to see the psychiatrist, he got up one morning, looked at the taxis and cyclists, told his mother that he had trodden on the toes of too many people and that, as a result, had no option but to go to Wales and kill himself. (His mother let him go out of disbelief.) At this point he went to Wales, buying paracetamol at the pharmacy on route, walked for six hours into the hills and took 100 paracetamol tablets and 25 of his Melleril. He began vomiting and, believing that the tablets would not work as a result, telephoned his parents to say he was coming home. They in turn, contacted the police who were able to locate Shaun and take him to hospital.

Cognitive therapy

Following the identification of problem and goal lists, Shaun prioritised working towards finding out more about what was going on with respect to his fears of conspiracy as his first goal.

We began therapy by examining one particular incident that had happened that morning which was bothering Shaun. In looking at the relationship between a particular event, Shaun's interpretation of it, and his resulting emotion, we were able to understand that rather than being a particular comment that caused him to feel anxious (see the example of the chemist's remarks in Fig. 3.3), it was the way in which he interpreted the situation. From that we were able to generalise the model into an understanding that interpretations affect the affective response to any given situation. Using the given example, we looked at the evidence that supported his thoughts that the chemist's words had been directed at him and the evidence, which did not fit with this.

Additionally, during this session we began to discuss the information processing biases that accompany mood changes. Shaun felt this to be highly relevant to his situation and felt that once anxious, he would remember negative interpersonal interactions, notice all personal glances and nuances of tone and intonation, and interpret everything as relating to him. We generalised this model to show how negative interpretations of situations caused him to become anxious and, once anxious, how he remembered negative information, noticed negative events in his environment, and interpreted ambiguous information with a negative bent. Once the model had been generalised and we had looked at the evidence regarding his main concerns of the morning, Shaun expressed some flexibility of his beliefs. He felt that it was possible (albeit a very low probability—about 1%) that it was thoughts rather than facts that led him to the conclusion the chemist was giving him a warning. See Fig. 3.1 for the initial model regarding information processing changes following mood change and the resulting impact on anxiety. See Fig. 3.2 for the personalised model (taken from Shaun's experience) of information processing changes following mood change and the resulting impact on anxiety.

Once some degree of doubt was introduced into the equation, Shaun was eager to look at the facts surrounding many of his past and present concerns. Therapy began by helping Shaun to examine the evidence surrounding some of his present concerns, which in turn, increased his conviction in his theories of conspiracy. Alongside this, we began to examine some of the processes that might affect the way in which information is processed once Shaun had

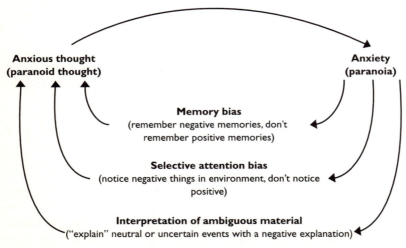

Figure 3.1 The generalised model of information processing changes following mood change.

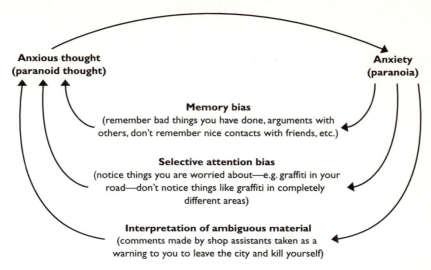

**Anxious thought
(paranoid thought)**

**Anxiety
(paranoia)**

Memory bias
(remember bad things you have done, arguments with
others, don't remember nice contacts with friends, etc.)

Selective attention bias
(notice things you are worried about—e.g. graffiti in your
road—don't notice things like graffiti in completely
different areas)

Interpretation of ambiguous material
(comments made by shop assistants taken as a
warning to you to leave the city and kill yourself)

Figure 3.2 The personalised model of information processing changes following mood
change.

become anxious. Shaun thought this to be highly relevant to his situation; he
felt that he was continually scanning his environment to look for clues as to
the conspiracy, and was therefore eager to look at the evidence for his
concerns.

Therapy proceeded by gaining more understanding of these attentional
and interpretative biases. We began to look at magazine horoscopes (which
Shaun did not believe in) and to discover how, if one was looking for significance, that one would be able to discover it in a vague paragraph of writing.
We used this to discuss how things could be perceived as significant in different ways by different meaning, but might be said or written without any
specific person in mind and not meant to convey hidden meaning.

The work helping Shaun to evaluate the evidence for his concerns and thus
their accuracy was done using standard forms designed in therapy. Two
standard forms were used for this process: (a) the adapted automatic
thoughts diary; and (b) adapted pie chart records.

Adapted automatic thoughts diary

This was used to allow Shaun to fully understand the process of therapy,
and thus to continue to implement such strategies outside of the therapy
situation. Shaun was first shown how to evaluate evidence supporting and not
supporting his beliefs. He was taught how to use only factual "court room"
observable evidence rather than interpretation, and to use this to reinterpret

the accuracy of his concerns and any effect this reinterpretation had on his anxiety (see Fig. 3.3).

Adapted pie chart records

These were used to allow Shaun to evaluate all possible explanations for an observed event and to rate all of these by relative probability. He was asked to write down his paranoid interpretation of the event and, in the later list of possible explanations, to place this interpretation as the final possibility. Following this, Shaun would generate alternative explanations for the event and, starting from the top, allocate a percentage of the pie chart (and thus total probability) that this interpretation would account for the event. He would then use the result to reinterpret his initial interpretation and anxiety (see Fig. 3.4).

These forms were also reassessed at the beginning of each session in order to create a metacognitive shift—that is to say, in order to challenge Shaun's belief that his interpretations of the situation were always correct and factual. Rather, a different belief—that, due to anxiety, he may interpret things in a more threatening manner than the reality of the situation—was tested as an alternative hypothesis.

The development of an historical perspective

Alongside the models and strategies used to evaluate the accuracy of his current concerns, therapy continued to look at the development of his difficulties and used this to create a developmental formulation. This was to allow Shaun to view another explanation for the creation of his problems rather than one that surrounded the events at the bookmakers.

The formulation (see Fig. 3.5), based on Beck's model of emotional disorders, looked at how earlier experiences had led to the development of beliefs and rules, which when triggered by a critical incident had led to the activation of these rules and, from there, to an upsurge of paranoid thoughts increasing his anxiety and further exacerbating his information processing biases. Shaun agreed that his early experience did somewhat "set him up" for becoming paranoid, and was adamant that his increased marijuana use played a large role in this (he had not smoked marijuana since his last admission, nor had he used any other recreational drugs). But he still believed that his previous employers and the bookmakers had been involved in a conspiracy against him due to his complaint about the odds given him on the bet.

However, once Shaun was able to consider present situations that caused him anxiety, he felt able to look at the events surrounding the development of his paranoid beliefs and the beliefs he held regarding the conspiracy against him. The process began similarly but continued with a series of behavioural

Event: Went to the chemist on the way to appointment. The chemist said "I'm getting a swing bin". She also sold Ribena.

Anxious or paranoid thought

> When she said "I'm getting a swing bin" she meant "You are rubbish—hang yourself". The bottles of Ribena were meant to be my blood and be a warning to me.

Belief at time 75%
Anxiety at time 75%

Evidence supporting the anxious or paranoid thought	Evidence NOT supporting the anxious or paranoid thought
She looked at me when she said it.	It's ignorant not to look at someone you are serving.
They had bottles of Ribena on the counter.	She might have been trying to be friendly.
They began to tidy up when I went	Staff tidy up the shop to keep it presentable or else people would go and shop elsewhere.
	Staff tidy up to look busy in case the boss comes.
	The chemist could have been saying I'm getting a swing bin to the other woman in the shop, but looked at me because I just walked in.
	Most chemist shops sell Ribena. It is a popular product.
	Popular products are often put on display.

How much do you believe the anxious or paranoid thought now? 60%

How anxious are you now? 60%

Do you think this was a fact or just a thought?   Thought

Is there another, better explanation for the situation?

Figure 3.3 Adapted automatic thoughts records used in therapy.

Event: Waiting for an appointment at surgery. Listening to receptionist on telephone.

Anxious or paranoid thought

People at the GP's surgery want me to leave their surgery and kill myself.

Belief at time 100%

Anxiety at time 100%

Evidence supporting the anxious or paranoid thought	*Evidence NOT supporting the anxious or paranoid thought*
They are abrupt with me.	It can be a very long day for them.
They talk on the phone using phrases I can relate to.	I often go in the afternoon.
They make me wait even when the surgery is empty.	Other patients ring the surgery up and those phrases could also be relevant to their questions.
They won't let me phone for a repeat prescription.	Doctors are very busy and they do see me when I need an appointment.
	Phone lines are for appointments and ill patients. Maybe they have to see me for a new prescription.
	They continue to see me and give me sick notes; they could force me to leave by not giving these to me.
	They have not asked me to leave the practice.
	They still always give me my tablets and check out how I am.

How much do you believe the anxious or paranoid thought now? 60%

How anxious are you now? 60%

Do you think this was a fact or just a thought?

Is there another, better explanation for the situation?

Figure 3.3—contd

Event: Doctor gets my prescription wrong.

Anxious or
paranoid
thought

> The doctor is doing this
> deliberately as the surgery
> no longer wants me as a
> patient.

Belief at time <u>65%</u>

Anxiety at time <u>65%</u>

Are there any other factors that might explain the actual event?

Write these down, leaving your initial explanation as the last one.

1. They have a lot of patients and can easily make mistakes.

2. I have to take a lot of tablets and this can be confusing.

3. My medication has gone up and down loads over the past few years.

4. If doctors want you to go they cannot do this by messing up your tablets.

5. Doctors don't discuss patients so mistakes are likely to be genuine.

6. The doctor is doing this deliberately because they don't want me as a patient any more.

For each explanation (starting
from number one), rate how
much (out of 100%) of what
happened could be explained by
that factor:

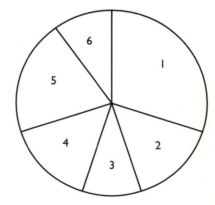

1 = 30%; 2 = 15%; 3 = 10%; 4 = 15%; 5 = 20%; 6 = 10%.

Figure 3.4 Adapted pie chart sheets used in therapy.

Event: People ask me how my parents and my dog are. They are always
very polite.

| Anxious or paranoid thought | They are telling me that something is going to happen to them. | Belief at time <u>50%</u>

Anxiety at time <u>50%</u> |

Are there any other factors that might explain the actual event?

Write these down, leaving your initial explanation as the last one.

1. They might just be being friendly.

2. Everyone in the neighbourhood knows our dog.

3. My mum and dad are popular in our area.

4. People know that I always walk the dog.

5. People often ask how elderly people are.

6. People who know I've been very ill probably don't
   know what to say to me.

7. They are telling me that something is going to happen
   to them.

For each explanation (starting from number one), rate how much (out of 100%) of what happened could be explained by that factor:

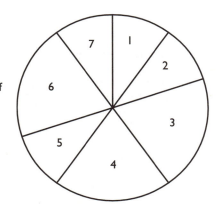

1 = 10%; 2 = 10%; 3 = 20%; 4 = 20%; 5 = 10%; 6 = 20%; 7 = 10%

Figure 3.4—contd

Event: Taxis, cyclists and people down my road, near my house.

Anxious or
paranoid
thought

> Handsel Trading want me to leave the city; they have sent taxis, hikers, cyclists and people with flowers down Stacy Road, near my house.

Belief at time 70%

Anxiety at time 70%

Are there any other factors that might explain the actual event?

Write these down, leaving your initial explanation as the last one.

1. Stacy Road is a main road.

2. Taxis are used by a lot of people.

3. It is the time of year for people to buy flowers.

4. I live near the country where hikers walk.

5. People cycle in warm weather.

6. Stacy Road leads to the whole estate.

7. It's directed at me, to get at me.

For each explanation (starting from number one), rate how much (out of 100%) of what happened could be explained by that factor:

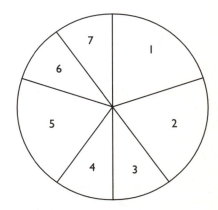

1 = 20%; 2 = 20%; 3 = 10%; 4 = 10%; 5 = 20%; 6 = 10%; 7 = 10%

Figure 3.4—contd

"Early" experience
Played truant, led by friends, no qualifications
"Sensitive" nature always; thought people out to get me
Difficult economic times, many youth opportunity schemes; did not work out
Early recreational drug use; turned to frequent drug use

Formation of beliefs
People are out to get me
The world is uncaring/watch your back

Formation of dysfunctional assumptions
If you "tread on people's toes", they will get you
If you don't keep your guard up, others will get to you
If you cause trouble for others, then they will get back at you

Critical incident
Increase in marijuana use; remember past
event where complained against an employee

Assumptions activated

Negative automatic thoughts

Information processing changes
Memory, selective attention and interpretation of ambiguity

Anxiety

Figure 3.5 Developmental formulation based on Beck's model of emotional
disorders.

experiments designed to further test this out. Shaun avoided all bookmakers
and other shops, which he believed to be involved in the conspiracy. He
thought that should he enter any of these premises he would be ordered out
of the shop and trouble would ensue. Once Shaun's conviction in such beliefs
had been reduced, he felt able (with the therapist present) to begin to frequent
these establishments to ascertain whether his feared catastrophe would occur.
This information would then be used to help Shaun decide on the accuracy of
his beliefs regarding the conspiracy against him.

Shaun began by drawing up a hierarchy of those premises that he would
find difficult and his predictions of what would happen in each of them. This
process was made more difficult by the fact that he felt that in many of them
his warning to leave would be in code and might only happen after he
had frequented the premises for a number of weeks. Descending from most
difficult to least difficult, Shaun's resulting hierarchy was as follows:

- Going to place a bet in a betting shop.
- Entering certain shops in the local area.
- Going into a busy pub.
- Going to a fast food chain.
- Going for a haircut.
- Speaking to someone I don't know.
- Going to the doctor's surgery.
- Answering the telephone.

At the time that this book was in preparation, this component of therapy (behavioural experiments) was just beginning (see Fig. 3.6). However, Shaun

Behavioural experiment

Feared situation:

What do you think will happen if you go into this situation?
How much do you believe this? __%

How could you test this out?

What might get in the way?
How could you prevent this from happening?

EXPERIMENT: What did you do?

What happened?
Did your prediction come true?
What can you learn from this about your concerns?

Figure 3.6 Behavioural experiment form.

was able to come up with specific predictions and, although fearful, had expressed a willingness to find out more about the accuracy of his predictions and thus the premises on which they were based. These behavioural experiments were, however, planned by client and therapist to begin in January. Unfortunately, Shaun took his own life over the Christmas holiday.

Retrospective discussion

Whether he had had a setback, the millennium experience had proved overwhelming, a specific incident had occurred exacerbating his paranoia, or the fight had become too difficult, we can only guess. However, in keeping with his pleasure at being asked to be written up as a case study, I have chosen to include this chapter in the book to remember an inspirational person.

REFERENCES

Beck, A.T. (1952). Successful outpatient psychotherapy of a chronic schizophrenic with a delusion based on borrowed guilt. *Psychiatry*, *15*, 305–312.

Beck, A.T. (1963). Thinking and depression: Idiosyncratic content and cognitive distortions. *Archives of General Psychiatry*, *9*, 324–333.

Beck, A.T. (1976). *Cognitive therapy and the emotional disorders*. New York: Meridian Books.

Beck, A.T., Rush, A.J., Shaw, B.F., & Emery G. (1979). *Cognitive therapy of depression*. New York: Guilford Press.

Chadwick, P., Birchwood, M., & Trower, P. (1996). *Cognitive therapy for delusions, voices and paranoia*. New York: Wiley.

Fowler, D., Garety, P., & Kuipers, E. (1995). *Cognitive behaviour therapy for psychosis: Theory and practice*. Chichester: Wiley.

Kingdon, D.G., & Turkington, D. (1994). *Cognitive behaviour therapy for schizophrenia*. Hillsdale, NJ: Lawrence Erlbaum Associates Inc.

Morrison, A.P. (1998). Cognitive behaviour therapy for psychotic symptoms. In N. Tarrier, A. Wells, & G. Haddock (Eds.), *Treating complex cases: A cognitive behaviour therapy approach*. Chichester: Wiley.

Chapter 4

Cognitive therapy for psychosis

Emphasising engagement

Hazel Dunn

INTRODUCTION

Cognitive therapy has been successfully used to treat a range of emotional disorders over the past 30 years. Beck et al.'s (1979) model of cognitive therapy highlights the way an individual's emotions and behaviours are largely determined by the way that person structures his world. Evaluative cognitions are based on the person's attitudes or core beliefs, which themselves are a product of previous experiences.

While cognitive models and therapy were experimentally used to explain and treat emotional disorders, there appeared to have been little activity in relation to schizophrenia. The reasons for this oversight are suggested by Chadwick, Birchwood, and Trower (1996) as centring on the validity of the concept of schizophrenia, which is traditionally characterised by pessimistic and baffling presumptions (see Bentall, 1990 for further discussion).

Current research into cognitive therapy for schizophrenia focuses more on a symptom model—particularly the positive symptoms—with most attention given to hallucinations and delusions. Developing and utilising a symptom model in the approach to cognitive treatments for schizophrenia begins to address an apparently complex and most certainly diverse group of symptoms that collectively attract the diagnosis of schizophrenia. Different symptoms require different models to both explain development and maintenance, and inform treatment. Some emerging models of specific symptoms (Morrison, 1998a) are not unlike existing models of specific anxiety disorders in that individuals misinterpret normal phenomena, which leads to distress and disability.

One of the cornerstones of cognitive therapy for psychosis is the normalisation of those phenomena and how the individual's previous experiences, attitudes, and core beliefs contribute to their misinterpretation.

CASE EXAMPLE

This case study describes a man (Tom) who misinterpreted phenomena and then went on to misinterpret the consequences of doing so. His delusional interpretations were similar to the catastrophic misinterpretation of symptoms of anxiety in panic disorder (as has been suggested to be common by Morrison, 1998b). His core beliefs, relating to self, and his dysfunctional assumptions led him to compound those misinterpretations of what were originally normal or benign experiences. Over time he thought, felt, and behaved in ways congruent with his delusional beliefs and encouraged his wife and daughter to collude and support him, while recognising that they did not share his beliefs.

Progress was achieved through the reinterpretation of experiences and testing out of delusional beliefs while normalising the development, maintenance and escalation of problems. Early symptom relief and a sense of hope increased Tom's willingness to be active in and out of sessions, and the use of idiosyncratic formulation and goals helped him "make sense of it all" and see the "bigger picture". This approach to treatment incorporates similar strategies to other cognitive behavioural approaches to delusions (e.g. Chadwick et al., 1996; Fowler, Garety, & Kuipers, 1995) but is based on a Beckian cognitive conceptualisation and emphasises the therapeutic relationship.

Referral information

Tom was a 32-year-old man with a 10-year history of psychotic symptoms and a 25-year history of obsessional thoughts and behaviours. There had been limited investigation of a possible neurological disorder with no conclusive evidence to confirm or negate the presence of any abnormality. His psychotic symptoms were causing increased distress and the multidisciplinary team felt there was significant risk of self-harm.

The assessment

Symptom profile

The following symptoms were assessed using the tests indicated:

- Positive and negative symptoms: PANSS (Kay, Opler, & Lindermayer, 1989).
- Auditory hallucinations: PSYRATS (Haddock et al., 1999).
- Delusions: PSYRATS.
- Anxious thoughts: AnTI (Wells, 1994).
- Depression: BDI (Beck, Ward, Mendelson, Mock, & Erbaugh, 1961).
- General psychopathology: PANSS.

Results

Tom experienced auditory hallucinations, almost daily, with a highly distressing content. He was convinced that they were from an identifiable external source and that he had no control over them at any time or under any circumstances. He was preoccupied with persecutory delusions and experienced intense distress as a consequence of his 100% belief in them. General psychopathology features included severe anxiety, feelings of guilt, lack of insight and active social avoidance. He scored 37 on the BDI, indicative of a severe level of depression. He believed he had nothing to look forward to and would like to kill himself. His auditory hallucinations included a voice that frequently gave him instructions to harm himself. High scores on the AnTI highlighted preoccupation with physical illness, thought control, and social acceptance.

General functioning

This was assessed using the Social Functioning Scale (Birchwood, Smith, Cochrane, Wetton, & Copestake, 1990) and scores reflected Tom's inability to function independently outside the home and therefore little social activity. Within the home he attended to self-care needs and engaged in two or three insular activities, such as gardening and reading.

Summary of assessment

Tom described the presence of both delusions and hallucinations. He believed that he had caused the King's Cross tube station fire, which killed a number of people, because he "did not do something correctly" or that he had "done the wrong thing". He spent a significant amount of time engaged in overt and covert neutralising behaviours but continually worried that they may not be effective in preventing harm happening to family, friends, and the world's population at large. The overt rituals focused on ensuring that "bad" numbers were avoided—these were 5, 7 and 13 (he cancelled a flight because it took place on the 5th of the month)—and attempting to introduce the number four into behaviours. He would pour out four cups of coffee when making it for three people, stir the drinks four times, and pour away the extra coffee in four tips of the cup. His most potent behaviours for averting disasters, he believed, were those that could reflect the number 16 (4×4) but he usually had to satisfy himself with achieving the number 4. Too much time spent in achieving the number 16 in behaviours might cause him to miss out on performing another behaviour completely, with dire consequences, he believed, for other people.

Tom may have been engaging in covert rituals but he did not disclose them at this stage. He was not working at keeping himself safe from harm and indeed believed himself to be a "bad person" because he was responsible for so many "bad things" happening to other people since he was five years old. He further worried that once the police realised that he was responsible for certain disasters he would be arrested, and this increased his anxiety and led to hypervigilance for the presence of police. There was a secondary benefit from having engaged in the rituals for so long. Tom had worked out that if he could stop "bad things" happening he could make "good things" happen, but he was selective in the use of that "power" and only used it to improve the performance of a particular football team.

He was experiencing auditory hallucinations (see the PSYRATS scores later in this chapter). He heard the voice of the devil, which always said "cruel things", telling him he was responsible for major national and international disasters and instructing him to harm himself. The other voice he heard was a woman who was always "nice" and may have been his grandmother or aunt (both dead), but he heard less of her voice than he did of the devil's. Tom also experienced high levels of anxiety and guilt feelings, mainly driven by the belief that he had been responsible for so many negative events and may be responsible for many more in the future.

Tom identified high levels of intrusive worrying thoughts related to social situations, health, and the meaning of having these thoughts. He was moderately depressed and felt he had nothing to look forward to. He engaged in very few social activities outside the home but spent time productively and enjoyed time in the company of his wife and daughter.

Finally, Tom lacked insight and judgement into his condition.

Medication

Tom was prescribed the neuroleptic medications, thioridazine and risperidone, but had not taken them for three months because "it wasn't working" and he experienced unpleasant side effects. He was restless, while at the same time lethargic, and described being in a "zombie-like" state most of the time.

History of the disorder

The obsessive-compulsive disorder appeared to have its origins in his childhood, when, shortly before his death, Tom's grandfather asked him to run an errand which Tom did not do. After the death he began to worry that he had caused it by not carrying out a specific action, and around the same time his mother told him, "one day, when you wake up, the devil will be beside you". Tom interpreted this as an indicator that he would be responsible for "something wrong or bad that would occur in the future". From this time he intermittently engaged in neutralising behaviours but was unable to identify circumstances or triggers for them.

A diagnosis of schizophrenia was made 10 years ago when Tom was 22 years old, but little attention appeared to have been given to the obsessive-compulsive features of his presentation and treatment was neuroleptic medication and acute hospital admission for the visual and auditory hallucinations he experienced. At that time there was concern that Tom may have a neurological condition, possibly temporal lobe epilepsy or narcolepsy, based on his presentation, but investigations were inconclusive. There did not appear to be any single critical incident for the onset of the psychotic symptoms, but rather an escalation of anxiety combined with family changes and relationship problems. Tom believed that working with certain chemicals while he was a gardener and a minor concussion prior to hospital admission may have contributed to his symptoms.

The visual hallucinations quickly subsided and the auditory hallucinations became less distressing and, after a short stay in the acute psychiatric unit, he was discharged and had been managed in the community on medication for 10 years. He was unable to work, lost confidence, was convinced he had a neurological disorder and refused to leave the house unaccompanied. He continued to engage in neutralising rituals but felt compelled to increase the range of behaviours, and tried to incorporate the number four into as many actions as possible. He worried that the rest of his life would be unchanged and about the effect that would have on his wife and daughter.

Personal background

Tom is the youngest of three children and was born and brought up locally. He left school at 16 and worked as a gardener until his first admission to hospital, but has not worked since. He lives with his wife and 14-year-old daughter. He had a warm and loving relationship with his grandparents but never felt his parents cared for him: he describes them as too selfish to care about anyone else and is always criticised by them for the "soft" side of his nature, while they attempt to take advantage of it. He has distanced himself from them recently and wishes he had done so years ago.

Presentation

Tom presented as nervous but cooperative, and desperate to find a way of making any improvement to his circumstances. He was very open about his experiences but carefully gauged my response to his disclosures before going further. He said, later, that he was concerned the therapist would judge him negatively or that she either might not understand or might trivialise his experiences. A further concern was that, because he was a "jinx", something "bad" would happen to the therapist because she had been in contact with him and had tried to help him, and he tried to reassure her by describing how many rituals he intended to carry out to keep her as safe as possible.

Suitability for cognitive therapy

The Safran and Segal (1990) Suitability for Short-Term Cognitive Therapy Rating Scale was used at session three to assess overall suitability for cognitive therapy and identify areas that could influence progress in therapy.

Tom scored 36 out of a possible total score of 50. The highest scores from the 10 items in the scale (the higher the score the more positive the prognosis) were in patient optimism, alliance potential, compatibility with the cognitive model, and acceptance of personal responsibility for change. Chronicity of the problems was considered a possible obstacle to progress and special attention was paid, collaboratively, to both the impact of experiencing psychotic symptoms over a prolonged period, and how would Tom deal with the possible realisation that he had "got it wrong for all those years, and missed out on so much in life".

The indications were that Tom would engage with and be active in therapy and, indeed, he had completed all the homework negotiated in sessions one and two. Assessing suitability helped identify the patient's strengths, and utilise them, and highlighted areas of weaknesses to tackle or work around.

Treatment

Initially six sessions of cognitive therapy were negotiated to establish a problem list, develop prioritised treatment goals, socialise Tom to the model, assess the quality of the therapeutic relationship, and assess Tom's suitability for cognitive therapy. Sessions, with agreed objectives, would then be negotiated in blocks of six.

Progress of therapy

Treatment was planned in three stages, to cover from problem list through to relapse prevention/management. The primary focus of stage one was to engage Tom both with the therapist and the therapy and develop an initial formulation. In stage two Tom was encouraged to become more active in the therapy (both within and outside therapy) in identifying and making appropriate changes. Stage three was the consolidation of the issues covered in stage one and the work done in stage two, and integrating the two into relapse prevention/management strategies.

Stage one

Just because an individual takes part in a cognitive therapy session doesn't mean that cognitive therapy takes place. This is as true for the therapist as it is for the patient. Cognitive therapy is an active, collaborative process between the patient and the therapist, like co-drivers of a vehicle that is the means to get to an identified destination by an agreed route observing appropriate speed limits. The driver changes at times but neither party is a passenger, no matter how pleasant or well behaved.

The first stage of therapy is not completed until the patient has engaged with the therapist and the therapy. Engagement is not just liking someone or something; it involves understanding and respect, a shared vision of goals and the way to achieve them, and hope fostered by the belief that change is both possible and probable. Being clear about what the problems are for *the patient* and what can be changed increases the patient's confidence that the therapist understands what he or she wants to gain from therapy, what the obstacles might be during the process, and that it is not a solitary journey.

The aims for this stage were to:

- establish a rapport;
- identify factors which may influence the process of cognitive therapy;
- normalise and decatastrophise Tom's experiences;
- socialise Tom to the cognitive model;
- identify a problem list; and
- develop and share an initial formulation.

Sessions one to three

Engagement is often perceived as a single concept in the therapy process, but there are two distinct areas of engagement to consider. One is the engagement of the patient with the therapist and the other is their engagement with the therapy, and the therapist needs to be aware of and address any issues that may interfere with either.

Blackburn and Davidson (1995) identify five qualities in a therapist to enhance engagement of both types:

1   To listen in an objective but empathic way, be totally other-focused and not self-conscious.
2   Be directive, enquiring and didactic. Questioning and giving feedback aid awareness/insight into experiences.
3   Enjoy the process of discovery, searching, and modifying a formulation.
4   Judicious use of a sense of humour to enhance the therapeutic relationship and elevate mood.
5   A creative mind, in order to adapt treatment strategies and employ colourful concrete images, analogies, stories, and vignettes.

It is not essential to establish engagement with the therapist *before* focusing on engagement with the therapy. They can be addressed concurrently, but if the therapeutic relationship is weak or even negative, one would expect a significant impact on the process of socialising the patient to the cognitive model.

"Selling" the cognitive model relies heavily on the concept of "persuasive communication" from social psychology literature. Essentially the approach consists of three elements that address the question of "who says what to whom with what effect?" The structure of the message (the cognitive model and therapy), characteristics of the source (the therapist) and the person it is aimed at (the patient) are evaluated to assess the effect on the patient's attitude and therefore motivation towards engaging in cognitive therapy.

Hovland, Janis, and Kelley (1953) have shown that the source (the therapist selling the model) is more likely to be effective if that person is seen as, for example, trustworthy, likeable, and having expertise and experience in the field. The more factors patients perceive they have in common with their therapist the easier it will be for them to consider and evaluate the possible usefulness and relevance of the cognitive model. Therapist and patient do not have to share age, sex, religion, culture, etc. for socialisation to take place, but common factors may reduce patient resistance.

The message (socialisation) is more likely to be acceptable if it appears believable. If the patient can understand the therapist's language, relate to case examples used and relate this to their own experiences then the likelihood that they will tentatively engage in therapy will be increased. Tom was easy to engage both interpersonally and with the therapy because he was looking for an alternative treatment to medication for his experiences. He valued the therapist's open, collaborative style, which did not make promises about outcome but engendered confidence and hope.

Tom was keen to embark on a treatment process that did not focus on neuroleptic medication and believed that a psychological intervention held the greatest hope for change. He had an open mind about the development and maintenance of his problems: this is not to say he had no thoughts on the possible factors, but rather that he had not yet come to a convincing conclusion. Although Tom was nervous at first, and concerned about the consequences to the therapist as a result of working with him, the fact that he was so open about past and current experiences and thoughts made it easier to pick up on significant issues that could have hampered engagement, and collaboratively explore them within that session.

The California Psychotherapeutic Alliance Scale (CALPAS) (Gaston & Marmar, 1994) was used to assess the quality of the therapeutic relationship/ alliance in the early, middle, and end stages of therapy. The CALPAS consists of four subscales and the alliance can be measured from three views: the patient, the therapist, and an external observer. The four scales address the separate contributions of the patient and therapist to the alliance, as well as their mutual agreement on therapeutic goals and how best to achieve them. They are:

- patient working capacity—disclosing information and deepening understanding;
- patient commitment—motivation and confidence in therapist/therapy;
- working strategy consensus—agreement on goals and process of achievement; and
- therapist understanding and interest.

In Tom's case the patient and therapist rated the therapeutic alliance at sessions three, nine, and fifteen. The session three measures indicated a high level of therapist understanding and interest and working strategy consensus by both parties but a lower level of patient commitment and working capacity. At session nine all four subscales were scored highly by both the patient and the therapist, with a similar scoring at session fifteen.

The quality of the therapeutic relationship enhanced the quality of the therapeutic process within and between sessions, with both parties being actively engaged within the session and in completing agreed homework tasks. Both the patient and therapist held their own sets of notes and had copies of all audiotapes made of sessions. Tom enjoyed the focused and structured approach of the sessions, was active in setting the agenda, and competent in summarising the content of the session and the conclusions reached.

Normalising and decatastrophising Tom's experiences while introducing the cognitive model was quickly achieved because he did not hold an alternative conflicting model. If anything, he was too eager to embrace the cognitive model and part of one session was to encourage him to be scientific in his evaluation of the model. Establishing Tom's problem list was not such an easy matter, largely because it appeared to be so huge, from his point of view, and so disparate that he was unable to make connections between factors. There also appeared to be a considerable number of factors relating to his physical state which added to the list. It was possible, however, to generate an extensive list, then group problems into obvious areas, and begin to explore the relationships between the groupings and the individual problems while attempting to identify the best approaches to each group of problems. The problems were identified and grouped as follows:

- Group one: Paranoia

  a   Believed he was responsible for the King's Cross underground station fire.
  b   Living in fear that the police would arrest him any day because he caused the fire.
  c   Believes he was responsible for his grandfather's death.
  d   Believes he was responsible for major global disasters—television newscasters told him this.
  e   Worried that criminals would harm him because he is an easy target.

f   Believes he is a "jinx"—bad things happen to people who are in contact with him.

- Group two: Auditory hallucinations

  a   Hears one male voice that tells him he is evil and should harm himself, even to the point of suicide. Tom believes this voice is the devil.
  b   Hears one female voice that is always "nice". Believes this may be his aunt or his grandmother, both of whom are dead.

- Group three: Compulsions/rituals

  a   Engages in numerous rituals involving significant numbers. Must avoid numbers five, seven and thirteen, while introducing the number four into as many activities as possible. This behaviour, he believes, will prevent harmful things happening.

- Group four: Physical health

  a   Feels very tired and quickly falls asleep after eating, and therefore does not eat during the day.
  b   Can fall asleep without warning—diagnosed as narcolepsy.

- Group five: Unusual experiences

  a   Experiences uncontrollable bouts of "laughter"—abdominal muscular spasm effecting breathing, which sounds like laughter. Feels weak and has to lie down.
  b   Worries that people will think he is strange or means to laugh at them.

An initial formulation was developed using Beck's (1976) cognitive model of the development and maintenance of emotional disorders as follows (and see Fig. 4.1):

- Early experience

  — Parenting style characterised by lack of affection and holding Tom responsible for negative events beyond his control.
  — Sexual assault by an adult male.
  — Low self-esteem, suspicious of others.

- Formation of conditional assumptions and schemas

  — Strange experiences are bad.
  — I'm a jinx.
  — Bad things happen to people around me.
  — If I don't look after people bad things will happen to them and me.

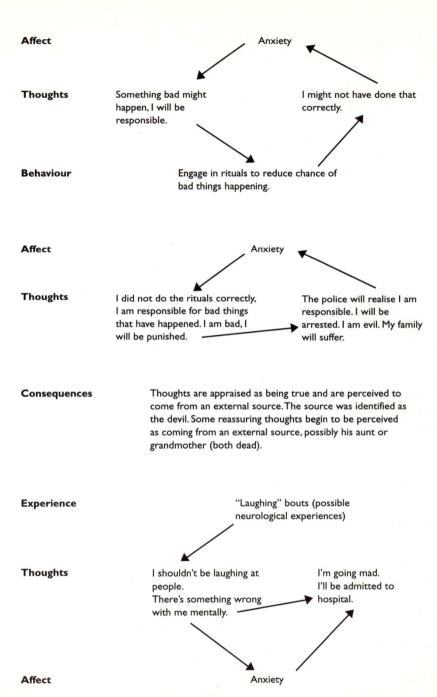

Affect   Anxiety

Thoughts   Something bad might   I might not have done that
happen, I will be   correctly.
responsible.

Behaviour   Engage in rituals to reduce chance of
bad things happening.

Affect   Anxiety

Thoughts   I did not do the rituals correctly,   The police will realise I am
I am responsible for bad things   responsible. I will be
that have happened. I am bad, I   arrested. I am evil. My family
will be punished.   will suffer.

Consequences   Thoughts are appraised as being true and are perceived to
come from an external source. The source was identified as
the devil. Some reassuring thoughts begin to be perceived
as coming from an external source, possibly his aunt or
grandmother (both dead).

Experience   "Laughing" bouts (possible
neurological experiences)

Thoughts   I shouldn't be laughing at   I'm going mad.
people.   I'll be admitted to
There's something wrong   hospital.
with me mentally.

Affect   Anxiety

Figure 4.1 Initial formulation maintenance cycles.

  — Not all people can be trusted.
  — Anxiety is bad for you.
  — I should be able to control my thoughts.

- Critical incidents

  — Birth of daughter.
  — Deterioration in relationship with wife.
  — Possible neurological disturbances.
  — Over-occupied with physical health.

Stage two

Problems identified and reflected in the formulation during stage one were re-framed in stage two into goals. It is essential to begin to focus on goals once the problem list has been identified for the following reasons:

- it clarifies the objectives of therapy and reduces deviation or distraction;
- goals can be divided into short, medium and long-term categories;
- goals will identify when therapy should end; and
- where problems focus on the negative and the past and distress, by attending to goals the focus is on the future, the positive and movement rather than helplessness.

The proposed route to goal achievement must be collaboratively negotiated at stage two but will usually incorporate information gathering, experiments and evaluation of change. Returning to the motoring analogy, this stage is where the following are negotiated:

- destination;
- route;
- speed;
- stops;
- progress checks; and
- maintenance of vehicle (patient).

Included in the route to goal achievement was the use of behavioural experiments to test out the accuracy of Tom's evaluation of his "powers". Both the relationships between his behaviours and negative experiences for other people, and his ability to read minds were explored. As Tom completed experiments and began to achieve some of his goals, an updated formulation was developed to reflect the changes that had taken place. The new formulation formed the basis for Tom's development and implementation of a relapse prevention/management plan.

The aims for stage two were to:

- establish a goals list;
- explore physical health problems;
- evaluate the impact of medication;
- undertake and evaluate behavioural tests;
- expand formulation; and
- begin relapse prevention/management work.

Sessions four to six

The goals list was established and items prioritised in a similar manner to the problem list but reversed, identifying general themes first then describing the specific goals within them. The list was divided into four areas to help the patient and therapist stay focused and structured, and encourage the use of experiments that would produce maximum effect across the individual goals in each area. The following goals were collaboratively identified:

- Physical:

    a   Remain free of neuroleptic medication.
    b   Adjust to changes brought about by prescribed amphetamines.
    c   Establish presence or absence of neurological disorder.
    d   Resolve other minor physical problems.

- Relationships:

    a   Be less dependent on wife and play a greater role in house and child care.
    b   Spend more time with his daughter, educationally and socially.
    c   Sever contact with parents.

- Responsibility beliefs:

    a   Stop being responsible for bad things happening.
    b   Stop having to engage in complicated rituals.
    c   Stop being suspicious.
    d   Be able to find rational explanations for unusual events.

- Auditory hallucinations:

    a   Be free of auditory hallucinations.
    b   Understand where they come from.

PHYSICAL HEALTH

Tom appeared to experience a range of unexplained physical disturbances. He would fall asleep after even a light meal or snack and so would starve himself during the day and eat a large meal at night. He had six or seven episodes a day and two or three at night where his diaphragm caused involuntary bouts of what sounded like laughter lasting ten minutes, which left him feeling weak and needing to lie down. Before this bout of "laughing" he felt "enlightened" and was aware of the smell of hot milk pudding. It was hypothesised that starving himself during the day may have caused some of the episodes of light-headedness he experienced and may have been a trigger for the "laughing" bouts. It was also possible that the "laughing" bouts were of a neurological origin, and the warning signs, lack of muscular control, and feeling weak afterwards made it worthy of further investigation.

These frequent episodes increased Tom's anxiety levels, disturbed his sleep pattern and his wife's, and put him at risk of making catastrophic misinterpretations of their origin. It was agreed that Tom would discuss these symptoms with his consultant psychiatrist. This would allow him to be more assertive in his relationship with the psychiatrist and give him a sense of empowerment that he was active in identifying problems and solving them. This interaction would then be the base for other problem-solving objectives related to medication.

BEHAVIOURAL TESTS

It was agreed to devise behavioural tests in two areas to make it possible for Tom to accurately evaluate his beliefs. While the outcome of these tests could have significant influence on the problems experienced in the defined areas, it could also provide him with information that would help him investigate other similar problems of faulty evaluation. The results of the tests would also enrich the formulation and be incorporated into the relapse work.

The objective for encouraging a patient to engage in behavioural experiments or reality-testing is to help him realise that his appraisal or evaluation of a situation is inaccurate. The experiments are designed to introduce doubt by producing contradictory evidence for further appraisal. It is important to set up the experiment so that the conclusions that can be drawn are accurate.

The first area agreed for testing was Tom's belief that he could read minds. The starting point was to gain peripheral information about when, where, with whom, why, and how this phenomenon occurred. The affective response to the belief that he could read minds was explored and the questions posed and addressed were:

• Did this make him special?
• What if it wasn't really true?
• What would it mean to discover he had been wrong all this time?

Tom rated his belief that he could read minds at 80%. He only used his ability to read minds with policemen but, as he spent a great deal of time avoiding them, he had very little data to examine. How or why the mind-reading occurred had never crossed Tom's mind, and he just accepted it as a fact. It was tempting at this point to focus discussion on how lack of evidence can lead to an inaccurate conclusion being drawn, but a more effective point to have that discussion would be after data had been collected and evaluated within a behavioural experiment. Highlighting faulty reasoning and demonstrating its role in the development and maintenance of distress in the wider formulation helps the person develop a normalised understanding of how they reached the inaccurate conclusion in the first place. Combining being wrong with the reason for it reduces negative affective responses. Normalising the person's experience in global terms of "most people misjudge or misinterpret experiences sometime" and specific in terms of "well if I'd had the experiences you did it's likely I would have drawn the same conclusions about mind-reading" minimises the effect of "getting it wrong".

A behavioural experiment to try and establish the extent of Tom's powers of mind-reading was collaboratively designed. There would be within and without session experiments. The object was not do decide whether he could or not, but to gather information about where and when. The expected result on the therapist's part would be the same, but the patient was being encouraged to be scientific and open-minded; a patient is more likely to engage in seeking information from an "interested in" perspective than a confrontational perspective.

Tom held a 40% belief that he could read the minds of people other than the police and that this applied to reading the mind of the therapist. To make things a little easier, the subject of her thinking was decided and, as it seems common to demonstrate mind-reading with playing cards, that was the selected topic. To make it easier again, the colour of suit was agreed and the therapist undertook to think "as hard as she could" of a specific card. Tom would attempt to read her mind by whatever means he could. After two or three minutes Tom declared that he had no idea what the card was and could only hazard a guess with a one in twenty-six chance of being right. He re-evaluated his belief in his ability to read the therapist's mind at 0%.

There are a number of responses the therapist can make at this point and the least productive is probably "so you were wrong then; and if you were wrong about that what else are you wrong about?" Let the patient make the connection, and say "umm, what do you make of that?" He might say "you weren't trying hard enough" or "well I'm having a bad day" or something similar. Encouraging further experimentation outside the session will furnish him with more evidence to re-evaluate his belief. Tom was puzzled that he could not read the therapist's mind, but concluded that it might be his 40% belief rating that was inaccurate rather than his belief about his ability. It was therefore agreed that he would conduct further experiments between sessions with a range of people but without telling them: he thought it would make him look foolish if he asked people to take part in experiments. At the next session he reported that he had been unable to read any person's mind accurately but he did know what some people were going to do or what they might be feeling. When these issues were examined in session Tom was able to appreciate the difference between interpreting non-verbal clues and reading minds. He was also able to see how anxiety, when in the presence of the police, might influence the conclusions he would draw. Information gained from this experiment was the basis for agreeing and evaluating further experiments.

The most significant change came from the second area of experimentation. One of Tom's problems was believing he was responsible for both global and local disasters, but he also had the belief that he could make some positive things happen, and he did not consider that a problem. He only used that power to enhance the match results for Manchester City Football Club and football clubs that he felt were the underdogs in any fixture. Discussion focused on Tom's ability to influence events, whether positive or negative in his eyes. The conclusion was that he both could influence and was responsible for events, or couldn't and therefore wasn't responsible. If he wasn't responsible and couldn't influence events then what was the point in the rituals he engaged in? The agreed experiment was to look, in session, at the Football Association fixtures scheduled for the coming Saturday and identify the team he considered was the underdog for each fixture and then spend dedicated time, up to Saturday, using his usual thought processes to ensure that the underdog won in each fixture. The approach was one of "going for bust", meaning that this was the definitive experiment of whether he could or he couldn't.

At the next session Tom reported that he had been unable to make either all the underdogs or Manchester City Football Club win their matches. His conclusion, reached without prompting, was "I can't do it". While it was a disappointment that his favourite team could no longer count on his influence in the future, he felt a huge relief that he could not influence or be responsible for negative events, whether personal, local, or global. This experience was the breakthrough that helped him to examine and challenge other conclusions/assumptions he had made that were causing him distress. Tom dealt with the realisation that these beliefs had caused huge practical and interpersonal problems with the response "well, at least it's over now and I can get my normal life back".

Information gained from the behavioural experiments and their evaluation was incorporated into a revised formulation. All new information realised in therapy was treated in the same way and was used to normalise Tom's experiences and inform the relapse prevention/management plan.

Sessions seven to ten

MEDICATION

Tom had stopped taking his neuroleptic medication (his own unilateral decision) three weeks prior to commencing therapy. It was hypothesised that the medication side effects were contributing to some of the problems identified and that not taking the medication had allowed him to think more clearly and be more active within and between sessions. Tom reported no worsening in his symptoms and indeed the removal of medication side effects was improving his functioning and mood.

Between sessions seven and eight Tom's consultant psychiatrist prescribed amphetamines for his narcolepsy. Initially he felt energised but, as the dosage was increased, he became more irritable, self-focused and overactive. His sleep reduced to three to four hours per twenty-four-hour period (sometimes during the day), his weight reduced dramatically, and preoccupation with physical health problems escalated. The amphetamines were reduced to a level that controlled the narcolepsy without disrupting other areas of his life. Incorporating this change in medication into the formulation and reflecting on how medications can change perceptions encouraged Tom to determine which experiences were a product of the medication and how to adaptively appraise and deal with them.

RELAPSE PREVENTION/MANAGEMENT

Having made significant gains in therapy, Tom was keen to develop strategies to prevent or shorten relapse. The initial and revised formulations were utilised to identify relapse triggers, early warning signs, and strategies known to be effective in dealing with emerging psychotic symptoms.

Many individuals are not aware of the initial signs of relapse, and it is only through a careful breakdown of each relapse episode that the patient can discover the idiosyncratic indicators, which, if unheeded, are likely to lead to relapse. The earliest indicators of change may become obvious to those close to the patient before he is aware of them himself. In Tom's case his wife could spot small changes in his manner and behaviour well before he could and so she was utilised as a key player in the identification of relevant, observable changes and their monitoring. Tom's wife also agreed to prompt and coach him in implementing appropriate identified strategies when early signs emerged.

The motoring analogy was used to help Tom understand and remember the value of responding quickly to warning signs and identify what he could do about them and when the help of others may be needed. Changes in engine noise, car performance, smoke and unusual smells, as well as the more obvious and less easily ignored red lights on the instrument panel were compared with the early warning signs that Tom identified from previous episodes of relapse.

EARLY WARNING SIGNS AND RESPONSE STRATEGIES

Six signs and strategies were identified as set out in Table 4.1. Tom's key worker was a community psychiatric nurse who continued to have contact and input throughout treatment with cognitive behavioural therapy, and it was agreed that if Tom was unable to prevent "lapse becoming relapse", through the above strategies, that he would consult with his key worker to decide the most appropriate steps to take.

Stage three

The final stage of treatment was a consolidation of gains made in therapy as highlighted in the relapse plan and final formulation. Outcome measures were taken and results compared with pre-treatment scores. The relapse plan had been implemented and its effectiveness was monitored to demonstrate to Tom the need to evaluate and revise, where needed, appropriate strategies. The aims for stage three were to:

- monitor effectiveness of relapse plan;
- share and evaluate the outcome data;
- develop a final formulation; and
- identify the gains made in therapy.

Sessions eleven to fifteen

These were the final treatment sessions and the number of sessions had been negotiated at sessions six and twelve. The aims were addressed in the following order: relapse plan; outcome data; final formulation; and gains made in therapy.

Table 4.1 Early warning signs of relapse and strategies to be implemented

Early warning sign	Strategy
"Obsessive/responsibility thinking"	Challenge thoughts, resist behaviours
Increased irritability	Use green-leaf tea, count to 10
Apathy, decreased interest, social withdrawal	Introduce activity scheduling, discuss with wife/ key worker
Becoming sceptical/paranoid	Scientifically evaluate the evidence
Preoccupation with physical health	Decide what is "real" and what is anxiety related
Negative thoughts related to self-worth	Challenge using evidence

RELAPSE PLAN

When monitoring early warning signs of relapse and implementing strategies Tom also monitored the effectiveness of the strategies. He noted how effective each was, and those that were the least effective were modified. This process of monitoring, evaluating, and modifying strategies was to become an integral part of relapse prevention/management and a process that Tom was comfortable with and adept at using.

OUTCOME DATA

The outcome data is set out in Table 4.2. Prior to treatment Tom experienced excessive levels of anxiety, which, in part, maintained his delusional beliefs and auditory hallucinations. His beliefs and experiences, and accompanying distress, led to levels of depression that were severe at times and put him at medium risk of committing suicide. Tom's level of social engagement and activity was fairly low, only leaving the house in the company of others and only socialising with others in his own home.

Following fifteen one-hour treatment sessions of cognitive behavioural therapy, Tom was not experiencing any positive or negative symptoms and his mood was almost within population norms. He was no longer preoccupied with his physical health and his overall level of anxiety had reduced significantly. There was an improvement in socialising within and outside the home, and Tom was more self-confident and assertive in dealing with the many professionals he was in contact with.

Table 4.2 Pre- and post-treatment data

	Pre-treatment	Post-treatment
PANSS		
Positive scale	25	10
Negative scale	14	7
General psychopathology	46	33
PSYRATS		
AHRS	35	0
DRS	20	0
AnTI	81	33
BDI	35	11
SFS	728	871.5

FINAL FORMULATION

Tom had learned to become scientific in his approach to evaluating unusual experiences. The "usual" experiences—i.e. anxiety and negative automatic thoughts—were resolved by using specific strategies for dealing with them. His vulnerability lay in the misinterpretation of unusual events, either related to his physical state or environmental. A generic strategy was developed that slowed down the process of evaluation and prevented him from jumping to conclusions. Tom questioned, where appropriate, the source of the experience, any meaning attached to it (if it involved the behaviour of others), and how the experience should be resolved in a way that minimised any negative affect (see Fig. 4.2 for examples).

The introduction in stage two of treatment of amphetamines to treat his narcolepsy exposed Tom to numerous physical effects he had not previously experienced. Without the ability to systematically evaluate the cause of these effects and deal with them appropriately, it is likely that they would have been misinterpreted and possibly have resulted in the return of anxiety and psychotic symptoms.

GAINS MADE IN THERAPY

The words "thank you for making things better; it if wasn't for you I wouldn't be where I am today", when spoken by a patient, should ring alarm bells for the therapist. From the outset of therapy the patient needs to understand that *they* will be doing the work that brings about change and *they* will take the credit for progress made. The therapist must play down their part in the process; yes they turn up when they say they will and yes they bring some

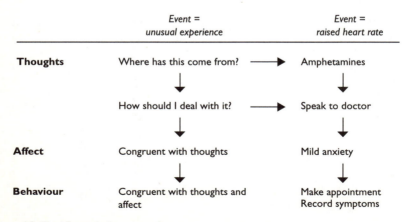

Figure 4.2 Final formulation examples.

expertise with them from a therapist's perspective, but change only occurs because the patient makes it happen.

When it comes to reflecting on gains made in therapy, patients need to be reminded of their own unique contribution to the process; for example, their ideas for experiments, or how they participated in therapy and homework even when it was painful to do so. If patients can believe that change is possible and achievable through their efforts then they are more likely to actively use the relapse prevention/management plan devised in the therapy.

Tom's gains were:

- insight into the development and maintenance of his symptoms;
- awareness of vulnerability factors in relation to relapse;
- ability to monitor various factors related to relapse;
- generation and implementation of a range of effective strategies to address symptoms;
- awareness of ineffective strategies and responses that worsen symptoms;
- knowledge of the actions and side effects of prescribed medication; and
- increased assertiveness with health professionals.

CONCLUSION

Tom is a man who prior to treatment had only been exposed to a medical model/explanation of the development and maintenance of symptoms. When presented with a believable alternative, which offered him the opportunity to explore and influence the origin and effect of these symptoms, he was highly motivated to engage in that process. Early success led to a high level of engagement with both the therapist and the therapy, and increased his motivation to attempt further experiments aimed at investigating and/or responding to unusual experiences.

The skills he learned during therapy better prepared him for dealing with vulnerabilities and triggers that he felt sure would be part of his future, and which he was confident could be resolved with minimum impact to his psychological well-being.

REFERENCES

Beck, A.T. (1976). *Cognitive therapy and the emotional disorders.* New York: International Universities Press.

Beck, A.T., Rush, A.J., Shaw, B.F., & Emery, G. (1979). *Cognitive therapy of depression.* New York: Guilford Press.

Beck, A.T., Ward, C.H., Mendelson, M., Mock, J., & Erbaugh, J. (1961). An inventory for measuring depression. *Archives of General Psychiatry, 4,* 561–571.

Bentall, R.P. (1990). The syndromes and symptoms of psychosis: Or why you can't play twenty questions with the concept of schizophrenia and hope to win. In R.P. Bentall (Ed.), *Reconstructing schizophrenia*. London: Routledge.

Birchwood, M., Smith, J., Cochrane, R., Wetton, S., & Copestake, S. (1990). The Social Functioning Scale: The development and validation of a scale of social adjustment for use in family intervention programmes with schizophrenic patients. *British Journal of Psychiatry*, *157*, 853–859.

Blackburn, I.M., & Davidson, K.M. (1995). *Cognitive therapy for depression and anxiety*. Cambridge: Blackwell.

Chadwick, P., Birchwood, M., & Trower, P. (1996). *Cognitive therapy for delusions, voices and paranoia*. New York: Wiley.

Fowler, D.G., Garety, P., & Kuipers, E. (1995). *Cognitive behaviour therapy for psychosis: Theory and practice*. Chichester: John Wiley and Sons.

Gaston, L., & Marmar, C.R. (1994). The California Psychotherapy Alliance Scales. In A.O. Horvath & L.S. Greenberg (Eds.), *The working alliance*. New York: Wiley.

Haddock, G., McCarron, J., Tarrier, N., & Faragher, E.B. (1999). Scales to measure dimensions of hallucinations and delusions: The psychotic symptom rating scales (PSYRATS). *Psychological Medicine*, *29*, 879–889.

Hovland, C., Janis, I., & Kelley, H.H. (1953). *Communication and persuasion*. New Haven: Yale University Press.

Kay, S.R., Opler, L.A., & Lindermayer, J.P. (1989). The positive and negative syndrome scale (PANSS): Rationale and standardisation. *British Journal of Psychiatry*, *155*, suppl. 7, 59–65.

Morrison, A.P. (1998a). A cognitive analysis of the maintenance of auditory hallucinations: Are voices to schizophrenia what bodily sensations are to panic? *Behavioural and Cognitive Psychotherapy*, *26*, 289–302.

Morrison, A.P. (1998b). Cognitive behaviour therapy for psychotic symptoms. In N. Tarrier, A. Wells, & G. Haddock (Eds.), *Treating complex cases: A cognitive behaviour therapy approach*. Chichester: Wiley.

Safran, J.D., & Segal, Z.V. (1990). *Interpersonal process in cognitive therapy*. New York: Basic Books.

Wells, A. (1994). A multi-dimensional measure of worry: Development and preliminary validation of the Anxious Thoughts Inventory. *Anxiety, Stress, and Coping*, *6*, 289–299.

Chapter 5

The search for meaning: Detecting congruence between life events, underlying schema and psychotic symptoms

Formulation-driven and schema-focused cognitive behavioural therapy for a neuroleptic-resistant schizophrenic patient with a delusional memory

Alison Brabban and Douglas Turkington

INTRODUCTION

Trying to understand or find meaning appears to be a fundamental aspect of humanity. From birth we are taking in our surroundings and reaching conclusions about the world and our position within it. In early years this search for meaning is at a very simple level. Babies will learn through countless experiments the relationship between their actions and the effect they have on the environment, and this leads to intentional actions where they realise their actions make a difference. So they may learn that pushing a food bowl at arm's length makes it disappear over the edge of the table, if they shake a rattle it makes a noise, and so on. As children grow older so their level of understanding becomes more sophisticated. By adolescence some have gone beyond concrete black and white thinking and can think in abstract terms, follow logical propositions, and reason by hypothesis (Piaget, 1952).

Making sense of our world serves as an essential survival strategy. Through both positive and negative experiences we learn what is safe and what is dangerous and to be avoided. Putting a hand in the fire makes it hurt, smiling at mum often results in a cuddle, and so on. This learning and understanding allows us to try to predict what is going to happen from one moment to the next and this provides some sense of control over our lives. In short it means that on a typical day when we go through the usual routines such as going to work, we will have a general idea of what will happen, how others will react to us, and how we will deal with the demands of the day. On a day when the routine is broken and we are faced with the unfamiliar such as meeting strangers or attending new situations then we are faced with less certainty. Our powers of prediction and knowing seem less certain and we are likely to feel either anxious or excited. Every new experience brings with it new information that can contribute to our internal representations of the world and increase our sense of understanding.

When evidence starts mounting that the model we have of the world or ourselves may be wrong in some way, then the mismatch between what we see and what we believe produces a state of discomfort as a result of cognitive dissonance (Festinger, 1957). Cognitive dissonance exists when two cognitions occurring together are inconsistent with each other according to the expectations of the person. For example, a man who has been abused as a child may have formed the belief that "people are no good and not to be trusted". If later in life that same man then meets someone who is kind, considerate, and seems genuinely concerned, it will be difficult for him to accommodate this new found behaviour within his existing belief structure and he will be left in a state of "not knowing".

To reduce dissonant states of this kind and the tension that accompanies them, existing belief systems need to be changed or alternatively there needs to be a change in perception (in terms of cognitive distortions) so that the world once again fits with personal core beliefs or schema. In terms of the man in our example, he must change his belief from "people *generally* are no good and not to be trusted" to "*some* people are no good and not to be trusted". Alternatively to reduce his dissonant state, he can change his perception of the other person's behaviour by minimising it "yes, but that's one time in a million" or by discounting it in some way "that wasn't genuine kindness". The process by which perceptions are distorted or shaped to fit in with original beliefs and thereby reduce cognitive dissonance has been called "hypothesis preservation" (Gorman, 1989). This process could be seen as operating to maintain a sense that we understand and can predict ourselves and our environment (even if, such as in the example, this results in a belief that the world is an unsafe or bad place).

Cognitive therapy of course is focused on the meaning that individuals attribute to events that happen around them. When a person comes into therapy it is often because their understanding of themselves, the world and the future is dysfunctional in some way. Either the meaning they have derived from events is having a negative effect upon their mood, or alternatively they are unable to use their current internal models to make sense of what is happening in their lives and are suffering the discomfort of "not knowing". "What is happening to me?", "Why am I like this?", "Why is he/she acting like that?" are all common questions that patients ask when they come for therapy. At times it seems the not knowing is causing as much discomfort as the situation itself.

Meaning and delusions

Although Strauss (1969) demonstrated the existence of a spectrum of belief from normal beliefs through overvalued ideation to delusions, the dominant view remains that delusional beliefs are separate entities from *normal* beliefs (Hamilton, 1978). With normal beliefs one can understand how they are formed based on a person's perception and reasoning. With delusions some believe that the same processes do not occur: they are caused entirely by deficits in normal cognitive processing. Jaspers (1963) wrote how delusions could not be understood in terms of the person's personality and experiences and, almost 20 years later, Berrios (1991) described delusions as "empty speech acts, whose informational content refers to neither self nor world". It seems that a significant cognitive bias has been operating to develop such a hypothesis because this theory appears to fly in the face of available evidence. Often it seems quite evident that the content of delusions reflects concerns the individual has about himself and how others perceive him.

More recently there has been a move away from this particular viewpoint, and research has been testing the hypothesis that cognitive biases implicated in the neurotic disorders may also operate within psychosis (Bentall, 1996). The results have been challenging the model that delusional beliefs are fundamentally different from normal beliefs and are without meaning. Instead there is mounting evidence that delusional beliefs can be understood in terms of biased processing within normal belief formation. This theory explains extreme beliefs as resulting from extreme biases in cognitive functioning.

The results from a number of studies have suggested the presence of a bias in probabilistic reasoning among people with delusional beliefs: in other words, they are more likely to miscalculate the probability of an event occurring (Garety & Hemsley, 1994; Garety, Hemsley, & Wessely, 1991; Huq, Garety, & Hemsley, 1988). However, this interpretation has now been disputed (Garety & Freeman, 1999). It seems that those suffering delusional beliefs *can* estimate probabilities; the bias is in the gathering of data that is gathered prior to making a decision. Those suffering delusions appear to collect and use less information before accepting an hypothesis than non-delusional individuals—they are more likely to jump to conclusions (John & Dodgson, 1994; Linney, Peters, & Ayton, 1998).

Hemsley and Garety (1986) showed that when a delusion is formed two factors appear to be important in relation to initiation and maintenance: expectation and current relevant environmental information. Delusion formation is often preceded by a period of delusional mood usually described as a feeling of foreboding. We postulate that the period of delusional mood predating the development of a primary delusion could be viewed in terms of a cognitive dissonance phenomenon. This is linked to the direct invalidation of a long held compensatory schema (i.e. one that is central to a person's self-worth but dysfunctional). This invalidation usually occurs due to an accumulation of unfortunate, traumatising life events that lead to the emergence of a new belief. Harrow, Rattenbury, and Stoll (1988) estimated that 70% of delusional ideas were overtly related to non-delusional ideas that predated the delusion. A delusion is therefore best defined as a false belief at one end of the spectrum of consensual agreement (Turkington et al., 1996). The delusion arises from the interaction of vulnerabilities (both genetic and schematic) and particular life events. Delusions then behave slightly differently from normal beliefs being held with more intensity due to their often bizarre content that elicits confrontational responses from others in society. This also leads paradoxically to a reduced disconfirmatory information search as confrontation always leads to an increased search for supportive material that will help to "win the argument". In short, it seems that delusions appear to represent an individual's search for meaning within his or her own personal world.

Cognitive therapy and the search for meaning

Cognitive therapy will hopefully improve insight, increase adherence, and empower the patient to engage in further detailed reality-testing. To have any chance of helping a patient to correct the distortions and affective disturbances/behavioural avoidance that maintain psychotic symptoms it would seem vital to proceed slowly, develop a rapport of joint working, and move to the development of a normalising explanation. The aim of this engaging process is always to end up at a shared and agreed individualised case formulation.

What a cognitive formulation aims to accomplish is to explain *how* the patient is interpreting events, *what* effect this is having on his or her mood, and *why* he or she is inclined to interpret events in such a way. Having produced a formulation or understanding of the problem, the goal is then to work collaboratively with the patient to find a shared alternative, more functional perception of events.

Developing a shared understanding of events is equally as crucial when working with how the patient has coped with aspects of psychiatric treatment. Patients can have experienced many extraordinary and frightening events—everything from intramuscular neuroleptic treatment under common law to hospitalisation under the Mental Health Act. It is part of human nature that individuals will try and make sense of events, and individuals suffering from psychotic symptoms are no different; they will also attribute meaning to their experiences. When looking at individuals' perception of their symptoms, Romme, Honig, Noordhoorn, and Escher (1992) found that among people experiencing auditory hallucinations, those who coped better perceived themselves as stronger than their voices and perceived the voices themselves in a positive sense. This was opposed to the poor copers who believed they were less powerful than their voices and who perceived their voices as generally negative. On a related theme, Chadwick and Birchwood (1994) found that individuals' beliefs about the power and meaning of their voices impacted upon their affect and behaviour. Those who believed their voices were "benevolent" attempted to engage them and found them generally reassuring or amusing compared with those who viewed their experiences as "malevolent", who felt distressed by their voices, and tried to eradicate them.

It is not just a person's perception of their symptoms that can cause distress, but also aspects of the diagnosis. Being given a diagnosis of schizophrenia with all of its negative connotations can in itself be traumatic unless delivered with much patience and explanatory information. A young woman during assessment for cognitive therapy reported interpreting her diagnosis of schizophrenia as meaning that she suffered from a "split personality". Although she had no personal evidence to suggest this was the case, to her this was even more worrying as she was convinced the worst was yet to come. Her "model" of schizophrenia was that if she lost control of her emotions then another, evil side of herself would take over and she would become an axe-wielding child killer. This belief system had major repercussions on her behaviour. Because she was desperate not to lose control of her emotions she avoided all potentially arousing situations, especially if there were children present. She also avoided talking about or finding out about her diagnosis because she felt that her worst fears would be confirmed. Many of this patient's behaviours were of course misinterpreted as being negative symptoms.

Turkington and Kingdon (1996) have described a number of cognitions that they have observed in patients who have been given the diagnosis of schizophrenia, including "I am mad", "I will be locked up", "I will be beaten and tortured in an asylum", "They will strap me down and give me electric shocks", and "They will give me very strong drugs and I will turn into a zombie". These typical beliefs are consistent with media representations of mental illness. Although the 1975 film *One Flew Over the Cuckoo's Nest* is often cited as being the epitome of anxiogenic psychiatric imagery, it is clear that very little progress has been made in diminishing these public myths when watching the likes of Channel 4's recent series *Psychos*. Unfortunately, beliefs of what will result from being ill can in themselves lead to increased anxiety and hopelessness and a general exacerbation of symptoms both neurotic and psychotic (Slade, 1973).

Understanding the patient's viewpoint and developing an individualised therapeutic formulation is therefore of vital importance. Not only will it help to provide a rationale to explain the patient's presenting problems, it will also serve as a guide to direct the therapeutic intervention. Of course formulations will differ depending upon the knowledge base of the individual creating the model. Present the same details of a case to a range of therapists from different therapeutic schools and each will produce a different rationale to explain the presenting problems. In the same way, each patient will have their own model of understanding the world which will be shaped by his or her own cultural, family, and personal belief system. For the person to need cognitive therapy there is an underlying assumption that this personal understanding is not working for the patient in some way and that an alternative perception of events would be more adaptive.

As well as there being a variety of different rationales that can be developed to interpret experiences, these explanations can provide varying depths of understanding. Offering a simplistic cognitive rationale to explain a patient's affect, one can propose that the person's feelings resulted from his or her thoughts or interpretations of an event. This does account for the person's affect at a basic level but it does not clarify *why* the individual is thinking erroneously. This requires a deeper level of understanding that utilises information processing models in conjunction with theories of schema formation and maintenance. Deciding what level of understanding or formulation is appropriate to be shared with the patient is an important aspect of therapy and is determined by a number of different factors. These include the ability of the patient to understand the proposed rationale, his or her concordance with the model, and his or her ego strength to be able to contain the distress that often accompanies in-depth schema level work. If these factors are not well judged the therapist risks a developing dissonance between therapist and patient. Without an apparent common understanding the possibility of the patient becoming disengaged from the therapist and the therapy increases. Without engagement the therapy is doomed to fail. Considering the sharing of a formulation therefore becomes a crucial aspect of therapy, especially when working with delusional beliefs; in this instance there is a delicate balance to be achieved between reaching a shared understanding without either colluding with the patient's misconceptions or rejecting his or her understanding of events.

TOWARDS A SHARED UNDERSTANDING

Cases can be formulated at a number of different levels and from a number of different viewpoints. The following models offer different perspectives on the same presenting problems.

The stress vulnerability model

A stress vulnerability model has been described by a number of different theorists but has been summarised and put in simple terms by Zubin and Spring (1977). The model incorporates identifiable personal vulnerability factors of both a biological (e.g. genetic predisposition, pre and peri-natal injury, etc.) and psychological (e.g. early experiences) kind. Stressful life events that the individual experiences prior to the onset of the psychotic symptoms are then incorporated into the model.

This type of formulation has two clear advantages. First, it offers a personalised view of the development of each person's symptoms that integrates the biological/medical perspective that he or she is likely to have been exposed to. Second, it provides a normalising rational (Kingdon & Turkington, 1991) that points to the idea that everyone has the potential to develop psychotic symptoms if put under sufficient stress. This normalising of symptoms helps to counteract alternative, terrifying models of madness that the patient may hold.

A simple cognitive model

Cognitive therapy proposes that emotions and behaviours do not result directly from events, but from the way the individual perceives or interprets these incidents. This theoretical model can also be explained to the patient to demonstrate that it is possible to have different ways of thinking about the same event and that divergent interpretations can modify mood. Within this rationale it should also be explained that it is normal for all people to have biases in their thinking in order to preserve their beliefs. Typical thinking errors such as dichotomous (black and white) thinking, arbitrary inference (jumping to conclusions), and selective abstraction (only seeing part of the picture) can also be explained to the patient in order to help them make sense of these biases.

The thought–mood connection can also be linked to the vulnerability stress model as explained above. Using cognitive therapy techniques the patient can reduce his or her level of stress and thereby lower the chance of relapse and, in turn, increase self-efficacy.

A schema level formulation

Understanding the roots of a problem will help the therapist to direct the therapy in an appropriate direction and to deal with core issues that can remain unresolved. Having an in-depth formulation should provide information on why the patient has developed delusional beliefs *of this kind* (as opposed to the stress vulnerability model, which simply provides a reason why the patient has developed delusions). Cognitive behavioural therapists will be familiar with typical schema or core dysfunctional assumptions; however, Fowler, Garety, and Kuipers (1995) encountered five main schematic themes among people with psychosis:

• The belief that the self is extremely vulnerable to harm—i.e. "I am fragile" or "I am unsafe" (core maladaptive schemas).

- The belief that one is highly vulnerable to losing self-control—i.e. "I am dangerous to others" (core maladaptive schema) and "I must strive to control all things at all times" (schema compensation).
- The belief that the self is doomed to social isolation—i.e. " I am utterly alone in the world" (core maladaptive schema).
- The belief in inner defectiveness—i.e. "I am damaged/deficient" (core maladaptive schema).
- The belief in unrelenting standards—i.e. "I must perform to the optimum standard in all areas at all times" (schema compensation).

Numerous other core maladaptive schemas are involved in the genesis and maintenance of psychotic symptoms—e.g. "I am different", "I am abandoned", and "I am special". Other compensatory schemas include "I must be approved of at all times" and "I should be rewarded as I am entitled to at all times". Often these dysfunctional assumptions can be identified within delusional themes or key concerns of the patient. This theory has been supported by research carried out by Raune, Kuipers, and Bebbington (1999) at the Institute of Psychiatry: they discovered links in the themes between the content of delusions and hallucinations and early psycho-social stressors. The therapist should also be able to identify *why* such assumptions should be present, because the identified schema should be congruent with the patient's early experiences. Overall one should expect there to be clear themes linking personal experience, schema *and* emergent psychotic symptoms (both in form and content). If this is not in evidence one should question the accuracy of the formulation and in turn the subsequent focus of the therapeutic intervention.

Delusions serving a defensive function

Within psycho-dynamic literature it has been postulated that delusional beliefs result from unconscious defence mechanisms (Bak, 1954; Schueler, Herron, Poland, & Schultz, 1982). These processes, fundamental to psycho-dynamic theory, are seen to operate in the person's thinking to protect from overwhelming emotions such as anger, guilt, shame, and anxiety, and to help maintain a delicate self-esteem. Traditionally, defence mechanisms do not tend to be afforded much discussion within the cognitive therapy literature and are seen as being part of another domain. Through research into apparent cognitive biases related to delusional beliefs, cognitive and psycho-dynamic models appear to be drawing closer. Kaney and Bentall (1989) looked at the attributional style of individual's experiencing persecutory delusions and discovered a self-serving attributional bias. Overall, this group was more likely to make excessively external attributions for negative events and internal attributions for positive events when compared with normal and depressed control groups. In short, the individuals were maintaining a positive view of themselves at the cost of having a deleterious view of others as a defence against depression.

Being aware of a possible defensive nature of a delusional belief is particularly important when formulating a case because there are obvious emotional repercussions to be considered. Directly challenging a delusion that is maintaining self-esteem is going to have a deleterious effect on the patient's emotional well-being. Therefore the ability for both patient and therapist to contain high levels of distress needs to be seriously considered before it is attempted. Whether a delusion has a defensive quality and the potential for distress when challenged should be evident from an accurate formulation.

THE CASE OF HELEN

The following case is presented to illustrate how the models of understanding discussed in the previous section can be integrated when producing an individualised formulation. The formulation should guide the therapist on a therapeutic course that will address the needs and vulnerabilities of each individual patient. It is our opinion that a formulation demonstrating coherence between life events, underlying schematic vulnerabilities, and resultant psychotic symptoms is the key principle guiding the course of cognitive therapy with a psychotic patient. This should lead to increasing adherence not only with the use of in-session cognitive techniques and homework experiments but also to increased adherence with neuroleptic medication. Patients whose key psychological concerns are being addressed within a collaborative therapeutic stance often become less antagonistic to medication partly through improved insight and partly through reduced alienation.

Presenting problems

Helen had been brought into hospital under Section 2 of the Mental Health Act. At the time she had complained that her brain was undergoing a haemorrhage and she had been seeking a priest to read her the last rites. She described blood running down her neck and believed she could feel her blood vessels splitting. At the time of her admission to hospital she believed she was being abducted by "anti-Christians" and was extremely frightened and upset.

She related her problems to a time in utero when she alleged her parents had held a transistor radio to her mother's stomach and increased the volume in an attempt to abort her. She believed she had been left with permanent brain damage as a result.

Helen came to our attention approximately three years later. She had insight into her admission and felt quite embarrassed about some of the views she had held at the time. However, she was still adamant that she had acquired brain damage whilst in utero. She believed this had resulted in many long-term adverse consequences and felt that these had prevented her from achieving her true potential. In particular she stated that her brain damage had affected her intellect and her ability to think, it prevented her from talking articulately to others, and caused her to get extremely anxious in certain situations. In addition, she believed that her brain damage was terminal, that she would not live beyond the age of 35, and she would therefore never have the opportunity to lead a normal life.

Helen described a time prior to acquiring the brain damage when as a foetus she could remember having a "marvellous intellect". She felt that had her brain not been harmed it would have been likely that she would have worked in the legal profession.

Helen was unsure how she could benefit from seeing a cognitive therapist, although she appreciated having someone with whom she could talk about her difficulties who would listen attentively.

Personal history

Helen was the youngest in a family of three siblings. Her father was a solicitor and her mother appeared to do a lot of voluntary work (though Helen had very little respect for her). Helen described an unhappy family life, she believed her parents had never wanted her and said that they had always made this clear. In particular she felt that her father had been emotionally abusive towards her as a child; he would be helpful one moment and then "would turn on her" the next. Always, however, he would make Helen feel inferior. Her mother was not so active in her reproach, but she would echo her husband's actions.

Helen felt that the relationship with her siblings had not been any better. She said that her eldest sister had bullied her both physically and emotionally for 24 years. This had stopped only when Helen had threatened to report her actions to the police. The relationship she had with her second sister had been more ambivalent, but lacked any nurturance.

School life for Helen was no happier than at home. Although academically bright, she had no friends and described being bullied from an early age until she left school at 18. Despite this, she achieved good exam results at O' and A' level and went on to do a degree course. After achieving a good mark in her degree she undertook a masters course.

It was while studying for her second degree that she had her first psychotic breakdown. She had been preparing for her exams and had been working continuously, having only about three hours of sleep each night. She also had been having problems with her landlord at the time and this had culminated in her being thrown out of her lodgings only days before her first exam. At this point Helen had felt her brain start to haemorrhage and had returned home to visit her local priest, only to end up being admitted to a psychiatric ward. Helen did not return to complete her degree following her hospital admission, but returned home to live with her parents.

Formulating the case

Helen had felt both unwanted and unloved as a child and throughout her life generally. She appeared to have made sense of this by personalising the rejection and believed unconditionally "there must be something wrong with me" (core maladaptive schema). It seemed the only area in her life that she believed she had been successful was within academia. This appeared to have been the mainstay of supporting her self-worth throughout years of bullying both at home and at school. Helen was aware that she was above average intellectually and this seems to have served as her only source of self-esteem. From these early experiences she developed the dysfunctional assumption that "to be of any worth I must achieve intellectually" (compensatory schema).

This conditional belief or schema appears to have helped Helen to some extent in that it served as a driving force while she was studying, but it left her vulnerable should her studies begin to fail. Motivated by this belief she studied hard and was able to achieve considerable academic success that led to her taking a masters degree. Unfortunately, in the period prior to her exams the pressure to succeed was so great that she focused on revision at the expense of everything else (schema activation—often the prelude to psychosis emergence in vulnerable individuals). She stopped going to bed in order to work through the night, her eating deteriorated, and she cut herself off from her peers.

Helen herself said that in retrospect she became quite "strange" during this period. It seems that her landlord also noticed that her behaviour was unusual and threw her out two days before her first exam. This event appears to be the final stressful life event that pushed her over the edge and led to her psychotic breakdown during which she developed the delusional belief that her brain was damaged. The emergence of Helen's delusion would therefore appear to fit the classification of an anxiety psychosis (Kingdon & Turkington, 1998). The delusion is robustly defended from change from two perspectives. First, it is expressed as a delusional memory, which to some degree reduces the possibility for reality-testing. Secondly, it reiterates an altered version of the core maladaptive schema—i.e. "there must be something wrong with me" is expressed as "I am brain damaged". Such a core maladaptive schema would only change very gradually through the use of schema-focused approaches, but the strong affect linked to the delusion would be liable to make this work even more difficult.

Helen's belief of having a damaged brain also serves two other functions. First, it has a defensive quality in that it excuses the fact that she did not succeed with her MA without feeling personally responsible for this apparent failure. Secondly, it seems that her belief about brain damage has a meta-phorical context (Bannister, 1983). She sees her parents as being responsible for her damaged brain through the use of very loud music in an attempt to cause an abortion that is perhaps seen as a righteous vehicle to express her anger about her upbringing which she can only do in relation to overt damage.

Fig. 5.1 provides a classic diagrammatic formulation of Helen's problems, with presenting problems represented at the bottom leading from the root causes at the top. Formulating a case in this manner is essential for ensuring the integrity of the therapeutic approach. To what degree this formulation is shared with the patient will depend upon the therapist's judgement. In this case it did not seem appropriate to be sharing the entire formulation with Helen because it was at odds with her own understanding that her problems resulted entirely from an acquired brain injury. To have divulged our own personal viewpoint would, I believe, have jeopardised the relationship with Helen who could have easily felt patronised and ignored. She was not open to exploring alternative explanations throughout the course of cognitive therapy.

Because Helen could see that she had suffered from a psychotic illness in

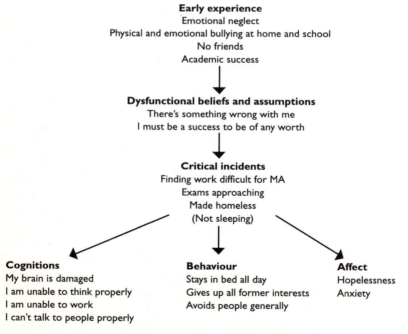

Figure 5.1 A classical cognitive formulation of Helen's problems.

the past this provided a good starting point in terms of sharing an integrated bio-psycho-social formulation. An analogy of a bucket being filled and over-flowing was used to describe the stress vulnerability model. This was put in terms that each person's biological make-up and past experiences shaped how the bucket would be formed, what capacity it had, and what weaknesses it had. Stressful life events were described in terms of water filling the bucket— with the bucket having only so much room before the water reached the top. Once the volume of water filling the bucket over-stretched the capacity, then the water overflowed—the individual became symptomatic (see Fig. 5.2).

Helen was able to identify a number of stressful life events that could have contributed to her illness. Interestingly she was not genetically predisposed to schizophrenia or any other psychotic disorder. She found this model quite revolutionary and was keen to tell her family. Unfortunately, however, she also felt that this model offered some support to her theory of brain damage, which she saw as being *the* "vulnerability factor". Whether this strengthened her delusional belief or not, it did have a positive effect upon the therapy. Helen felt that this model gave some credence to her own belief system and felt she was being taken seriously within the therapy. The shared formulation therefore served as a major contributory factor to Helen becoming actively involved in a collaborative therapeutic approach.

Leading from the stress vulnerability model, the therapy focused on stress-inducing events. For Helen these centred on times when she lacked confidence, especially in social situations and when driving her car. This

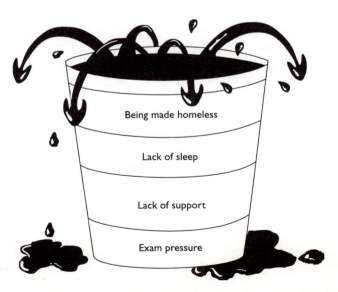

Figure 5.2 The bucket-filling analogy describing the stress vulnerability model.

appeared to be an appropriate stage to introduce a simple cognitive model of the thought–feeling link. Once again, Helen felt this model was particularly helpful and was enthusiastic to identify and start to challenge some of her most anxiogenic beliefs. Helen believed that because of her brain damage she was unable to carry out "normal" activities such as engaging in a conversation with a neighbour. Challenging some of Helen's negative predictions such as what would happen if she did talk to another person, served a secondary purpose. The cognitive model not only provided an alternative understanding of why she found such activities difficult, it also started to change many of her behaviours and beliefs that she had used as evidence to support her claim of brain damage.

Milton, Patwa, and Hafna (1978) discussed the importance of modifying delusions as opposed to confronting them in order to avoid them becoming more entrenched. During cognitive therapy with Helen, her delusional belief about brain damage was never challenged directly (though she had had a CT scan prior to entering therapy). Instead, therapy continued to focus on beliefs "peripheral" to the delusion (Kingdon & Turkington, 1994). Helen was convinced her brain damage had a number of effects, and in fact she blamed her brain damage for all aspects of herself that she saw as less than perfect, including her black and white thinking when it was highlighted. Many of these peripheral beliefs were evident as routine, negative, automatic thoughts and were coherent with her core maladaptive schema that she was in some way defective. Peripheral beliefs included:

- "I am unable to talk to others".
- "I am unable to concentrate".
- "I get pains in my head when my brain needs to work hard".
- "People see me as odd".

Continuing with this straightforward cognitive approach did have an impact upon Helen's delusional belief. After several sessions she reported that her brain damage was getting better—though she remained absolutely convinced that she did have brain damage. When asked why she thought this, she replied "because my way of thinking has changed". This improvement can be explained at two levels based upon the formulation. It is likely that by challenging Helen's peripheral beliefs there was less evidence to support her core schema and the related, externalised delusional belief. Put another way, it is possible that the cognitive work had a beneficial impact upon her self-esteem and this reduced the need for the delusion, which was serving as a protective defence.

Helen continues to this day to be convinced of her brain damage, but this belief is much less prohibiting. Whereas at one point she had given up on life and felt there was no point in doing much other than staying in bed most of the day, she now is much more active and wants to have a normal life. She now lives independently in her own house, has a fitness programme, and is doing a work rehabilitation course and is aiming for an office job.

CONCLUSIONS

Cases can be formulated at a number of different levels and from a wide range of perspectives. The purpose is to pull all the details of each individual case together and make sense of them as a whole in a collaborative manner. Having this understanding should be central in guiding the therapeutic approach. Specific vulnerabilities that the patient may have should be highlighted by the formulation and, in turn, this should explain the functionality and content of psychotic symptoms in relation to particular accumulations of schema threatening life events. In all cases coherence between life events, schematic vulnerability, and psychotic symptoms will guide the therapist in relation to the correct order of application of techniques. Schema change is vital to ensure durability of effect and is the main approach to a delusion when presented with no insight, when systematised, grandiose (Turkington & Siddle, 1998), or when, as in this case, it is presented as a delusional memory or as a restated core maladaptive schema. The most effective techniques in this case were therefore the development of a collaborative, trusting, therapeutic relationship, the generation of a formulation, and the use of schema-focused techniques that allowed several parameters of the impact of the delusion to begin to change. As Helen started to believe less in her own deficiency as a person she reported that her brain damage was improving. To gradually allow the delusion to shift towards the status of an overvalued idea meant that she had to be allowed to process in her own way the sadness and embarrassment linked to her academic failure and to her years of dedication to the brain damage hypothesis. This emotional change was handled sensitively within session using a variety of supportive techniques.

Research has shown (Gilhooly, 1983) that once we have formed a belief we are not very good at looking for evidence that might refute it (as is also the case in those holding delusional beliefs). However, as therapists we must remain mindful that our formulations are indeed just that—*our* formulations. We are as able to come up with a faulty model as the next. Realising that we can get it wrong as well as understanding that the process of formulating is a dynamic one of gathering new information and adapting previous models, should help us to be good therapists. It should also help us to listen to and appreciate alternatives, including, most importantly, the models that our patients bring with them. Overall, the principle of coherence between past experience, schema, and psychotic symptoms should guide us in our understanding. However, no matter how sophisticated the formulation we produce, only once the patient feels he or she has been heard and understood can therapy truly progress.

REFERENCES

Bak, R.C. (1954). The schizophrenic defence against aggression. *International Journal of Psychoanalysis, 35*, 129–134.

Bannister, D. (1983). The psychotic disguise. In W. Dryden (Ed.), *Therapists' dilemmas*. London: Harper & Row.

Bentall, R.P. (1996). From cognitive studies of psychosis to cognitive behaviour therapy for psychotic symptoms. In G. Haddock & P.D. Slade (Eds.), *Cognitive-behavioural interventions with psychotic disorders*. London: Routledge.

Berrios, G. (1991). Delusions as "wrong beliefs": A conceptual history. *British Journal of Psychiatry, 159*, Suppl. 14: 6–13.

Chadwick, P., & Birchwood, M. (1994). The omnipotence of voices: A cognitive approach to auditory hallucinations. *British Journal of Psychiatry, 164*, 190–201.

Festinger, L. (1957). *A theory of cognitive dissonance*. Stanford, CA: Stanford University Press.

Fowler, F., Garety, P., & Kuipers, E. (1995). *Cognitive behaviour therapy for psychosis*. Chichester: Wiley.

Garety, P.A., & Freeman, D. (1999). Cognitive approaches to delusions: A critical review of theories and evidence. *British Journal of Clinical Psychology, 38*, 113–154.

Garety, P.A., Hemsley, D.R., & Wessely, S. (1991). Reasoning in deluded schizophrenic and paranoid patients: Biases in performance on a probabilistic inference task. *Journal of Nervous and Mental Disorder, 179*, 194–201.

Garety, P.A., & Hemsley, D.R. (1994). *Delusions: Investigations into the psychology of delusional reasoning*. Hove, UK: Psychology Press.

Gilhooly, K. (1983). *Thinking*. London: Academic Press.

Gorman, M.E. (1989). Error, falsification, and scientific inference: An experimental investigation. *Quarterly Journal of Experimental Psychology, 41*, 385–412.

Hamilton, M. (1978). *Fish's outline of psychiatry* (3rd edition). Bristol: John Wright.

Harrow, M., Rattenbury, F., & Stoll, F. (1988). Schizophrenic delusions: An analysis of their persistence, of related premorbid ideas, and of three major dimensions. In F. Oltmanns & B.A. Maher (Eds.), *Delusional beliefs* (pp. 185–211). New York: John Wiley.

Hemsley, D.R., & Garety, P.A. (1986). The formation and maintenance of delusions: A Bayesian analysis. *British Journal of Psychiatry, 149*, 51–56.

Huq, S.F., Garety, P.A., & Hemsley, D.R. (1988). Probabilistic judgements in deluded and non-deluded subjects. *Quarterly Journal of Experimental Psychology, 40A*, 801–812.

Jaspers, K. (1963). *General psychopharmacology* (J. Hoenig & M.W. Hamilton, trans.). Manchester: Manchester University Press.

John, C.H., & Dodgson, G. (1994). Inductive reasoning in delusional thinking. *Journal of Mental Health, 3*, 31–49.

Kaney, S., & Bentall, R.P. (1989). Persecutory delusions and attributional style. *British Journal of Medical Psychology, 62*, 191–198.

Kingdon, D.G., & Turkington, D. (1991). The use of cognitive behaviour therapy with a normalising rationale in schizophrenia. *Journal of Nervous and Mental Disease, 179*, 207–211.

Kingdon, D.G., & Turkington, D. (1994). *Cognitive behavioural therapy of schizophrenia.* New York: Guilford Press.

Kingdon, D.G., & Turkington, D. (1998). Cognitive behavioural therapy of schizophrenia. In T. Wykes, N. Tarrier, & S. Lewis (Eds.), *Outcome and innovation in psychological treatment of schizophrenia.* Chichester: Wiley.

Linney, Y., Peters, E., & Ayton, P. (1998). Reasoning biases in delusion-prone individuals. *British Journal of Clinical Psychology, 37,* 247–370.

Milton, F., Patwa, V.K., & Hafna, R.J. (1978). Confrontation vs belief modification in persistently deluded patients. *British Journal of Psychiatry, 51,* 127–130.

Piaget, J. (1952). *The origins of intelligence in children.* New York: International Universities Press.

Raune, D., Kuipers, E., & Bebbington P. (1999). *Psycho-social stress and delusional and verbal auditory hallucinatory themes in first episode psychosis: implications for early intervention.* Presented to The Third International Conference of Psychological Treatments for Schizophrenia, Oxford, England.

Romme, M.A.J., Honig, A., Noordhoorn, E.O., & Escher, A.D.M.A.C. (1992). Coping with hearing voices: An emancipatory approach. *British Journal of Psychiatry, 16,* 99–103.

Schueler, D.E., Herron, W.G., Poland, H.V., & Schultz, C.L. (1982). Defence mechanisms in reactive and process schizophrenics. *Journal of Clinical Psychology, 38,* 486–489.

Slade, P.D. (1973). The psychological investigation and treatment of auditory hallucinations: A second case report. *British Journal of Medical Psychology, 46,* 293–296.

Strauss, J.S. (1969). Hallucinations and delusions as points on continua function: Rating scale evidence. *Archives of General Psychiatry, 147,* 1587–1595.

Turkington, D., John, C.H., Siddle, R. et al. (1996). Cognitive therapy in the treatment of drug resistant delusional disorder. *Clinical Psychology and Psychotherapy, 3,* 118–128.

Turkington, D., & Kingdon, D. (1996). Using a normalising rationale in the treatment of schizophrenic patients. In G. Haddock & P.D. Slade (Eds.), *Cognitive-Behavioural Interventions with Psychotic Disorders.* London: Routledge.

Turkington, D., & Siddle, R. (1998). Cognitive therapy for the treatment of delusions. *Advances in Psychiatric Treatment, 4,* 235–242.

Zubin, J., & Spring, B. (1977). Vulnerability: A new view on schizophrenia. *Journal of Abnormal Psychology, 86,* 103–126.

Part II

Specific cognitive therapies for psychotic symptoms

Chapter 6

The use of coping strategies and self-regulation in the treatment of psychosis

Nicholas Tarrier

INTRODUCTION

The use of coping strategies to treat the symptoms of psychotic disorders has developed over the past 10 to 15 years. The origin of this approach has its basis in a number of sources. First, the way people deal with aversive experience and events has long been of interest in general psychology and there is an extensive literature on such coping mechanisms (Zeidner & Endler, 1996). Central to the idea of coping is the process of appraisal whereby the person evaluates a set of circumstances or experience as a problem and attempts to cope, subsequently evaluating the success or otherwise of these attempts. Similarly important has been the concept of self-efficacy (Bandura, 1977).

Secondly, it has long been recognised that the use of personal resources such as coping strategies is important in buffering against psychotic decompensation leading to exacerbations or relapse of positive psychotic symptoms. For example, in the Nuechterlein (1987) stress vulnerability model of psychosis, coping and self-efficacy are cited as important personal protective factors.

Thirdly, has been the influence of theoretic positions that have developed to underpin cognitive behaviour therapy. The seminal paper by Kanfer and Saslow (1965) advanced the position that clinical problems could best be understood by a detailed analysis of the contextual circumstances and the applied behavioural analysis of the antecedents and consequences of the defined problem, rather than psychiatric classification into diagnostic groups. The use of behaviour analysis of positive psychotic symptoms was central to the development of a case formulation on which coping interventions were based. With the development of cognitive models of other disorders, mainly anxiety and affective disorders, the understanding of cognitive mechanisms and the inclusion of these in behavioural analysis has been advanced (Lowe & Higson, 1981).

Fourthly has been the work on self-regulation of Kanfer, Karoly, and others (Karoly & Kanfer, 1982) in which target behaviour is identified as undesirable or inappropriate and monitored with the purpose of implementing alternative learned responses through a process of self-regulation. This approach has also been shown to be effective with schizophrenic patients (Breier & Strauss, 1983). Clearly, there is considerable overlap between coping and self-regulation. Furthermore, self-regulation and coping may improve executive functioning by increasing control over basic processes such as attention, response inhibition, and response initiation.

Lastly are the empirical findings that schizophrenic patients do make effortful attempts to overcome or cope with persistent positive psychotic symptoms. This was initially based on the observation that the majority of patients who experienced persistent hallucinations and delusions made active attempts to cope with their symptoms with at least some success (Tarrier, 1987). This observation was in accord with other reports (e.g. Breier & Strauss, 1983; Brenner, Boker, Mueller, Spiching, & Wuergler, 1987; Carr, 1988; Cohen & Berk, 1985; Falloon & Talbot, 1981; Romme & Escher, 1987). It was reasoned that since many patients used coping strategies naturalistically they would further benefit from systematic training in coping skills combined with an awareness of the antecedents and context of their symptoms. Further research indicated that patients' beliefs about their symptoms and their appraisal were important in determining whether and how they coped (Kinney, 1999).

MODEL

Optimally, treatment or intervention for a clinical disorder should be based on a testable theoretical position. There are no unifying theories of schizophrenia, although the stress-vulnerability model advanced by Zubin and Spring (1977) was an attempt to produce an overarching second order model of schizophrenia that could accommodate within it different theoretical positions. We have attempted to produce an explanation of the determinants of psychotic symptoms as a clinical heuristic (Haddock & Tarrier, 1998) that will guide cognitive behavioural interventions, represented in Fig. 6.1.

It was speculated that psychotic experience could be a response to a combination of internal or environmental antecedents that may operate through a common mediating pathway, such as a dysfunction in the arousal system or in its regulation (Tarrier & Turpin, 1992). These internal factors could be biological or psychological and could be inherent or acquired. An example of inherent biological factors would be the transmission of genetic heritability, and an example of acquired would be damage resulting from birth trauma. Inherent psychological factors would be cognitive deficits, and acquired would be cognitive biases or certain beliefs or schematic representations. The model is basically a threshold model in which interacting internal vulnerabilities and external stresses culminate in precipitating and possibly maintaining psychotic symptoms. There is little attempt to explain what psychotic

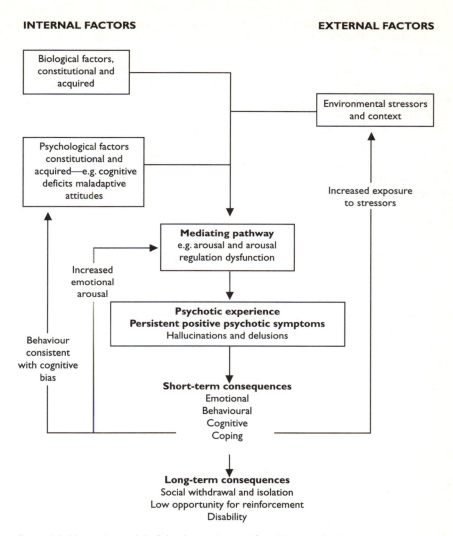

INTERNAL FACTORS   **EXTERNAL FACTORS**

Biological factors, constitutional and acquired

Environmental stressors and context

Psychological factors constitutional and acquired—e.g. cognitive deficits maladaptive attitudes

Increased exposure to stressors

Mediating pathway
e.g. arousal and arousal regulation dysfunction

Increased emotional arousal

Psychotic experience
Persistent positive psychotic symptoms
Hallucinations and delusions

Behaviour consistent with cognitive bias

Short-term consequences
Emotional
Behavioural
Cognitive
Coping

Long-term consequences
Social withdrawal and isolation
Low opportunity for reinforcement
Disability

Figure 6.1 Heuristic model of the determinants of positive psychotic symptoms.

symptoms are, other than to understand the conditions in which they occur. It is proposed that the experience of hallucinations and delusions has its consequences. Such psychotic experiences may well evoke emotions; they may be perplexing or frightening, disgusting or annoying, and so on. Furthermore, psychotic experience will almost inevitably have cognitive and behavioural consequences as the person attempts to explain or understand what is happening to them. They may make various attributions about the origins or nature of the voices or ideas that they have. The work of Birchwood and colleagues on the valence, omnipotence, and control of hallucinations (Chadwick & Birchwood, 1994) is evidence of this.

Symptoms can be maintained by the activation of feedback loops. Thus emotional responses to the psychotic experience, such as anxiety, fear or anger, would initiate a feedback loop and increase the severity of psychotic symptoms by contributing through increased levels of activity within the arousal system (Barrowclough & Tarrier, 1992, p. 161; Haddock & Tarrier, 1998). Similarly, cognitive responses and biases—such as misinterpretation, attention to perceived threat, selective attribution, and failure to reality-test—would also produce emotional sequelae and activate feedback. Behaviour could further serve to reinforce these cognitive responses if it was consistent with cognitive process or content, so that behaviour that was congruent with beliefs (belief-congruent behaviour) or resulted in confirmation of specific interpretations (hypothesis protection) would be likely to reinforce and maintain psychopathology. Further, behavioural responses could increase the patient's exposure to various environmental antecedents or stressors that would increase the probability of symptoms occurring.

The effects of the psychotic disorder will change over time and there may well be a build up of long-term consequences, such as social withdrawal, isolation and loneliness, decreasing opportunities for reward, ineffectual social skills, and so on. These in turn will perpetuate disability by restricting the patient's social networks, decreasing the opportunity for purposeful behaviour, and lowering motivation to initiate goal directed behaviour.

The aims of teaching coping strategies to patients would be to decrease exposure to powerful antecedents and triggers of their symptoms or improve tolerance to them, and to provide an alternative set of coping responses that would deactivate the feedback loops into the arousal system and produce more constructive behaviours. However, because of the multiple effects of a psychotic illness it would be anticipated that the many needs of patients would require multi-agency case management or a similar comprehensive treatment approach.

The model outlined earlier attempts to combine factors from general psychological models with an understanding of the specific nature of schizophrenia. Simply applying to schizophrenia a generic Beckian cognitive model that has been developed for other disorders, such as depression, may be misleading (Patience, 1994). For example, adopting Beck's cognitive model, such as that used to explain depression, would suggest that schizophrenogenic schema pre-date the onset of the disorder, and symptoms of hallucinations and delusions arise solely from these schema. There is no evidence to support this position. Thus, there are specific pathological processes that appear central to schizophrenia that need to be considered, such as the nature of arousal and arousal regulation dysfunction, or cognitive deficits and deficits in executive function (Dawson, Nuechterlein, & Adams, 1989; Frith, 1994; Hemsley, 1994). Thus lack of clarity in transporting explanatory models could result in theoretical confusion and misplaced interventions. The therapist also needs to be aware of a number of problems that may be associated with psychotic disorders that affect the procedure and process of therapy. Features that need to be assessed and possibly taken into consideration in cognitive behavioural therapy for psychotic patients include:

- Psychological

  — interference, disrupted or slowed thought processes;
  — difficulty discriminating signal from noise;
  — restricted attention;
  — hypersensitivity to social stressors and social interactions;
  — difficulty processing social stimuli and acting appropriately;
  — flat and restricted affect;
  — elevated arousal or dysfunctional arousal regulation;
  — hypersensitivity to stress and life events;
  — high risk of suicide;
  — stigmatisation;
  — risk of depression and hopelessness;
  — high risk of substance abuse;
  — onset in late adolescence/early adulthood interfered with normal developmental processes.

- Psycho-social

  — hypersensitive to family environments and social relationships;
  — risk of perpetrating, or being the victim of, violence;
  — integration of cognitive behavioural therapy with other interventions: e.g. family interventions.

- Social

  — conditions of social deprivation;
  — poor housing;
  — downward social drift;
  — unemployment and difficulty in competing in the job market;
  — restricted social network;
  — psychiatric career interferes with utilisation of other social resources.

EFFICACY

A method known as Coping Strategy Enhancement (CSE) was developed as a cognitive behavioural treatment that: (a) attempted to use established coping strategies already in the patient's repertoire; (b) used an array of different techniques, behavioural and cognitive; (c) practised coping in response to actual or simulated psychotic symptoms; and (d) included homework procedures and emphasised in vivo utilisation of coping strategies (Tarrier, Harwood, Yusupoff, Beckett, & Baker, 1990). A small, randomised, open, controlled trial compared CSE with problem-solving training in medicated patients suffering persistent positive symptoms (Tarrier, Beckett, Harwood, Baker, Yusupoff, & Ugarteburu, 1993a). The results indicated that both CSE and problem solving resulted in a significant decrease in positive symptoms compared with a waiting list control period. There was some evidence that CSE was superior to problem solving in reducing symptoms, especially delusions and anxiety. Hallucinations and depression showed less improvement. In some patients there was an increase in depressed mood associated with improvements in positive symptoms, although this was not statistically significant. Thus the effect of cognitive behavioural therapy on some types of symptoms in schizophrenic patients was unclear. Changes in measures of coping skills and problem-solving skills were also examined. The coping skills group showed significant increases both in the number of positive coping skills used and in their efficacy, whereas the problem-solving group showed a decrease in these measures during treatment. Both groups showed significant improvements in problem-solving skills. Improvements in coping but not problem solving were significantly related to decreases in psychotic symptoms during treatment (Tarrier, Sharpe, Beckett, Harwood, Baker, & Yusupoff, 1993b).

A second study, which recruited a geographical cohort rather than a convenience sample, investigated whether a combination of Coping Strategy Enhancement, problem solving and relapse prevention, as an adjunct to routine care including neuroleptic medication, would be efficacious when compared with supportive counselling and routine care, and routine care alone. Supportive counselling was used to control for therapy contact and social interaction, and the non-specific factors of such contact, and to provide general emotional support. An intention-to-treat analysis indicated that even when refusers and drop-outs were included in the analysis, cognitive behavioural therapy was superior to supportive counselling, which in turn was superior to routine care alone in reducing positive symptoms. Significant differences, however, were mainly between cognitive behavioural therapy and routine care alone, and there were some improvements in patients receiving supportive counselling. Analysis by means of logistic regression indicated that the receipt of cognitive behavioural therapy resulted in almost 8 times (odds ratio: 7.88) the chance of showing a 50% reduction in positive symptoms compared with receiving routine care alone (Tarrier, Yusupoff, Kinney, McCarthy, Gledhill, Haddock, & Morris, 1998a). In evidence-based medicine the benchmark with which to judge treatments is the number of patients needed to treat (NNT: Sackett, Richardson, Rosenberg, & Haynes, 1997). This is the number of patients that are required to be treated to result in one more successful outcome than the control or comparison treatment. Using an improvement of 50% or more in positive symptoms as the outcome at post-treatment, the NNT for cognitive behavioural therapy over routine care was 5, for cognitive behavioural therapy over supportive counselling it was 6, and for supportive counselling over routine care it was 25. An NNT of 5 and 6 is a very positive benefit in these terms (Sackett et al., 1997).

A more detailed analysis of the changes in different symptoms is an analysis-to-protocol—that is of patients who completed the treatment programme and demonstrated that both delusions and hallucinations responded to cognitive behavioural therapy (Tarrier, Kinney, McCarthy, Wittkowski, Yusupoff, Gledhill, Morris, & Humphreys, 2001). There were indications that delusions generally responded better to treatment and that patients who experienced hallucinations alone, without secondary delusions, did not respond at all. Delusions also responded significantly to supportive counselling but hallucinations did not. Patients suffering persecutory delusions showed greater symptomatology at pre-treatment but a greater change over treatment. Negative symptoms and thought disorder also showed improvement with cognitive behavioural therapy, although affective symptoms and social functioning did not. Depression showed a modest positive correlation with changes in positive symptoms and there was no indication that patients became depressed with the loss of their positive symptoms.

An investigation was made of why patients drop out of treatment (Tarrier, Yusupoff, McCarthy, Kinney, & Wittkowski, 1998b). The most common reason given was that the patients did not perceive the treatment as suitable for their problems. Patients who dropped out of treatment were more likely to be male, unemployed, and unskilled, single, with a low level of educational attainment and low pre-morbid IQ. They had a lengthy duration of illness, although at the time of discontinuation they were not necessarily severely ill and they were able to function at a reasonable level. They suffered both hallucinations and delusions and were likely to be depressed and moderately hopeless. They were as likely as not to be paranoid, although not necessarily suspicious of the therapist.

Follow-up at one year after the end of treatment showed that the differences between cognitive behavioural therapy and supportive counselling had decreased, but routine care alone did significantly worse on both positive and negative symptoms (Tarrier, Wittkowski, Kinney, McCarthy, Morris, & Humphreys, 1999). At two-year follow-up a significantly greater number of patients who received routine care alone now showed a deterioration from baseline of over 20% (Tarrier, Kinney, McCarthy, Humphreys, Wittowski, & Morris, 2000). Patients who received routine care alone had higher relapse rates and a shorter time to relapse over the 27-month treatment and follow-up period, although these differences did not reach significance.

COPING STRATEGIES

Coping is a natural process whereby an individual attempts to mobilise resources to deal with aversive experience. Here we define coping as an active attempt to control, overcome, or master the positive symptoms of psychosis or the distress that they cause. Kinney (1999) has found that the patient's appraisal of their symptoms is important in determining whether and how they cope. Symptoms that are regarded as taxing, that are burdensome, are most likely to elicit effortful attempts to cope, while those that are not are less likely to be appraised as requiring coping.

Coping can include strategies that involve cognitive processes, behavioural actions, and attempts to change sensory input or physiological states. An important aspect of this approach is that patients use appropriate methods of coping in a process of self-regulation. Thus coping skills refer to a process of response acquisition, where certain responses, either overt or covert, that do not exist within the patient's repertoire, or do so only partially or in an incomplete form, are acquired and utilised. Further, it can be speculated that coping methods result in improvement in executive functioning because they involve increased regulation of basic psychological processes such as attention, response inhibition, and response initiation.

ENGAGEMENT AND RATIONALE

Engagement is an extremely important issue in treating patients with schizophrenia. Most studies show that once a person has been engaged in therapy drop-out is relatively infrequent (e.g. Tarrier et al., 1998b). The relative success of supportive counselling would indicate that the non-specific aspects of therapy and the interpersonal processes are important and potentially beneficial (Tarrier et al., 1999, 2000). The therapist should take time to engage the patient, be careful to explain the rationale of therapy and proceed at a pace that suits the patient rather than rushing to deliver a protocol. Various specific problems associated with schizophrenia have been outlined in the lists at the end of the "Model" section earlier in this chapter, and the procedure of therapy, such as the duration of therapy sessions, should be geared to the patient's capabilities. With some patients the initial sessions may be aimed at the patient developing a tolerance of the therapist and the potentially stimulating effects of the therapeutic process.

ASSESSMENT

As with many cognitive behavioural approaches, intervention is based on a comprehensive and idiographic assessment and formulation, in this case known as the Antecedent and Coping Interview (ACI). This interview is based on a model of psychotic experience, which attempts to integrate explanations derived from general cognitive behavioural models of psychopathology, such as applied behavioural analysis and cognitive models of emotional disorders, and problems that are specific to psychosis, such as cognitive deficits and arousal system dysfunction. See Fig. 6.1 for an account of the model and also the lists of associative features at the end of the "Model" section earlier in this chapter, which need to be taken into account when providing psychological treatment with schizophrenic patients.

The ACI is a semi-structured interview that should provide adequate information to be used as a basis for intervention. It assumes knowledge and skills in being able to elicit psychotic symptoms and in being able to conduct a cognitive behavioural analysis. It consists of the five stages examined in the following sub-sections, namely:

1   the nature and variation of psychotic symptoms;
2   the emotions that accompany each psychotic symptom;
3   antecedent stimuli and context;
4   consequences; and
5   coping.

The nature and variation of psychotic symptoms

Each psychotic symptom needs to be elicited, and the Present State Examination (Wing, Cooper, & Sartorius, 1974) interview schedule is a useful tool to help do this, giving very good examples of questions that can be used. The interviewer needs to enquire about all psychotic experience—e.g. the types and nature of hallucinations, the types of delusions, and the nature of any interference with thought processes. Once each symptom has been identified the interviewer should elicit the frequency of the symptom. The interviewer should start with general questions such as "how often do you hear the voices?" and then be more specific: "how often did you hear them yesterday?"

The interviewer needs to elicit the various dimensions of each symptom, such as the severity or intensity of hallucinations or delusional thought, the physical characteristics of the voices, etc. There are now specialist rating scales, such as PSYRATS (Haddock, McCarron, & Tarrier, 1999) which provide scales for rating these various dimensions. The interviewer should be particularly alert to variations and patterns in the experience of the symptoms.

If the patient hears voices, it is important to know to whom or what they attribute them and where the patient thinks the voices are coming from, their level of power and control, and whether they are positive or negative, supportive, neutral or hostile.

The emotions that accompany each psychotic symptom

For each symptom or psychotic experience the interviewer should elicit the emotional reaction that accompanies the symptom. The interviewer should start with general questions such as "how do you feel when this happens?" and "how does this affect you?", then moving on to probe for more specific emotions such as, "do you feel frightened/nervous/angry/sad/fed up/guilty/ashamed/down . . .?" It is often a good idea to use a number of different descriptors for the same emotion—e.g. sad, down, fed up, moody, etc.

Once the interviewer has elicited the emotional reactions to the symptom in global terms they should attempt to break down the emotion into three systems—cognition (subjective experience), behaviour, and physiological reaction (self-report). Thus detailed questions about a specific emotion should be asked, such as "when you feel angry about the voices what type of thoughts go through your head?" Simulation exercises can assist this questioning if necessary: for example, "imagine you were hearing the voices now and you are getting angry, what would be on your mind, what thoughts would you be having?" Similarly, questions can be asked about the behavioural components of the emotion: "what do you do when you feel anxious?", and physiological reactions: "how do you feel inside, in your body?" Here probe questions about the type of physical reactions can be used, such as probes about increased heart rate, sweating, muscle tension, etc. At the end of this section the interviewer should have a good picture of the psychotic symptoms and the emotions they elicit.

Antecedent stimuli and context

The interviewer is searching for triggers or precipitators that determine the context for the symptoms. Patients may be very aware of these. Sometimes they are unaware of any pattern but one does unfold with questioning, while other patients, even with detailed questioning, are unable to identify any obvious context to their symptoms. Patients can be asked to monitor their symptoms and keep diaries to establish cues and patterns.

The interviewer should ask about each symptom in turn and question whether there are any triggers, or will the symptom occur in certain circumstances, or whether the patients knows a symptom is going to "come on". Sometimes this can be asked in a different way: e.g. "are there any situations in which you always hear the voices?" Besides location and circumstances the interviewer should enquire about situations such as the time of day and especially any social context.

Once the interviewer has asked about potential external stimuli they should then ask about internal stimuli such as internal feelings or specific thought patterns. The interviewer should also enquire about potential links between internal and external stimuli. For example, being with people makes the patient aware of feeling tense and a throbbing sensation in their head that makes them have the thought that something has been implanted in their head.

Particular attention should be paid to chains of stimuli and responses, especially where these relate to misidentifications or misattribution, such as misattribution of physical sensations or misidentification of noises or olfactory cues. Also, situations that the patient finds stressful need to be enquired about including situations that are characterised by deficits or absence of purposeful behaviour such as periods of inactivity, insomnia, etc.

Consequences

The interviewer should enquire about the consequences of the symptoms. These can apply to a number of areas of long-term behavioural change such as severe avoidance and social withdrawal, isolation, and loneliness, and also the consequence of persistent symptoms and psychotic disability such as poor employment prospects, restricted social networks, and deprivation. The patient can be asked: "how have these problems (voices/fears/illness) affected you/your life?"; "how would things be different if these problems hadn't happened?"; "how would you like to change things in you life/daily routine/ circumstances?" and similar questions that investigate the effect of schizophrenia on the person. Enquiry should also be made about behaviour that protects or encourages particular types of thought or attitudes, such as would support delusional thinking or acting in a way that reinforces negative self-esteem.

Besides these overt consequences of symptoms and psychosis there is also the opportunity to establish reactions to the psychotic experience that may feed back and maintain the psychosis. This line of enquiry is particularly important and can include behaviour change that further exposes the patient to stressful or difficult situations, such as exposure to arguments or hostile social situations, increased inactivity or disengagement, and thought patterns about their experience. Here it is useful to ask about how they interpret their experience and why it has happened, or what they make of the voices, or how they think about themselves, particularly in terms of their own self-worth.

Coping

Having established a comprehensive picture of what the patient experiences and how it affects them, it is now important to find out about how they deal with it. Questions can be asked about each symptom concerning how the patient manages that particular experience, such as "how do you cope with that?"; "is there anything you can do to make that better or easier (or anything that makes it worse)?"; "what do you do when that happens or you feel like that?"

It is also useful to evaluate how successful the coping method is. This can be done by ranking the coping strategy on a three-point scale: zero equals no or little use or moderately effective for a very short time; one equals moderately effective for a reasonable time or very effective for a short time; and two equals very effective for an extended period of time.

Many of these areas covered in the ACI will overlap and some of the areas are artificially divided, but this breakdown provides a comprehensive and over-inclusive structure for obtaining information about the experience of psychotic symptoms, their effects, and how the patient reacts.

INTERVENTION

Once a comprehensive picture of the patient's psychotic experience has been built up, this can be discussed with the patient and the rationale for coping training put forward. There may well be patients who are completely convinced of their delusional thoughts and who will not accept any alternative view, in which case coping with distress should be advanced as a suitable goal.

The characteristics of coping training are as follows:

- It emphasises a normal and general process of dealing with adversity.
- It is carried out systematically through over-learning, simulation, and role-play.
- It is additive in that different strategies can be added together in a sequence that progresses to in vivo implementation.
- It is based on providing a new response set that will be a method of coping with an ongoing problem rather than being curative.
- The learning of cognitive coping skills is through a process of external verbalisation, which is slowly diminished until the required procedure is internalised under covert control (cf. Vygotsky, 1962). This is analogous to a developmental process through which children acquire internal control.
- The learning of behavioural coping skills is through a process of graded practice or rehearsal.

Intervention should be based upon the detailed and comprehensive set of information provided by the assessment interview. This should produce an overall intervention strategy, which will include a number of possible tactics for reducing symptoms and distress.

Coping methods

These methods include changes in cognitive processes, content, and behaviour such as those discussed in the following sub-sections.

Attention switching

This is a process whereby a patient actively changes the focus of their attention from one subject or experience to another. This involves inhibiting an ongoing response and initiating an alternative. Patients are trained to switch attention on cue through rehearsal, often to a set of positive images, within the session. For example, one patient who was asked to choose a positive scene to which to attend, chose a restaurant in Blackpool where he had had an enjoyable meal. He was trained to be able to elicit a visual image of the restaurant by describing the scene, furniture, decorations, and such like in great detail. He was then asked to remember the experience of the meal in all senses—the visual memory of the food, its smell and taste, the feel of the knife and fork, the experience of eating, and so on. He then continually rehearsed the memory of the meal in the restaurant until he was able to elicit it at will. He then rehearsed switching his attention away from delusion thoughts to the images of the meal.

Attention narrowing

This is a process whereby the patient restricts the range and content of their attention. Many patients talked about "blanking" their mind or focusing their attention as a method of coping. Evidence suggests that one problem that schizophrenic patients face is an inability to adequately filter information input, to distinguish signal from noise (Shakow, 1962). Training to focus their attention and improve attentional control may assist them in overcoming this difficulty.

Modified self-statements and internal dialogue

Patients use self-statements, and that this can be incorporated successfully into intervention has been known for some years (Meichenbaum & Cameron, 1971). The use of self-statements and internal dialogue can take on a number of functions: in emotion control such as teaching the patient to overcome negative emotions associated with their voices; in cueing goal-directed behaviour; and in cueing and directing reality-testing. In each case the patient is taught statements that direct the appropriate response, such as "I don't need to be afraid", "I need to keep going and get on the bus", or "why do I think that man is looking at me when I've never seen him before?" Within the session the patient is first asked to repeat the set of statements out loud when given the appropriate cue. The verbalised statements are then gradually reduced in loudness until they are internalised. Patients then practise these in simulated situations within the session.

Reattribution

Patients are asked to generate an alternative explanation for an experience and then practise reattributional statement when that experience occurs. When we started coping training we used reattributions that were illness-related, such as "it's not a real voice, it's my illness", but we have since abandoned this as unhelpful. We would now try to use alternative explanations like "it may seem like a real voice but it's just my own thoughts". If patients do make changes that increase their control over their symptoms or circumstances, or challenge the omnipotence or infallibility of their voices, then these changes can be evidence for a reattribution concerning the nature of their symptoms or the patient's ability to exert control.

Awareness training

Patients are taught to be aware of and monitor the onset of their positive symptoms. Thus there are similarities here between self-monitoring in the self-regulation processes described by Karoly and Kanfer (1982) and the treatment of hallucinations, termed focusing by Haddock, Bentall, and Slade (1996) and exposure by Persaud and Marks (1995).

De-arousing techniques

Because high levels of arousal have been implicated in the psychopathology of schizophrenia (Dawson et al., 1989) and frequently occur as both antecedents (Slade, 1972) and responses to psychotic experience, teaching patients to cope with these is important. These coping strategies can be simple, passive behaviours to avoid agitation, such as sitting quietly instead of pacing up and down, or more active methods of arousal control, such as breathing exercises or quick relaxation. We have not favoured lengthy relaxation training such as traditional progressive relaxation exercises, because these are time consuming and off the point.

Increased activity levels

Many patients appear vulnerable to delusional thought or hallucinations during periods of inactivity, and this is a problem to which schizophrenic patients appear particularly prone. Many patients report that finding something to do is helpful. Simple activity scheduling can be a powerful coping strategy, especially if implemented at the onset of the symptom and thus creating a dual task competing for attentional resources.

Social engagement and disengagement

Although many patients tolerate social interactions poorly, surprisingly many also find social engagement a useful method of coping. It is beneficial to be able to titrate the amount of social stimulation involved in any interaction with the tolerance level of that particular patient, and also to teach patients that there are levels of social disengagement that can be used to help develop tolerance of social stimulation. Social withdrawal and avoidance is the common response to experiencing overstimulation from social interaction. However, patients can learn less drastic methods of disengagement, such as leaving the room for a short period and then returning, temporarily moving away from the social group, and functional disengagement by not conversing for short periods or lowering their gaze. By use of these methods social stimulation can be controlled and tolerated. Patients may also feel more confident to initiate social interaction as a method to reduce the impact of their symptoms. Simple training in specific skills for interaction and role-plays can facilitate this.

Belief modification

Patients can learn to examine their beliefs and challenge them if they are inappropriate by examination of the evidence and the generation of alternative explanations. Many patients do this to some extent already, but the level of arousal experienced or the level of isolation and avoidance conspires to make these attempts largely unsuccessful. These methods are very similar to those used in traditional cognitive therapy, except that the patient may need more prompting and the goal is to incorporate the skills of belief modification into a self-regulatory process. Patients can be encouraged to ask questions of their beliefs as they occur, such as what would the purpose be of someone spying on them; how much effort and cost would it take; how would this be resourced and organised; and for what gain?

Similarly, patients can be encouraged to look for inconsistencies and to use these to make challenges. For example, the patient who was involved in a fight 15 years earlier and still avoids young men because he fears that the same group of young men is out to get revenge, may be asked to reflect on the fact that the members of the gang will now be in their mid to late thirties and he has been vigilant for the wrong age group. This can be used to challenge his fear that he needs to be vigilant to stay safe.

Patients can also learn to examine evidence to challenge their beliefs about their voices. Where voices are seen as omnipotent and truthful, evidence can be investigated to see if they have been wrong or incorrect. For example, the patient whose voices told him he had committed a murder and a rape were believed because he could not remember not doing it, and so concluded that the voices must be true. However, the voices also told him that he was Russian, but as he could find no supporting evidence for this assertion he decided it was untrue. However, he had never thought to challenge the voices veracity concerning the murder and rape accusations. Remembering that he was not Russian, as the voices had asserted, helped him challenge the idea that he was a murderer and rapist by doubting the truthfulness of the voices and look for further, supporting, objective evidence, which was not forthcoming.

Reality-testing and behavioural experiments

Probably the strongest way of testing beliefs is to test them out in reality by some type of action, behaviour change being probably the best way to produce cognitive change. Patients will sometimes do this naturally, although a tendency to bias interpretation and for hypothesis protection will lead them to erroneous conclusions. Patients can learn to identify specific beliefs and generate competing predictions that can be tested. The failure to do this in real life usually leads to patterns of avoidance, which can be reversed to challenge the beliefs upon which they are underpinned.

Coping strategy enhancement

Coping methods have developed over time and vary in their complexity, from simple and direct attempts to control cognitive processes, such as attention, to more complex self-directed methods that modify cognitive content and inference. Frequently, combinations of different coping strategies are built up, for example the use of attention switching and de-arousing techniques helps to dull the strength of a delusion so that reality-testing can be implemented. Without these initial coping methods the patient would not be able to undergo reality-testing. Furthermore, the initial coping strategies can be used to challenge the strength of the delusion of the omnipotence of the voices and provide an increase in self-efficacy. Questions can be asked such as "You've used these attention switching methods to cope effectively with your voices; what does that tell you about them being all powerful and you being helpless?" The patient may well make statements that indicate the voices have been demonstrated as fallible and he had some control over the situation, which can then be used as self-statements or a modified internal dialogue to further enhance self-efficacy and coping.

CASE EXAMPLE

The following case example will give some indication of how coping strategy enhancement can work. John was a 36-year-old man who had 12 years previously been diagnosed as suffering from schizophrenia. He lived with his elderly parents in their bungalow and had few social contacts other than rather superficial interactions with relatives and neighbours. In the past he had attended day hospital and drop-ins, but had discontinued attendance and now rarely ventured far from his house.

He experienced true auditory hallucinations, which were voices of a number of people talking about him in the third person. These voices were male, hostile, and threatening. The voices' content consisted of such comments as "there's the bastard now, he's in there . . . we're going to get him . . . let's do him now . . . he's an ugly sod isn't he . . .?" and such like. The voices varied in their intensity and loudness, invariably starting quietly and then becoming louder as time went on. John would mainly experience these voices when inactive, usually in his bedroom while lying on his bed, which he did a lot of the time especially in the afternoon and evenings. He would also hear them when he was in the lounge, where he spent some time with his parents watching television. On these occasions the voices would be less intense and usually only a whisper, more fragmented and would last for a shorter duration. On further analysis it was found that although he spent time in the lounge with his parents he was rarely engaged in any interaction with them. Frequently, he would not be concentrating on the television but would be functionally detached from what was going on in the room, lost in his own thoughts. It was at these times that the voices were more likely to occur and be more intense. If he was enjoying watching the television the voices were less intense, more fragmented, and easier to dismiss.

John believed that the voices emanated from a gang of Hell's Angels who were out to harm him. Many years previously he had been subject to a period of harassment by a group of youths who used to loiter near where he caught the bus to the day hospital. There had been no physical threat to him but the episodes had worried him significantly. This experience was one reason why he spent most of his time at home. At another time he had seen a film about a motorcycle gang, which he had connected, quite spuriously, with his own experience. He was now convinced that a gang of Hell's Angels were stalking him with the intention of attacking him in his home. These delusions of persecution were secondary and explanatory to the experience of auditory hallucinations. The voices, especially when heard in his room, were interpreted by John as signifying that the gang were outside the house and preparing to break in and attack him. Thus the belief of imminent threat was substantiated by the content and threatening nature of the voices. However, considerable generalisations of interpretation had occurred so that extraneous noise outside the house, such as creaks, noises in the bushes, footsteps, talking from people passing by, and motor-engine noises were now all perceived as evidence for the presence of the gang. John would be vigilant for these noises and listen for them with growing apprehension and anxiety. His fear would increase once he became aware of the voices, and with their increasing loudness his anxiety would accelerate until he started to shout back at the voices to leave him alone and to go away. His fear at this point would reach a crescendo and he would continue to shout at the voices until, after a while, he became aware that the voices were no longer present. As time passed he came to believe that he had only escaped harm because he had shouted at the gang of Hell's Angels outside the house. This he believed had unsettled them in their attack and they had left, to return again at another time. This reinforced his belief that he had been in danger and that only his own actions of shouting at the gang had saved him from that danger. He further believed that he would be in increasing danger in the near future as the Hell's Angels would become increasingly violent as a result of being thwarted.

Formulation and intervention

There were two inter-linked symptoms—the auditory hallucinations and the delusions of persecution. The hallucinations were most likely to occur when John was inactive and not engaged in any task. This was most probable when he was alone in his bedroom, but could also happen if he was functionally disengaged while sitting in the lounge. The experience rarely occurred during the morning when he tended to be more active and mobile. The delusion occurred in response to the hallucinations. Delusions could also be triggered by real sounds, but this only happened at times and in situations during which John hallucinated.

The first phase in the intervention was to reduce John's exposure to situations that triggered hallucinations, such as spending long periods alone and inactive in his bedroom, and being functionally disengaged when sitting in the lounge. This was dealt with in two ways. First, via simple activity scheduling whereby John would spend the afternoon and early evening out of his bedroom and by using this time to engage himself in purposeful activity and externally focusing his attention rather than being lost in his thoughts (internal focus). Two activities were suggested: (a) to engage his parents in conversation and (b) to concentrate on watching the television and absorb what he was watching. Both were achieved by encouraging self-instruction to carry out the relevant tasks, with rehearsal in a simulated situation during a treatment session. Interaction with his parents, especially initiating conversation, was practised by role-playing, while attention directed towards the television was achieved by self-instructional statements, such as "What is this programme about? What are the characters speaking about? What setting are they in?" and similar descriptive questions to maintain his concentration.

The second phase of the intervention was to address the more difficult problem of the experience of hallucinations and delusional interpretations that were now restricted to occurring in the later evening when John retired to his bedroom. This was achieved in a number of stages. First, John was taught awareness training to identify the onset of his hallucination, which was achieved through a simulation in session where the therapist very quietly verbalised the voices and John indicated their onset, thus focusing solely on the physical characteristic of the voices (cf. Haddock et al., 1996). Secondly, John was taught reattributional statements immediately the voices started, which allowed an opportunity to suggest an alternative explanation of the voices other than that they were real in time and space. This was that they could be a misidentification of John's own thoughts (this point is returned to later). Following this, John was taught to switch his attention to alternative images and subjects.

The next stage was to teach John some method of coping with the cascade of arousal that was precipitated by hearing the voices. Reattribution and attention switching would be insufficient in themselves to counter the high levels of arousal that were associated with the psychotic symptoms. To this end John was instructed in a method of quick relaxation. Finally, a reality-test was formulated to counter John's symptom congruent behaviour. This was his action of shouting back at the voices and belief that only this had prevented the attack. Thus it was proposed that if he did not shout back and if nothing catastrophic occurred, this would provide evidence contrary to his fear. In this case the aforementioned stages could be combined so that John identified the onset of the voices when they were at their weakest and before his arousal levels were too high, immediately started reattributing statements followed by attention switching. Quick relaxation was then used to cope with the increasing fear, and self-instruction to guide the required behaviour in the reality-test, such as "I don't need to shout back, I can come to no harm, nothing will happen". All these strategies were chained together by self-instruction, previous practice sessions and were now practised in vivo. John had instructions written on flash cards to help him remember the various strategies and how to perform them. Frequently over a week the strategies were only implemented once or twice and the next session involved enquiring from John what he felt he had learnt from the experiment and how this could be further substantiated.

Once John had had some success in not responding to his voices the alternative explanation that the voices were a misidentification of his own thoughts could be expanded upon. He could be prompted for reasons why he might have thoughts about gangs threatening him that would elicit his previous experiences in being threatened, and being frightened by the film he had seen on Hell's Angels.

Patients vary in how many sessions they require to acquire coping skills and this will also be affected by the severity of their symptoms. In John's case 10 sessions were required. However, there are many factors (see the lists at the end of the "Model" section earlier in this chapter) that may affect the speed and pacing of therapy, so that no hard and fast rules about its duration should be assumed. For example, John at first found the social interaction within the therapeutic context difficult to tolerate so sessions were initially kept short.

PREVENTION OF RELAPSE

An important part of the treatment approach is to plan for the future, especially potentially stressful events that may occur, and how to be aware of emerging symptoms and relapse.

Life stresses

As far as possible it is useful to try to predict what stresses will be a problem in the future. It is known that both life events (Bebbington & Kuipers, 1992) and difficult interpersonal relationships (Butzlaff & Hooley, 1998; Kavanagh, 1992) can be precursors for relapse. The problem-solving format can be used to generate ways of coping with these difficulties and stresses and once a strategy has been mutually decided upon it can be broken down into its constituent parts and thoroughly rehearsed. Again, over-learning is important if a coping strategy is to be successful because retention will decay with time and changes in circumstances.

Re-emergence of symptoms

Building on the knowledge that patients frequently experience a prodromal period prior to relapse (e.g. Tarrier, Barrowclough, & Bamrah, 1991), it is possible to construct a strategy of coping to deal with the various stages of the prodrome and re-emerging psychotic symptoms. Because memory and motivation are likely to be reduced as time passes it may well be helpful to have this plan written down, with various levels of action required by an increasing proximity to relapse. A similar intervention has worked well with manic-depressive patients (Perry, Tarrier, Morriss, McCarthy, & Limb, 1999).

Coping with feelings of low self-worth

Patients suffering from schizophrenia frequently have a poor perception of themselves and low self-esteem. These global concepts can be hypothesised to be manifest in terms of a negative self-schema. This is postulated as being a consequence of suffering from a severe mental illness and all that goes with it. The factors that potentially impact upon and maintain negative self-schema are represented in Fig. 6.2, and it can be seen that they are strong, multiple, and relentless. The consequence of suffering a severe mental illness is the formation of such negative self-schema, which then serves to bias the way information is assimilated so that these schema are maintained and strengthened rather than being challenged and modified.

The onset of a psychotic breakdown will be a traumatic experience. In fact there is evidence that this trauma is sufficient to result in Post-Traumatic Stress Disorder (Williams-Keeler, Milliken, & Jones, 1994), although it could be debated whether the nature of the trauma is consistent with original ways of thinking about PTSD. Within the PTSD literature much is made of the dramatic effect that trauma has on a person's views of the world and how their beliefs about issues such as safety, trust, vulnerability, and justice can completely change (Janoff-Bulman, 1985). Thus, in an analogous way, the onset of psychosis may totally change a sufferer's views about themselves, the world, and the future. This, in conjunction with the persistent effect of

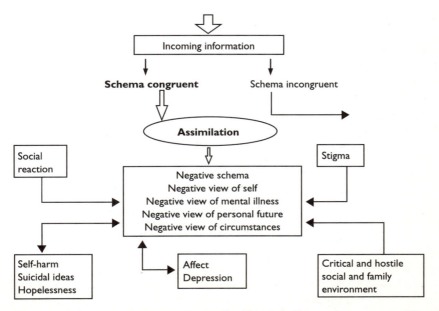

Figure 6.2 Factors that maintain negative self-schema in sufferers of severe mental illness.

stigmatisation of the mentally ill, probable downward social drift, feelings of hopelessness, and the known effects of critical and hostile family members is most likely to instil and maintain negative self-schemas.

Low feelings of self-worth can inhibit the effective use of coping strategies as well as increase the risk of depression and self-harm. Take the case presented in Fig. 6.3, which provides a diagrammatic representation of a common problem. The patient, Dave, has paranoid delusions and is very sensitive to the actions—real and interpreted—of others, so that he is vigilant and constantly scanning and searching for other people's behaviour. Two events trigger off a reaction: the first when he looks out of the window and sees a man walking by the house, and the second while he is travelling on the top deck of a bus he notices a pedestrian looking in his direction. Both these incidents capture his attention and he becomes locked on to these stimuli. He makes specific and personalised inferences of these people's behaviour, which are experienced as causal explanations about their behaviour, and which also trigger thoughts about the possible threat to himself. This results in a sudden cascade of emotions that have in the past caused him to act in an inappropriate and aggressive manner towards others. This type of behaviour elicits social sanction varying from the disapproval of others to arrest and prosecution. Although at the time of referral Dave was not acting on his delusional thoughts and interpretations, the fact that he had in the past reinforced his view of himself as "bad and mad". This also strengthened the idea that people and society were against him and confirmed his vague ideas of a plot against himself. These ideas maintained a state of increased sensitivity, vigilance, focused attention and heightened arousal. This is an example of a positive feedback loop as indicated in Fig. 6.1.

By using the methods described earlier it was possible to teach Dave to cope adequately with this type of situation, as represented on the right side of Fig. 6.3. Dave was taught to be aware of his vulnerabilities and the antecedent situations that were likely to trigger his paranoid thoughts. He was taught to use these antecedent stimuli as cues for readiness so that he could broaden his range of attention to other stimuli and switch his attention away from focusing on the behaviour of others. He learnt to challenge his automatic interpretations by generating alternatives and also how to defuse the emotional cascade by the use of these coping responses.

It was anticipated that Dave's success in coping with his paranoia and the improved level of functioning that he attained would generalise so that he would feel more in control and thus have increased self-esteem and self-efficacy. These generalised positive attributes would be incongruent with his negative self-schema, which would thus be weakened and a more positive view of himself reinforced. This did not happen. No new information about himself and his capabilities was integrated. It appeared that his negative schema were protected, remained active, and even reinforced. Dave declared that although he realised he could cope much better and that his life was now

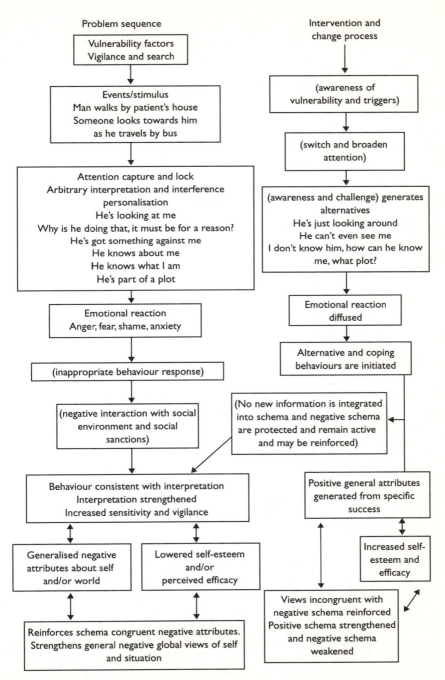

Figure 6.3 Problem and intervention sequences indicating coping methods and belief maintenance.

richer and he was less isolated, this did not change his circumstances. He was, he said, "still bad and mad", even if other people were unaware of this. The fact that he had to expend such an amount of energy on coping with an everyday event, such as a bus ride, depressed him and strengthened his view that he was worthless.

The risk here is that Dave will feel increasingly hopeless and abandon his attempts to cope with his symptoms. And that his feelings about himself may lead to clinical depression and increased suicide risk. Thus low self-esteem in cases such as Dave's is being viewed as an increased vulnerability for relapse and action needs to be formulated to reduce this risk. A possible approach to this is outlined in the next section.

Improving the patient's self-esteem

The aim of this set of techniques is to produce generalisations of positive attributes, challenge negative self-schema, and to improve global self-esteem. The procedure is as follows:

- Ask the patient to produce 10 positive qualities about themselves (the number can be varied dependent on the patient's capabilities, and it is important not to have the patient fail in generating the required number).
- Once the patient has produced a list of these qualities ask them to rate each one on how much they actually believe it to be true, on a 0 to 100 scale (where 0 = not at all and 100 = completely).
- Ask the patient to produce specific examples of evidence of each quality, prompt specifically for actions that have occurred recently and can be time linked such as "last week", and also use your knowledge of the patient to elicit examples. Prompt as many examples as possible and list them.
- Ask the patient to rehearse the list of examples for each quality—this can be done through verbal description and mental imagery of the event— and then to re-rate their belief that they possess this quality. (Usually the belief rating changes to show an increase. It should be emphasised to the patient that their belief can change depending on what evidence they focus their attention upon.)
- The patient is set a homework exercise of monitoring their behaviour over the next week and recording specific evidence to support the contention that they do have these qualities. The aim is to produce generalisation and experiential learning of a number of positive attributes (cf. Teasedale, 1999).
- At the next session provide feedback on examples and prompt further examples. Again ask the patient to re-rate their belief that they actually do have these qualities and further point out any changes in these beliefs.
- Ask the patient to reflect on the effect eliciting and focusing on specific

behaviours and evidence has on their beliefs about themselves and the qualities that they have, and how this could effect their general opinion of themselves. Reinforce all positive attributes and the process whereby the patient comes to a more positive view of themselves.

• Continue to repeat the above procedure. Continually emphasise that beliefs about themselves vary depending on what is the focus of attention, and that self-esteem can be greatly affected by belief and is thus amenable to change.

An example of this procedure being implemented is as follows. Dave had very successfully learnt to cope with his symptoms, which had been markedly reduced, and he had significantly improved his level of functioning. Dave produced a number of attributes that he thought he might have, comprising "helpful", to which he gave a belief rating of 60 out of 100; "friendly", which he rated 50; and "a good father" which he rated as 30. He was then asked to suggest concrete and specific evidence to support all of these. For "helpful" he cited having lent money to a friend some months before, opening a door to someone the previous week, and helping his father in the garden that week. He re-rated this belief as 90.

For "friendly" he cited that he had had many friends of 10 to 20 years standing; his friends contacted him regularly and enjoyed his company; and he could talk comfortably to people in pubs or on buses. Next, he got on well with the friends of his parents. Also, he thought he got on well with the therapist and enjoyed speaking to them, and cited that he could talk to different types of people from different backgrounds without difficulty or reserve. He re-rated this belief as 100.

For being a "good father" he cited that he enjoyed taking his son and daughter out every week (he was divorced from their mother who had custody). He was upset when he did not see them. He liked to buy them presents. He was happy for them to decide on activities, rather than doing things purely for convenience, and this in itself gave him pleasure. He re-rated this belief as 60. However, at this point he introduced some negative evaluations. He said that he felt that he could not be a good father as he did not live with his children. He did not get on with their mother. He said that it was always easier for absent fathers who saw their children for short periods of time and tended to spoil them. This was not responsible parenting in his view. At this point it was helpful to go through the model of how negative views such as this are maintained (see Fig. 6.2). To discuss these thoughts as being negative schema-congruent and indicate that the statements were over-generalisations, a process by which negatives are maximised and positives minimised. Further, that these thoughts and beliefs have a depressing effect on his mood and maintain negative beliefs about himself, but do not accurately reflect circumstances. To challenge his views of himself as a bad father various exercises where undertaken: he was asked to define a "bad father" in explicit terms and then objectively compare his behaviour with this definition. He was asked to compare his behaviour with others in similar circumstances. Lastly, he was asked to give a realistic and objective appraisal of his performance and circumstances. While carrying out these exercises the potential for negatively biased self-appraisals was emphasised, along with strategies for coping with this in the future.

At the time of writing, these methods, or any schema-focused therapy for that matter, have not been evaluated. In the case of Dave there was an independent but anecdotal report that after treatment he was expressing very positive feelings about himself. Other general methods for addressing low self-esteem are described by Fennell (1998).

FUTURE DIRECTIONS

There is well-established research demonstrating that family intervention has significant long-term clinical benefits, especially on reducing relapse rates (Tarrier, Barrowclough, Porceddu, & Fitzpatrick, 1994). Given the great importance of schizophrenic patients' social environment (Mueser & Tarrier, 1998) it is likely that social interactions and environments will exert a power-ful influence over the outcome of individual therapy. Thus combining cognitive behavioural therapy and family intervention would seem a logical development in non-drug treatment. There is also emerging evidence that the attitudes and behaviour of formal carers—that is professional staff—can have a similar effect on the course of schizophrenia as that of family members and informal carers (Tatton & Tarrier, 2000). Therefore, interven-tions that focus on the psycho-social environment created by the behaviour and attitudes of professional carers, as well as those created by relatives and informal carers, could also be constructively combined with cognitive behavioural therapy approaches with the individual patient.

The Manchester trial indicated that supportive counselling as a treatment showed increasing benefit with the passage of time; thus there may be a place for formulating a Social Cognitive Behaviour Therapy for psychosis. This would include sessions of the unstructured supportive counselling, focusing on developing social relationships and general issues, interspersed with the much more structured cognitive behavioural therapy approach focusing on symptom reduction and schematic self-esteem issues (Tarrier et al., 2000).

REFERENCES

Bandura, A. (1977). Self-efficacy: Towards a unifying theory of behavior change. *Psychological Review*, *84*, 191–215.

Barrowclough, C., & Tarrier, N. (1992). *Families of schizophrenic patients: A cognitive-behavioural intervention*. London: Chapman & Hall (reprinted in 1997).

Bebbington, P., & Kuipers, L. (1992). Life events and social factors. In D. Kavanagh (Ed.), *Schizophrenia: An overview and practical handbook* (pp. 126–144). London: Chapman & Hall.

Breier, A., & Strauss, J.S. (1983). Self-control in psychotic disorders. *Archives of General Psychiatry*, *40*, 1141–1145.

Brenner, H.D., Bokker, W., Mueller, J., Spichtig, L., & Wuergler, S. (1987). Autoprotective efforts among schizophrenics, neurotics, and controls. *Acta Psychiatrica Scandinavica*, *75*, 405–414.

Butzlaff, R.L., & Hooley, J.M. (1998). Expressed emotion and psychiatric relapse: A meta analysis. *Archives of General Psychiatry*, 55, 547–552.

Carr, V. (1988). Patients' techniques for coping with schizophrenia: An exploratory study. *British Journal of Medical Psychology*, *61*, 339–352.

Chadwick, P., & Birchwood, M. (1994). The omnipotence of voices: A cognitive approach to auditory hallucinations. *British Journal of Psychiatry*, *164*, 190–201.

Cohen, C.I., & Berk, B.S. (1985). Personal coping styles in schizophrenic outpatients. *Hospital & Community Psychiatry*, *36*, 407–410.

Dawson, M.E., Nuechterlein, K.H., & Adams, R.M. (1989). Schizophrenic disorders. In G. Turpin (Ed.), *Handbook of clinical psychophysiology* (pp. 393–418). Chichester: Wiley.

Falloon, I.R.H., & Talbot, R.E. (1981). Persistent auditory hallucinations: Coping mechanisms and implications for management. *Psychological Medicine*, *11*, 329–339.

Fennell, M. (1998). Low self-esteem. In N. Tarrier, A. Wells, & G. Haddock (Eds.), *Treating complex cases: The cognitive behavioural therapy approach*. Chichester: Wiley.

Frith, C. (1994). Theory of mind in schizophrenia. In A.S. David & J.C. Cutting (Eds.), *The neuropsychology of schizophrenia* (pp. 147–163). Hove, UK: Lawrence Erlbaum and Associates Ltd.

Haddock, G., Bentall, R., & Slade, P.D. (1996). Psychological treatment of auditory hallucinations: Focusing or distraction. In G. Haddock & P.D. Slade (Eds.), *Cognitive behavioural interventions with psychotic disorders* (pp. 45–70). London: Routledge.

Haddock, G., McCarron, J., & Tarrier, N. (1999). Scales to measure dimensions of hallucinations and delusions: The psychotic symptom rating scales (PSYRATS). *Psychological Medicine*, *29*, 879–889.

Haddock, G., & Tarrier, N. (1998). Assessment and formulation in the cognitive behavioural treatment of psychosis. In N. Tarrier, A. Wells, & G. Haddock (Eds.), *Treating complex cases: The cognitive behavioural therapy approach*. Chichester: Wiley.

Hemsley, D. (1994). Perceptual and cognitive abnormalities as the bases for schizophrenic symptoms. In A.S. David & J.C. Cutting (Eds.), *The neuropsychology of schizophrenia* (pp. 97–118). Hove, UK: Lawrence Erlbaum and Associates Ltd.

Janoff-Bulman, R. (1985). The aftermath of victimisation: Rebuilding shattered assumptions. In C.R. Figley (Ed.), *Trauma and its wake*. New York: Brunner-Mazel.

Kanfer, F.H., & Saslow, G. (1965). Behavioral analysis: An alternative to diagnostic classification. *Archives of General Psychiatry, 12*, 529–538.

Karoly, P., & Kanfer, F.H. (1982). *Self-management and behaviour change: From theory to practice*. New York: Pergamon.

Kavanagh, D. (1992). Recent developments in expressed emotion and schizophrenia. *British Journal of Psychiatry, 160*, 601–620.

Kinney, C.F. (1999). *Coping with schizophrenia: The significance of appraisal*. Unpublished Ph.D. thesis, Faculty of Medicine, University of Manchester.

Lowe, C.F., & Higson, P.J. (1981). Self-instructional training and cognitive behaviour modification: a behavioural analysis. In G. Davey (Ed.), *Applications of conditioning theory* (pp. 162–188). London: Methuen.

Meichenbaum, D., & Cameron, R. (1971). Training schizophrenics to talk to themselves: A means of developing attentional control. *Behavior Therapy, 4*, 515–534.

Mueser, K., & Tarrier, N. (1998). *Handbook of social functioning in schizophrenia*. Boston, MA; Allyn & Bacon.

Nuechterlein, K.H. (1987). Vulnerability models for schizophrenia: State of the art. In H. Hafner, W.F. Gattaz, & W. Janzarik (Eds.), *Search for the cause of schizophrenia* (pp. 297–316). Heidelberg: Springer-Verlag.

Patience, D.A. (1994). Cognitive behaviour therapy for schizophrenia. *British Journal of Psychiatry, 165*, 266–267.

Perry, A., Tarrier, N., Morriss, R., McCarthy, E., & Limb, K. (1999). A randomised controlled trial of teaching bipolar disorder patients to identify early symptoms of relapse and obtain early treatment. *British Medical Journal, 318*, 149–153.

Persaud, R., & Marks, I. (1995). A pilot study of exposure control of auditory hallucinations in schizophrenia. *British Journal of Psychiatry, 167*, 45–50.

Romme, M.A.J., & Escher, A.D. (1987). Hearing voices. *Schizophrenia Bulletin, 15*, 209–216.

Sackett, D., Richardson, W.S., Rosenberg, W., & Haynes, R.B. (1997). *Evidence-based medicine*. Edinburgh: Churchill-Livingstone.

Shakow, D. (1962). Segmental set: A theory of the formal psychological deficits in schizophrenia. *Archives of General Psychiatry, 6*, 600–612.

Slade, P.D. (1972). The effects of systematic desensitisation on auditory hallucinations. *Behaviour Research and Therapy, 10*, 85–91.

Tarrier, N. (1987). An investigation of residual psychotic symptoms in discharged schizophrenic patients. *British Journal of Clinical Psychology, 26*, 141–143.

Tarrier, N., Barrowclough, C., & Bamrah, J. S. (1991). Prodromal signs of relapse in schizophrenia. *Social Psychiatry and Psychiatric Epidemiology, 26*, 157–161.

Tarrier, N., Barrowclough, C., Porceddu, K., & Fitzpatrick, E. (1994). The Salford family intervention project for schizophrenic relapse prevention: Five and eight-year accumulating relapses. *British Journal of Psychiatry, 165*, 829–832.

Tarrier, N., Beckett, R., Harwood, S., Baker, A., Yusupoff, L., & Ugarteburu, I. (1993a). A controlled trial of two cognitive behavioural methods of treating drug-resistant residual psychotic symptoms in schizophrenic patients: 1. Outcome. *British Journal of Psychiatry, 162*, 524–532.

Tarrier, N., Harwood, S., Yusopoff, L., Beckett, R., & Baker, A. (1990). Coping Strategy Enhancement (CSE): A method of treating residual schizophrenic symptoms. *Behavioural Psychotherapy*, *18*, 283–293.

Tarrier, N., Kinney, C., McCarthy, E., Humphreys, L., Wittkowski, A., & Morris, J. (2000). Two-year follow-up of cognitive behaviour therapy and supportive counselling in the treatment of persistent positive symptoms in chronic schizophrenia. *Journal of Consulting and Clinical Psychology*, *68*, 917–922.

Tarrier, N., Kinney, C., McCarthy, E., Wittkowski, A., Yusupoff, Y., Gledhill, A., Morris, J., & Humphreys, L. (2001). Are some types of psychotic symptoms more responsive to cognitive behaviour therapy? *Behavioural and Cognitive Psychotherapy*, *29*, 45–55.

Tarrier, N., Sharpe, L., Beckett, R., Harwood, S., Baker, A., & Yusupoff, L. (1993b). A controlled trial of two cognitive behavioural methods of treating drug-resistant residual psychotic symptoms in schizophrenic patients: II. Treatment specific changes in coping and problem solving. *Social Psychiatry and Psychiatric Epidemiology*, *28*, 5–10.

Tarrier, N., & Turpin, G. (1992). Psycho-social factors, arousal, and schizophrenic relapse: A review of the psychophysiological data. *British Journal of Psychiatry*, *161*, 3–11.

Tarrier, N., Wittkowski, A., Kinney, C., McCarthy, E., Morris, J., & Humphreys, L. (1999). The durability of the effects of cognitive behaviour therapy in the treatment of chronic schizophrenia: Twelve months follow-up. *British Journal of Psychiatry, 174*, 500–504.

Tarrier, N., Yusupoff, L., Kinney, C., McCarthy, E., Gledhill, A., Haddock, G., & Morris, J. (1998a). A randomised controlled trial of intensive cognitive behaviour therapy for chronic schizophrenia. *British Medical Journal*, *317*, 303–307.

Tarrier, N., Yusupoff, L., McCarthy, E., Kinney, C., & Wittkowski, A. (1998b). Some reasons why patients suffering from chronic schizophrenia fail to continue in psychological treatment. *Behavioural and Cognitive Psychotherapy*, *26*, 177–181.

Tattan, T., & Tarrier, N. (2000). The expressed emotion of case managers of the seriously mentally ill: The influence of EE and the quality of the relationship on clinical outcomes. *Psychological Medicine*, *30*, 195–204.

Teasedale, J.D. (1999). Emotional processing three modes of mind and the prevention of relapse in depression. *Behaviour Research and Therapy*, *37* (*suppl. 1*), 53–79.

Vygotsky, L.S. (1962). *Thought and language*. New York: Wiley.

Williams-Keeler, L., Milliken, H., & Jones, B. (1994). Psychosis as precipitating trauma for PTSD: A treatment strategy. *American Journal of Orthopsychiatry*, *64*, 493–498.

Wing, J., Cooper, J., & Sartorius, N. (1974). *Measurement and classification of psychiatric symptoms*. Cambridge: Cambridge University Press.

Zeidner, M., & Endler, N.S. (1996). *Handbook of coping: Theory, research, and applications*. Chichester: Wiley.

Zubin, J., & Spring, B. (1977). Vulnerability: A new view of schizophrenia. *Journal of Abnormal Psychology*, *86*, 103–126.

Chapter 7

Shame, humiliation, and entrapment in psychosis

A social rank theory approach to cognitive intervention with voices and delusions

Max Birchwood, Alan Meaden, Peter Trower, and Paul Gilbert

INTRODUCTION

Recent cognitive research on positive symptoms of psychosis has revealed an unexpected finding with regard to hallucinations; namely that the distress and behaviour linked to voice activity may be understood in terms of the nature of patients' *relationship* with their voices, and in particular their personification of it and their appraisal of voices' power and omnipotence. Social rank theory (Gilbert, 1992; Gilbert & Allan, 1998; Price, Sloman, Gardner, Gilbert, & Rohde, 1994) is particularly suited to understanding these links as it provides a general theory of how humans respond under conditions of dominance and entrapment by another. The experience of voices exemplify this type of relationship. The theory has guided our recent development of a form of cognitive therapy intervention for hallucinations in general and command hallucinations in particular. We also propose that the theory is applicable to other symptoms, particularly delusions and some negative symptoms. Furthermore, clear evidence is emerging that these symptoms commonly reflect a core self-perception of low social rank; that is, the person sees themselves as being in an unwanted subordinate position and subject to other people's control and derogation, particularly family and peers but also community at large. In this chapter we outline the theory as applied to voices, draw out the more general implications for symptoms and core beliefs, review some of the recent research that supports the approach, describe some of the basic principles of assessment and intervention, and provide case examples that illustrate different facets of cognitive assessment and intervention from this perspective.

THE COGNITIVE APPROACH TO VOICES

Cognitive theory of psychopathology has developed rapidly within the last decade from its origins in depression (Beck, 1963) and has found wide application in a range of psychiatric disorders (Clark & Fairburn, 1997). The application of the cognitive approach to psychosis has been a relatively recent development led by groups in the UK. A major specific component of this development has been the application of cognitive theory and therapy to hallucinations.

SUBORDINATION AND ENTRAPMENT TO VOICES AND SIGNIFICANT OTHERS

A number of studies have shown that the distressing affect and behaviour arising from auditory hallucinations may be understood not simply as a function of the content or topography of voice activity, but voice hearers' appraisal of their meaning (Birchwood & Chadwick, 1997; Chadwick & Birchwood, 1994). One of the key insights from this research has been to view the auditory hallucination as an "activating event" (A), the significance of which is appraised by the individual in terms of their belief system (B), and which largely gives rise to characteristic emotional and behavioural consequences (C). There is now substantial evidence for cognitive mediation in the genesis of beliefs about voices because in many cases the content of these beliefs were "at odds" with voice content, suggesting that meanings were constructed by individuals rather than directly voice driven, and indeed patients disclosed "compelling" evidence for their beliefs that only occasionally drew upon voice content (Chadwick & Birchwood, 1995).

A second discovery from this body of research has, we believe, thrown radical new light on the nature of the appraisal of voices. This is our finding that the distress and behaviour linked to voice activity may be understood in terms of the nature of patients' perceived *relationship* with their voices, in particular their personification of them, their appraisal of voices' power and omnipotence, and whether the voice is malevolent or benevolent (Chadwick & Birchwood, 1994).

This pattern can perhaps be most clearly seen in command hallucinations—those potentially dangerous voices that can, in their most extreme form, instruct the patient to kill themselves or others. As we will show, the perceived power of the voice is one of the most important predictors of acting on such commands. Among those with voices, between 40% and 60% will report what they believe to be instructions and commands (Birchwood & Chadwick, 1997; Hellerstein, Frosch, & Koenigsberg, 1987; Nayani & David, 1996).

THEORETICAL MODELS

A number of cognitive theories have recently been formulated that provide leads towards a theoretical model for hallucinations in general and command hallucinations in particular. However, while these may account for the fact that appraisals of voice activity substantially lead to characteristic emotional and behavioural consequences, they do not account for the relationship aspect of voices. An approach that does help to understand these phenomena is that of social rank theory (Gilbert, 1992; Price et al., 1994). Social rank theory argues that various mental mechanisms evolved within the context of social hierarchies. In these contexts those with superior strengths/skills were able to threaten, attack, or intimidate those less able, and those in subordinate positions would defend themselves by escaping, fleeing, and submitting. These two mechanisms, which operate as "attack the weaker and submit to the stronger" are played out internally in patients who hear hostile voices. Hence, the attacking voice is normally derogating and controlling (just as any hostile dominant would be to a subordinate) and the person experiences these internal signals as requiring submission or appeasement. However, the consequences of the low social rank that these strategies entail have severe consequences in terms of low self-esteem, humiliation and entrapment, anxiety and depression, and submissive behaviour, including complying with the demands of dominant others.

Social rank theory has been developed to explain features of depression (Gilbert 1992) and social anxiety (Trower & Gilbert, 1989) and has empirical support in both these areas (Brown, Harris, & Hepworth, 1995; Hope, Sigier, Penn, & Meier, 1998; Trower, Sherling, Beech, Harrop, & Gilbert, 1998). We also believe the theory can be used to explain the nature of the relationship to the powerful voice. Indeed, research has shown that powerful voices evoke just these types of consequences in voice hearers. The findings from a number of studies can be summarised as follows:

1   Voice hearers construct the link between themselves and their voice as having the nature of an intimate interpersonal relationship, and often one that is inescapable (Benjamin, 1989). In a cross-sectional study Junginger (1990) found that recent compliance was more likely where the individual personified the voice (i.e. attributed it to an identity).

2   Over 85% of voice hearers saw the voice as powerful and omnipotent, whereas the hearer is usually weak and dependent, unable to control or influence the voice (Birchwood & Chadwick, 1997).

3   More than two-thirds of voice hearers were at least moderately depressed, which was directly attributable to the interpersonal appraisal of power and entrapment by the voice (Birchwood & Chadwick, 1997).

4   The greater the perceived power and omnipotence of the voice, the greater the likelihood of compliance (Beck-Sander, Birchwood, & Chadwick,

1997), though this relationship is not linear and is moderated by appraisal of the voice's intent and consequences of resisting.

5   Voice hearers perceive the voice as omniscient (e.g. know the person's present thoughts and past history, was able to predict the future, etc.) and this was seen as evidence of the voice's power.

6   Some voice hearers construed their voice as benevolent, others as malevolent and persecutory (Birchwood & Chadwick, 1994, 1997).

7   Those with benevolent voices virtually always complied with the voice, irrespective of whether the command was "innocuous" or "severe" (Beck-Sander et al., 1997) whereas those with malevolent voices were more likely to resist, and this resistance increased if the command involved major social transgression or self-harm (Chadwick & Birchwood, 1994). However, subjects predicted the malevolent voice would inflict harm whenever they resisted, and, if they continued to resist, felt compelled to appease the voice by carrying out an alternative action (Beck-Sander et al., 1997).

Given a sound empirical base for a social rank understanding of the relationship between voice hearer and voice, we next explored the idea that the same type of dominant-subordinate rank may characterise other key relationships, particularly parents and siblings, and possibly from childhood onwards. This would follow from social rank theory, which says that the appraisal of social subordination to another comes from a *general* process of social comparison serving the formation of social ranks (Gilbert & Allan, 1998). Moreover, social rank not only involves a comparison of relative strength and power, but social attractiveness and talent, perceived belonging, or "fit" with a social group is also considered to be involved in the process of social comparison (Gilbert, Price, & Allan, 1995).

We therefore predicted that those who perceive themselves to be entrapped in a subordinate and inferior position with regard to their voice, will also perceive themselves that way in their significant social relationships. To test this we carried out a study in which we examined whether the relationship with the voice is a paradigm of social relationships in general, in accordance with the prediction of social rank theory (Birchwood, Meaden, Trower, Gilbert, & Plaistow, 2000). In a sample of 59 voice hearers, measures of power and social rank difference between voice and voice hearer were taken in addition to parallel measures of power and rank in wider social relationships. We found that subordination to voices was closely linked to subordination and marginalisation in other social relationships. This was not the result of a mood-linked appraisal. Distress arising from voices was linked not to voice characteristics but to social and interpersonal cognition.

This study confirmed our prediction—that voice hearers who perceive their voices as higher in social rank and more powerful than themselves perceive a similar difference in social rank and power between self and others in their social world. Thus the subordinate relationship is mirrored in other social relationships and suggests the operation of anomalous interpersonal schemata subserving both. In further research we examined the genesis of these schemata in early caregiver relationships (Drayton, Birchwood, & Trower, 1998) and in social marginalisation.

We can now with reasonable confidence assume that powerful voices (hallucinated relationships) and powerful others (actual relationships) have a common theme—they both generate social signals and stimuli (activating events) that trigger the involuntary subordination response and the dysfunctional cognitive, emotional, and behavioural consequences so far discussed. However, we can extend this still further and include important other social stimuli that can set the subordination response in train. Such activating events are the actual and/or perceived life events—the onset of psychosis, possible compulsory hospitalisation, loss of roles and goals, and the stigma of schizophrenia. In one study (Rooke & Birchwood, 1998) we found that these can all lead to actual and/or perceived low social rank, particularly marked by loss of social attractiveness and talent, of belonging, or "fit" with a social group. In a word, they can lead to marginalisation and loss of a sense of self.

In summary, among the various signals and stimuli that communicate low social rank to the individual are the voices, the family milieu—specifically the relationship to the parents and siblings, such as is commonly found in high expressed emotion (EE) environments—and psychosis-related life events, which, in the context of the wider community, stigmatise and "down-rank" the individual.

The application of social rank theory to psychosis has clear implications for cognitive assessment and intervention, and the authors are in the process of adapting cognitive therapy assessment and intervention strategies to take this into account. This approach uses our ABC framework (Chadwick, Birchwood, & Trower, 1996) to guide the search for and organise activating events (A), beliefs, including automatic thoughts, assumptions, and images about the activating events (B), and the emotional, behavioural, and physiological consequences (C) that follow from B given A. Within this framework we divide activating events into three types: symptoms and "internal" events (including voices and descriptions of other experiences at the phenomenological level); descriptions of interactions with significant others, particularly parents and siblings; and significant life events, such as diagnosis, hospitalisation, and social stigma. Beliefs include inferences (automatic thoughts) about the activating events (including delusional inferences), and evaluations including core beliefs or assumptions about self, others, and the world. In interview we focus particularly on beliefs around the theme of low social rank (loss of status, worth, entrapment, loss). An outline of this model is given in Table 7.1. We then employ interventions aimed at modifying the activating events where possible (e.g. significant others and life events), dysfunctional beliefs, and self-defeating patterns of behaviour and emotional distress.

Table 7.1 The ABC model

Activating events (internal or external)	Beliefs (thoughts, images, assumptions)	Consequences (emotional and behavioural)
Symptoms: Voice activity (critical, commanding)	Beliefs, including delusions, concerned with low social rank (loss of status, humiliation, entrapment)	Depression, anxiety, anger Flight/flight Submit/comply
Other people: High EE critical family members		
Life events: Diagnosis, hospitalisation, stigma		

In the following sections we provide three illustrative cases. The first demonstrates an approach to assessment for a person with command hallucinations, and implications for intervention are spelled out. The second case illustrates a more complex delusional problem that emerges from a broader social context, and this shows different levels of cognitive and psycho-social assessment and intervention. The final case shows a complete assessment and intervention of a person with voices and delusions.

CASE ONE: KAREN

Background

Karen is in her late 30s. She began experiencing psychotic symptoms some 20 years ago. Symptoms have remained constant in their content but vary in their intensity. Karen describes the onset of her symptoms as occurring in her late teens following an extremely stressful period at home. Currently Karen lives independently in the community. Her symptoms show only a modest response to neuroleptic medication. Karen has had many admissions to hospital, usually at times of increased family tension.

Assessment

We routinely administer the Beliefs About Voices Questionnaire (BAVO) (Chadwick & Birchwood, 1995). As well as providing information on antecedents, behaviours, and emotional consequences, the scale also provides scores for the degree of engagement and resistance with the voices and beliefs about their purpose and power.

Karen reported hearing up to 10 voices. Her most dominant (and distressing) voice she identified as her sister Louise. Karen completed the BAVO in relation to this voice, which was rated as predominantly benevolent producing similar amounts of resistance and engagement. The Power Scale developed by Birchwood and Meaden (Birchwood et al., 2000) comprises seven dimensions of power (powerfulness, strength, confidence, respect, ability to harm, equality, and knowledge). Voice hearers are asked to rate how they feel in relation to their voices on each of these seven dimensions on a five-point scale. We have used this clinically to determine power relationships both between the voice hearer and their voice and (in an adapted version of the scale) between the voice hearer and other people). Karen again completed the scale in relation to her most dominant voice. She rated her voice as being overwhelmingly stronger, more confident, and more knowledgeable than herself. She also felt that the voice lacked respect for her. However, she felt equal to the voice and more able to harm it than be harmed by it. Overall Karen considered that she had about the same amount of power as the voice.

These findings were closely paralleled when rating herself in relation to others generally, producing similar ratings for power, strength, confidence, and equality. However, significantly different ratings were obtained on dimensions of respect, ability to harm (others being seen as much more able to harm her), and knowledge.

The Power Scale highlights the importance of assessing the different dimensions of power, as opposed to obtaining a more general rating of power. While in some respects Karen sees her voice as more powerful, this is not universally so. Moreover, while there are some parallels in how she views herself in relation to others there are some key differences.

Symptoms

During interview Karen revealed that she currently experiences up to ten voices, two of which being especially persistent and troublesome. Karen identifies these voices as belonging to those of her sister and mother. She experiences collateral visual hallucinations, which she links with the two main voices and converses freely with them.

Delusional beliefs are also associated with the content of these two voices. These centre upon themes of jealousy and betrayal: "My boyfriend is having an affair with my sister". Karen reports increased conviction in these beliefs at times of increased voice activity. She reports feeling angry at these times and often acts on her increased conviction and angry feelings, accusing others of various infidelities. Karen often reports feeling depressed afterwards.

Self-referent beliefs

Karen's predominant view of herself is that of being unlovable, unlikeable, and incompetent. These she noted were partly the result of her illness and were constantly being reinforced by her experience as a person with schizophrenia living in the community. However, she also felt that they were long-standing beliefs about herself, borne out of emotional neglect and constant comparison between herself and her sister.

Family relationships

Karen perceived her mother as critical and rejecting. She felt unwanted as a child and considered that she did not get the support and love that she needed. In contrast, Karen felt that her sister Louise was the favourite. Louise was viewed as being much more confident and generally a stronger person than Karen. Despite these difficulties, Karen maintained close links with her family—especially her sister, whom she often found to be supportive.

Formulation

Karen's relationship with her voices presents strong parallels with her relationships with both her sister and her mother. Most notably, the identity of the voices is given as those of her mother and sister. Perhaps more important clinically, voice activity is triggered by increased criticism and perceived rejection by her sister and mother.

Clear links were evident between childhood themes of neglect and criticism, and voice content: "Everybody hates you!" Moreover, Karen's beliefs about her voices—"They hate me" and "They keep me company and try to help me"—closely parallel her ambivalent feelings towards her family.

As regards Karen's secondary delusional beliefs, "My boyfriend is having a relationship with my sister" can be connected to Karen's self-evaluative thinking: "I am unlovable". The formulation is outlined in Fig. 7.1.

Opportunities for intervention

The close parallels between Karen's power relationships with her voices and those with her family (as well as wider interpersonal ones) suggest new avenues for intervention. Formulating cases in this way suggests that working on power issues in interpersonal relationships may have beneficial reciprocal effects on power relationships with voices. Building on areas of strength in relation to others (as identified from the Power Scale) and addressing issues of dominance should produce benefits in relation to voice-power differentials. The next case study in this chapter addresses these interventions in more detail.

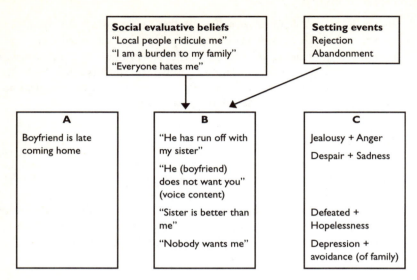

Figure 7.1 Karen's delusional beliefs: Formulation.

CASE TWO: HARJINDER

Background

Harjinder is a 24-year-old second generation Indian of the Sikh religion. Living with his parents he was referred after a period of two to three years of increasing social isolation following two terms at university. He received a diagnosis of paranoid psychosis due to ongoing delusions about a facial disfigurement. He attempted suicide on one occasion.

The presenting problem

Harjinder spends 90% of his time at home and does not communicate with his parents. He finds all form of social contact difficult, believing that people take unusual notice of him in the street and pass adverse comment. He believes that he suffers from a major facial disfigurement involving protrusions of his upper jaw bone, which is so prominent and ugly as to attract derision from perfect strangers. This causes him to feel humiliated and despairing most of the time.

He feels life is not worth living without somehow reversing his "disfigurement". He feels guilt because he believes that he brought this upon himself by distorting his jaw bones when, three years previously, he clenched his teeth hard together for a number of minutes which forced the bones to distort. He brought several pictures of himself to the sessions "before" and "after" the disfigurement. He is of very slim build and facially his cheeks are what may be described as "hollow". All who know him, including his GP concur that there is no deformity, but he cites as evidence the pictures and "comments" from people. He visits his GP frequently and has been sent to neurologists and orthopaedic specialists who, he believes, "condemn" him as mentally ill, which has inflamed his anger towards people, and professionals in particular.

A linked belief suggests that the clenching of his jaw bones has compressed his brain, which has resulted in changes to his feelings ("mental numbness"), a detached feeling, and an inability to focus visually. Again, specialised opinion could not detect visual or brain dysfunction that might account for such reports.

In desperation Harjinder attempted "DIY surgery" on the basis that "what goes up must come down", and assembled a crude set of levers attached to his teeth and jaw bones to pull it down. The experience was extremely painful and failed, leading him to further despair and marked him as a major risk to himself.

Assessment

Delusional beliefs

1   "I distorted my upper cheek bones by clenching my teeth together". Evidence: Pictures of himself before and after. Comments from people.
2.   "My jaw bones have compressed my brain". Evidence: Loss of feeling. Detachment (derealisation). Inability to sustain visual focus.
3.   "People notice and pass adverse comments on me in the street". Evidence: "Looks" from people.

Secondary beliefs

Using thought chaining the question was posed, "If the facial disfigurement you believe you suffer from remains unchanged what do you feel might happen?" This line of discussion eventually elucidated two beliefs: (a) "Unless my appearance returns to normal this will prevent me from achieving an acceptable quality of life"; and (b) "My disfigurements prevent me from being liked and accepted by others".

Harjinder has high expectations for himself—he wanted to succeed and felt that he had something to prove to his parents. Harjinder presented as angry and felt that he was not taken seriously by health professionals and was particularly resentful of the mental illness label. He saw it as his task to prove them wrong and to rectify his disfigurements, if necessary without medical help. He had been prescribed antidepressants and neuroleptics but declined both and was referred for cognitive therapy for his delusions.

The intervention

Engagement

Harjinder's state of mind was not ideal for cognitive therapy. He had been told that he would receive cognitive therapy for his delusions and this, in the context of considerable anger towards professionals, immediately created an adversarial atmosphere—the very opposite of what is considered essential for cognitive therapy. He was nevertheless motivated to receive help partly in order to convince someone that there was indeed a change in his face, but secondly he felt demoralised that his future well-being depended on something that was not being taken seriously. How to create a working alliance?

The approach taken was to sidestep attention to the delusion and to create an alliance with his own goals. Essentially the question was posed, "I don't know if there has been a change to your face—I didn't know you before; if there has, it is unlikely to be reversed in the near future. . . . What concerns me at the moment is whether it is possible for you to achieve an acceptable quality of life in spite of what you feel has happened to your face". Thus considerable attention was paid to the assumption that the perceived changes to his face were incompatible with a fulfilling life.

There was considerable anxiety about a further attempt at what he called his "DIY surgery", which he repeatedly mentioned. This anxiety would have led to the implication that these beliefs were wrong and dangerous. It was suggested that "DIY surgery is an option for you; that's up to you. Meanwhile you and I should try to work towards your goal of improving your quality of life. . . . If we fail then at least we know what we're up against".

Harjinder was also invited to consider whether other people had achieved a reasonable quality of life in spite of extreme disfigurement. Various people with disfigurements were discussed, including the Falklands war veteran, Simon Weston. Did he have a poor quality of life? He was married, with family, and maintained an active life.

As Harjinder was so well defended, his presentation was difficult to fully formulate at this stage so the intervention focused on the secondary beliefs.

First steps

The initial manoeuvre involved attempts to improve his quality of life by taking action with a low perceived risk of failure or rejection. Harjinder was particularly keen to work and develop his career. A work preparation scheme operated by the mental health service offered basic experience in skills such as computing, interviews, preparation of CVs, etc. This took place alongside other people with a mental health problem. His experience in the vocational group was a very positive one, he felt everyone was in the same boat, and the focus of the group was not mental health but a vocational one. He also felt the activities were well within his ability and progressed to another training setting, growing in confidence.

The programme ran alongside occasional sessions with the therapist, which were supportive and steadily addressed his secondary belief that he could not be accepted by others or succeed with his "deformity". There was accumulating evidence, which he acknowledged, that he could indeed develop his life in spite of the disfigurement. From time to time the therapist asked if he had received any adverse looks from others in his group. He had not; he put this down to others being tolerant of him because they had their own problems.

Social evaluative beliefs: Loss of social status and group identity

After eight weeks in the vocational group the delusional beliefs remained unchanged but Harjinder's confidence grew. At this point therapy returned to the question posed at the outset: "What would other people think if they were to take notice of his face?" It was by now clear that he was at ease in the company of a number of people, including the therapist, his colleagues in the group, and also his brother-in-law. It was suggested that once people got to know him, his social anxiety decreases alongside sensitivity about his face. He acknowledged that once he was satisfied that he would not be humiliated, his concern did indeed fall.

At this point it emerged that he was particularly sensitive to fellow Sikhs' comments on his face; such comments did not come from Muslims (Pakistanis) or other groups. He described incidents in which he had been mistaken for a Muslim by other Sikhs. Harjinder described himself as a Sikh but was not a practising member of his faith and did not wear a turban. What was worse for Harjinder was the possibility that he might be mistaken for a Muslim by his own community (Sikhs). He described the long-standing enmity between Indian and Pakistani peoples and was particularly apprehensive that he would be rejected by his own cultural group.

When Harjinder was young he lived with his family in a Sikh area of Birmingham, which he described as extremely happy. He moved at age 10 to a white area and to a new, predominantly white school where he was subjected to racial taunts and abuse. He blamed his father for his unhappiness and at age 14 he rejected his parents and their cultural expectations of the "servile Punjabi son", which nevertheless he said was the "cornerstone of his identity". Thus Harjinder was extremely sensitive to cues from members of his own community that he was being evaluated and possibly rejected.

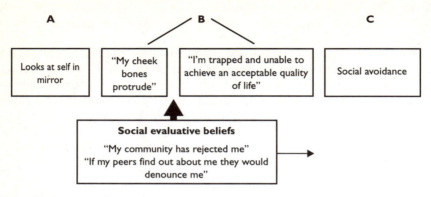

Figure 7.2 Harjinder: Formulation.

ABC formulation

At this stage, the social evaluative beliefs had emerged and a formulation was made. This is summarised in Fig. 7.2. The formulation essentially proposed that the delusional (inferential) beliefs were underpinned by "other-self" evaluation beliefs that concerned the shame of his rejection of his cultural identity and social affiliation. This recruited a bias towards evidence of rejection—in other words that he was being mistaken for a Muslim.

Working with the social evaluative beliefs

Harjinder recalled many occasions where he had been mistaken for a Pakistani. Together with the therapist the advice was sought of a practising Sikh about racial identity and racial confusion. Harjinder heard from him that the Sikh and Muslim races in northern India are drawn from common genetic stock and that he himself had at one time been mistaken for a Pakistani when not wearing his turban. One way of asserting his cultural identity was suggested, which was to wear a Sikh bracelet (*Karrah*) openly: he felt he could do this without sacrificing his principles. This simple manoeuvre helped Harjinder to feel accepted and to reduce any ambiguity about his group identity without, at the same time, sacrificing his wish to assert his own independence from his parents. This simple manoeuvre helped to affirm his social and group identity and was not of course a direct test of his delusional beliefs.

Outcome

Further evaluation with the power measures (see the appendices at the end of this chapter) revealed a dramatic improvement in Harjinder's perceived social inclusion. He still maintained that his face was disfigured but had "learned to cope" with it and, most importantly, his level of distress

12 months later was substantially reduced. He was subsequently successful in obtaining employment in local government in an administrative capacity.

Comment

The meaning of Harjinders's delusional beliefs lay in the ambiguity about his social identity and group "fit". The key to the intervention lay in uncovering this ambiguity and asserting his group identity without compromising his long held principles. It was theoretically significant that the delusions themselves had not changed but the distress was substantially improved through attention to these core social evaluations and also to the "hard" evidence that he could achieve something that he valued. The intervention was also unusual in that it deliberately sidestepped focus on the core delusions, but dealt mainly with the evaluative beliefs concerning failure and lack of achievement.

CASE THREE: ALTAF

Altaf is a 28-year-old British born Pakistani man living at home with his wife and four children, father, mother, two brothers, sister, brother-in-law, and nephew. He was referred to services due to risk associated with suicidal thinking. He presented with a variety of psychotic experience that subsequently proved largely resistant to conventional treatment, including ECT. Forensic assessment regarded him as a major risk and was managed through an assertive outreach team for individuals in the early phase of psychosis.

Presenting problems

Altaf described multiple voices commanding himself to harm self and others. Voices also comprised third person commentary including various inconsequential, banal commands. He also described visual hallucinations including members of another family who were "living" in his home and communicated with him through the voices. He also subscribed to persecutory and linked grandiose delusions in which he believed that a holy war was taking place in which he regarded himself as a key figure. He believed some individuals were part of a conspiracy to take over the world and that he had the power to detect who these individuals were and received instructions from his voices to slay them. He worked part-time helping his brother out in the family shop and reports that on occasions he had confronted customers whom he believed to be members of the evil power.

Background

At age 16 he described losing confidence in himself at school. He was subjected to bullying and developed aggressive fantasies. His father described that on occasions he got into playground fights. At 17 he left school, the aggressive fantasies ceased, and he worked happily as a carpet layer. At age 20 he sustained a knee injury and retired from this job and acquired work in a factory and also the family shop. Around this time he described the onset of voices in which he was kicked in a nightclub and broke his leg. At age 21 he was married in Pakistan and reported hearing voices during his stay. On his return from Pakistan at age 22 he described this as his best period living with his wife and baby and being relatively untroubled by symptoms.

At age 23 he was laid off from work due to an industrial accident and his family noted his decreased motivation and his increased isolation. In the context of increased social isolation he described the development of various (passivity) phenomena including persecutory thinking and increasing hallucinations. Altaf's family history was quite unremarkable. He was an observant Muslim and was the third of five children. There was no history of physical or sexual abuse and he was living in a large extended family in a single house with four children under seven. He was initially treated as an outpatient with conventional treatment. A crisis occurred where he lost tolerance for the voices that were commanding him to hurt others and self, and was found to have been yelling at his voices in public. He attempted an overdose.

Presentational puzzles

Altaf's level of distress seemed to fluctuate markedly from day-to-day. Some days he would be able to tolerate and contain his voices and the linked delusional system and to work effectively in the shop; yet on others his days would be characterised by yelling and making gestures with knives, describing an intent to harm himself and others. This was disclosed to mental health professionals rather than members of his family. There had been a number of attempts to move out of the home; for example, on one occasion he had packed his bags and demanded that his father take him to a hotel. There was also a general impression that family factors could also be influencing his presentation—for example, the family were largely unaware of his delusional world or voices and reported that he was behaving normally in spite of clear evidence to the contrary. Altaf also refused permission for the therapist to speak to his wife.

The voices

The ABC analysis essentially revealed that Altaf was locked into a subordinate power relationship with the voices and what they represented, and engaged in various forms of appeasement in order to reduce the need, as he saw it, to comply with commands to harm people, which he understood would have calamitous consequences for him and his family. His central belief in this relationship was that he had been chosen by a powerful but essentially benevolent agency on whose behalf he was fighting a holy war against evil. He believed he had been chosen because he himself was evil and was given commands to kill and slay evil people. His compliance belief was along the lines of "I must obey or I will be killed", yet he believed that it was wrong to kill. His resolution of this dilemma involved various forms of appeasement, which took essentially two forms. First, he would engage in a form of partial compliance, which involved acting on the commands in imagination including images and fantasies of slaying individuals. Secondly, he would repeat the command out loud or (subvocally) as if to affirm his intention to comply. This gave rise to some short-term relief but was quickly replaced by guilt that he should have complied; this was felt to feed back again into the cycle. The antecedents to his beliefs were the voice itself, but also of particular interest were the social triggers.

Social antecedents

These were individuals whom he felt he often met in the course of his work in the family shop. He felt they were not treating him with respect ("messing me about") or he felt they might be a threat. His attribution was that they were weak and vulnerable and that he could dominate them. This would trigger off a voice instructing him to slay (dominate) them, which he appeased by acting this out in his imagination.

Thus his behaviour towards the voice, the images of slaying, and his shadowing of the commands could be understood entirely within the context of the subordinate role he had with the powerful voice. This was confirmed on assessment using the Power and Social Rank Scales (see the appendices at the end of this chapter) showing that the power differential between self and voice was in the top 5% of our validation sample (i.e. large power differential), paralleled by low power and rank in relation to others in his social context, including notably his family. His low social power and social rank were mirrored in his relationship voices and in the nature of the social triggers.

The family context

There were a number of strands of evidence indicating significant tension in the home setting, which was hypothesised to be linked with his fluctuating difficulties with his voices. Altaf was unemployed, and was at one point a partner in the family shop, but was now a part-time helper. His brother wanted to sell the shop, which Altaf was very keen for him to do as he regarded working there as a potential threat to himself and his brother. However his brother changed his mind on several occasions without consulting Altaf, which caused him considerable frustration. He felt that he was unable to assert himself with his brother given that he was a "sick" member of the family who in effect was being looked after by the others. His wife wanted to leave the home and live in her own house nearby but he refused feeling that it would be disloyal to do so. His father was the patriarch of the family: Altaf handed over all his benefits to him, which he used with other forms of income to run the extended family household. In Altaf's view, to move house would be to challenge his father's position in the household. There were frequent confrontations between his wife and father. Altaf dealt with these conflicts in two ways. First, he avoided the conflict by hiding in his bedroom ("under the duvet") and it was significant that on many occasions when his voices were at their worst he had attempted to move out of the house. Secondly, he appeased the dominant members of the household by attempting to work in the shop and also by handing over his benefits.

Our analysis in essence argued that Altaf was in a "down-ranked" position within the household; his role had changed with little prospect, as he saw it, of escape. His relationship with the voice mirrored precisely his subordinate role in this key social structure in his life and when these conflicts were brought to a head he lost tolerance for his voices and the appeasement trap he had entered into.

Intervention

Changing the family power structure

The intervention proceeded at two levels. The first involved attempts to work with Altaf and his family to provide some relief to the subordinate and disempowered position he had found himself trapped in. In the family context, there were two foci. The first involved working in the system to enable him to gain greater control over key areas of concern. These were control over income and benefits and to counter his wife's sense of entrapment in her relationship within the family. Altaf's father was persuaded to allow the couple to move to living space that provided some privacy and autonomy, particularly in view of the overcrowded conditions in which they lived. Work with his brother was undertaken to emphasise the importance of involving

Altaf in all decisions that would impact upon him, in particular the decision to sell the shop. The second focus encouraged Altaf to resume activities that were valued in the family, particularly regular visits to the mosque for prayer, which he eventually managed to do. An opportunity was found for his wife to find support and contact outside of the family (she spoke no English) through an Asian Women's Resource Centre and contact with a Pakistani member of the mental health service. The cumulative effect of this family work was to provide Altaf with greater autonomy, more control over resources in the family, and greater respect.

Cognitive therapy

Cognitive behavioural therapy with his voices proceeded in parallel and focused on the subordinate power relationship with his voices. Beliefs about compliance and control were addressed first. Altaf was asked to consider why it was that, although he had instructions from the voice on well over 5000 occasions, he had resisted it and yet the consequences he feared had not occurred. Occasions were highlighted where he had neither obeyed the commands nor attempted to appease them—e.g. where he had heard the command but had been too busy in the shop to respond to it and had to leave the matter until a later time. It was suggested that this would be a useful strategy to develop to enable him to get things done without at the same time challenging the voice. He developed a strategy in which he told the voice that he would deal with matters later and reserved a particular time of the day to do so in his usual way. His evaluative belief that he was evil which was why the voices had chosen him was addressed, and the evidence identified for this proposition was outlined. It was suggested to him that in spite of intense provocation from the voice he had resisted all this time—why? He readily accepted that killing was an evil act and had therefore resisted it, but did this not imply therefore that he was not evil? His support for his children and his desire to help in the family shop in spite of his difficulties was also juxtaposed against his stated view that he was evil.

These manoeuvres to challenge the power of the voice, to assert his intellectual mastery of it, and to challenge his negative self-evaluation led to significant shifts in the power balance between himself and the voice. At this point the meaning behind the purpose of the voice was gently questioned. If the voice was so powerful why had it needed a mere mortal such as himself to wage this holy war, particularly as it was apparent that attempts to work through him were clearly not working?

Outcome

Simultaneous attention to his subordination to the voice and to that of his family dramatically improved the frequency of crises and general distress. The level of voice activity diminished only marginally but his relationship with it changed considerably. In essence, the formulation was that his lowered social status and inability to reassert his identity held the key to understanding his social schema and hence the relationship with the voice.

CONCLUSION

In this chapter we have demonstrated how new theoretical insights from social rank theory (Gilbert, Price, & Allan, 1995) and research based upon this can be applied to voices and other psychotic phenomena in clinical practice, in a modified form of cognitive therapy. Recent research has given strong support to the application of social rank theory to psychosis and shows that apparently disparate aspects of the psychotic experience—from voices to family relationships to diagnosis and hospitalisation—are all facets of the same process. This process involves a catastrophic loss of status in social rank terms, resulting in involuntary subordination, humiliation, and loss of self-esteem, and entrapment by powerful others. This can lead to anxiety, depression, and relapse in an ever worsening decline in social status. In this chapter we began by outlining the theory as applied to voices, drew out the more general implications for symptoms, relationships, and life events, reviewed some of the recent research that supports the approach, described some of the basic principles of assessment and intervention, and offered case examples that illustrate different facets of cognitive assessment and intervention from this perspective. We are engaged in a trial of cognitive therapy with command hallucinations drawing on this perspective, which aims to evaluate this approach under randomised controlled trial conditions.

Appendix A: Social Comparison Rating Scale: To Voices

We are now interested in how you compare yourself to *your voices*.
If you understand the above instructions please proceed. Circle
one number on each line according to how you see yourself in
relation to your voices.

* In relation to my voices I feel

Inferior	1	2	3	4	5	6	7	8	9	10	Superior
Incompetent	1	2	3	4	5	6	7	8	9	10	More competent
Unlikeable	1	2	3	4	5	6	7	8	9	10	More likeable
Left out	1	2	3	4	5	6	7	8	9	10	Accepted
Different	1	2	3	4	5	6	7	8	9	10	Same
Untalented	1	2	3	4	5	6	7	8	9	10	More talented
Weaker	1	2	3	4	5	6	7	8	9	10	Stronger
Unconfident	1	2	3	4	5	6	7	8	9	10	More confident
Undesirable	1	2	3	4	5	6	7	8	9	10	More desirable
Unattractive	1	2	3	4	5	6	7	8	9	10	More attractive
An outsider	1	2	3	4	5	6	7	8	9	10	An insider

Source: Adapted from Allan and Gilbert (1995).

Appendix B: Power Scale (Voices)

A list of statements follow. Please circle the number that best describes how you feel in relation to your voices.
.... name or description of voices.

Thank you for your help.

1	2	3	4	5
I am much more powerful than my voice	I am somewhat more powerful than my voice	We have about the same amount of power as each other	My voice is somewhat more powerful than me	My voice is much more powerful than me

1	2	3	4	5
I am much stronger than my voice	I am somewhat stronger than my voice	We are as strong as each other	My voice is somewhat stronger than me	My voice is much stronger than me

1	2	3	4	5
I am much more confident than my voice	I am somewhat more confident than my voice	We are as confident as each other	My voice is somewhat more confident than me	My voice is much more confident than me

1	2	3	4	5
I respect my voice much more than it respects me	I respect my voice somewhat more than it respects me	We respect each other about the same	My voice respects me somewhat more than I respect my voice	My voice respects me much more than I respect my voice
I am much more able to harm my voice than it is able to harm me	I am somewhat more able to harm my voice than it is able to harm me	We are equally well able to harm each other	My voice is somewhat more able to harm me than I am able to harm it	My voice is much more able to harm me than I am able to harm my voice
I am much more superior to my voice	I am somewhat superior to my voice	We are equal to each other	My voice is somewhat superior to me	My voice is much more superior to me
I am much more knowledgeable than my voice	I am somewhat more knowledgeable than my voice	We have about the same amount of knowledge as each other	My voice is somewhat more knowledgeable than me	My voice is much more knowledgeable than me

REFERENCES

Allan, S., & Gilbert, P. (1995). Social Comparison Scale, psychometric properties in relation to psychopathology. *Personality and Individual Differences*, *19*, 293–299.

Beck, A.T. (1963). Thinking and depression: 1, Idiosyncratic content and cognitive distortions. *Archives of General Psychiatry*, *9*, 324–333.

Beck-Sander, A., Birchwood, M., & Chadwick, P. (1997). Acting on command hallucinations: A cognitive approach. *British Journal of Clinical Psychology*, *36*, 139–148.

Benjamin, L.S. (1989). Is chronicity a function of the relationship between the person and the auditory hallucination? *Schizophrenia Bulletin*, *15*, 291–310.

Birchwood, M., & Chadwick, P. (1997). The omnipotence of voices: Testing the validity of a cognitive model. *Psychological Medicine*, *27*, 1345–1353.

Birchwood, M., Meaden, A., Trower, P., Gilbert, P., & Plaistow, J. (2000). The power and omnipotence of voices: Subordination and entrapment by voices and significant others. *Psychological Medicine*, *30*, 337–344.

Brown, G.W., Harris, T.O., & Hepworth, C. (1995). Loss, humiliation, and entrapment among women developing depression: A patient and non-patient comparison. *Psychological Medicine*, *25*, 7–21.

Chadwick, P., & Birchwood, M. (1994). The omnipotence of voices I: A cognitive approach to auditory hallucinations. *British Journal of Psychiatry*, *164*, 190–201.

Chadwick, P., & Birchwood, M. (1995). The omnipotence of voices II: The beliefs about voices questionnaire (BAVQ). *British Journal of Psychiatry*, *166*, 773–776.

Chadwick, P., Birchwood, M., & Trower, P. (1996). *Cognitive therapy for hallucinations, delusions, and paranoia*. Chichester: Wiley.

Clark, D., & Fairburn, C. (1997). *Science and practice of cognitive behaviour therapy*. Oxford: Oxford Medical Publications.

Drayton, M., Birchwood, M., & Trower, P. (1998). Early attachment experience and recovery from psychosis. *British Journal of Clinical Psychology*, *37*, 269–284.

Gilbert, P. (1992). *Depression: The evolution of powerlessness*. Hove, UK: Lawrence Erlbaum Associates Ltd.

Gilbert, P., & Allan, S. (1998). The role of defeat and entrapment (arrested flight) in depression: An exploration of an evolutionary view. *Psychological Medicine*, *28*, 585–598.

Gilbert, P., Price, J., & Allan, S. (1995). Social comparison, social attractiveness and evolution: How might they be related? *New Ideas in Psychology*, *13*, 149–165.

Hellerstein, D., Frosch, W., & Koenigsberg, H.W. (1987). The clinical significance of command hallucinations. *American Journal of Psychiatry*, *144*, 219–221.

Hope, D.A., Sigier, K.D., Penn, D.L., & Meier, V. (1998). Social anxiety, recall of interpersonal information and social impact on others. *Journal of Cognitive Psychotherapy*, *12*, 303–322.

Junginger, J. (1990). Predicting compliance with command hallucinations. *American Journal of Psychiatry*, *147*, 245–247.

Nayani, T.H., & David, A. (1996). The auditory hallucination: A phenomenological survey. *Psychological Medicine*, *26*, 177–189.

Price, J., Sloman, L., Gardner, R., Gilbert, P., & Rohde, P. (1994). The social competition hypothesis of depression. *British Journal of Psychiatry*, *164*, 309–315.

Rooke, O., & Birchwood, M. (1998). Loss, humiliation, and entrapment as appraisals of schizophrenic illness: A prospective study of depressed and non-depressed patients. *British Journal of Clinical Psychology, 37,* 259–268.

Trower, P., & Gilbert, P. (1989). New theoretical conceptions of social anxiety and social phobia. *Clinical Psychology Review, 9,* 19–35.

Trower, P., Sherling, G., Beech, J., Harrop, C., & Gilbert, P. (1998). The socially anxious perspective in face-to-face interaction: An experimental comparison. *Clinical Psychology and Psychotherapy, 5,* 155–166.

Chapter 8

Cognitive therapy for drug-resistant auditory hallucinations: A case example

Anthony P. Morrison

INTRODUCTION

Auditory hallucinations are defined in *DSM-IV* as being "a sensory perception that has the compelling sense of reality of a true perception but that occurs without external stimulation of the relevant sensory organ" (American Psychiatric Association, 1994, p. 767). The prevalence of auditory hallucinations in schizophrenia has been calculated as occurring in over 60% of such patients (Slade & Bentall, 1988), and they are often found to be the most common symptom observed in schizophrenia. Patients commonly identify the experience of auditory hallucinations as the most distressing aspect of their psychosis.

COGNITIVE MODELS OF AUDITORY HALLUCINATIONS

Early studies found that auditory hallucinations are accompanied by subvocalisation or covert movements of the speech musculature (Gould, 1950), which also accompanies normal thinking or inner speech. Studies have also found that verbal tasks that block subvocalisation also inhibit the occurrence of auditory hallucinations (Margo, Hemsley, & Slade, 1981). Such findings have led to agreement among theorists that auditory hallucinations are internal cognitive events that are misattributed to an external source (Bentall, 1990).

Some theorists have suggested that auditory hallucinations (externally attributed thoughts) result from biases of normal functioning. Bentall (1990) has argued that a hallucinator's tendency to misattribute internal events to an external source may reflect a bias, rather than primarily a deficit, in the monitoring of internal events. Bentall argues that this bias may be influenced by top-down processes (patients' beliefs and expectations about what kinds of events are likely to occur), and that reinforcement processes (particularly anxiety reduction) may facilitate the misclassification of certain kinds of internally generated events (for example, negative thoughts about self) as externally generated. This type of account explains why cultural differences in the experience of hallucinations are observed, because expectations about what kind of events are likely to be "real" are related to cultural practices. Morrison, Haddock, and Tarrier (1995) outline an account that proposes that metacognitive beliefs inconsistent with intrusive thoughts lead to their external attribution as auditory hallucinations, and that such a misattribution is maintained by reducing cognitive dissonance. This would explain a number of similarities in form and content between intrusive thoughts and auditory hallucinations.

There appears to be reliable empirical support for the notion that auditory hallucinations occur as a result of a cognitive or perceptual bias. Morrison and Haddock (1997a) showed that subjects experiencing auditory hallucinations had a bias towards externally attributing their thoughts in a word association task when compared with delusional patients and normal controls (a result replicated by Baker & Morrison, 1998). Bentall and Slade (1985) found that hallucinators showed a greater bias towards detecting signals, Heilbrun (1980) showed hallucinators are poorer than controls at recognising their own thoughts, and Bentall, Baker, and Havers (1991) found that subjects experiencing hallucinations exhibited an external attributional bias in a reality-monitoring study. Taken together, these findings suggest that auditory hallucinations do result from a bias in normal information processing.

There are currently a number of authors who suggest that interpretations of auditory hallucinations may be involved in the maintenance of such experiences and the distress associated with them. Kingdon and Turkington (1993) state that "the meaning invested in hallucinations may also be of importance—whether a person says to himself, 'The devil is talking to me' or 'I must be going crazy', or dismissively, 'That was a strange sensation, I must have been overtired'" (p. 78). Chadwick and Birchwood (1994) suggest that "affective, cognitive, and behavioural responses evolve together and are always meaningfully related" (p. 200), and they have found a strong positive relationship between appraisals of malevolence and resistance of the voices and between appraisals of benevolence and engagement with the voices (Chadwick & Birchwood, 1995).

Morrison (1998) has suggested that auditory hallucinations are normal phenomena, occurring in response to certain internal and external events, and that it is the misinterpretation of such phenomena that cause the distress and disability that are commonly seen in patients experiencing hallucinations with a diagnosis of schizophrenia. It is also proposed that these interpretations of auditory hallucinations are maintained by safety seeking behaviours (including hypervigilance). Relatively little investigation has been conducted regarding the role of hypervigilance in the maintenance of auditory hallucinations. However, Frith (1979) has argued that the symptoms of schizophrenia can be interpreted as the result of excessive self-awareness, and Morrison and Haddock (1997b) have shown that patients experiencing auditory hallucinations exhibit higher levels of private self-consciousness than psychiatric and normal control subjects, and self-focus was found to predict whether or not subjects experienced hallucinations in a logistic regression analysis.

When considered together, such models and experimental findings suggest the following: that auditory hallucinations are externally attributed thoughts; that interpretations of hallucinations account for at least some of the resulting distress; and that increased self-focused attention is associated with hearing voices. These assumptions readily translate into a clinical approach to hearing voices that involves: challenging the content of voices in a similar way to the challenging of negative automatic thoughts; challenging dysfunctional misinterpretations of voices; and modifying focus of attention or increasing flexible control of attention. A case example illustrating this approach, in the context of cognitive therapy, is outlined later in this chapter.

Effectiveness

Recent studies examining cognitive behaviour therapy (CBT) with psychotic patients have shown it to be effective in reducing residual positive symptoms on an outpatient basis, and maintaining these gains at follow-up (Chadwick & Birchwood, 1994; Garety, Kuipers, Fowler, Chamberlain, & Dunn, 1994; Kingdon & Turkington, 1991; Tarrier et al., 1993). CBT has been shown to be superior to other psychological treatments such as supportive counselling (Tarrier, Yusupoff, Kinney, McCarthy, Gledhill, Haddock, & Morris, 1998), to treatment as usual involving case management and antipsychotic medication (Kuipers et al., 1997), and to routine psychiatric care (Tarrier et al., 1998). A reduced stay in hospital (by 54% in comparison with control group) has also been shown for CBT of acute schizophrenic patients (Drury, Birchwood, & Cochrane, 1996) and recovery time for symptom reduction was also improved, suggesting that CBT is of benefit for in-patients as well as outpatients. Therefore, it appears that CBT methods can be used to promote symptom reduction and reduce time spent in hospital, as well as promoting relapse prevention.

While CBT has been shown to be superior to standard psychiatric care, the specific benefits that it yields are less clear; this is particularly the case for patients experiencing auditory hallucinations. Kuipers et al. (1998) found that global symptomatology was significantly better at end of treatment, but that hallucinations and delusions did not become significantly better until 18-month follow-up. Tarrier et al. (1993) found that hallucinations did not improve significantly whereas delusions did, and this is consistent with the difficulties found in another study examining CBT for hallucinations (Haddock, Slade, Bentall, Reid, & Faragher, 1998). However, Chadwick and Birchwood (1994) reported encouraging findings using cognitive therapy for voices, and Tarrier (1999) reported that CBT produced a greater change in hallucinations than delusions in comparison with supportive counselling. The delivery of such services and approaches to psychosis is consistent with service users' views as identified by Hansson, Bjorkman, & Svensson (1995) and current healthcare policy regarding promotion of choice for service users.

THE CASE OF STEVEN

Initial assessment

Steven was offered an initial appointment following self-referral to a service delivering cognitive therapy for psychotic individuals (he had learnt of the service from information for patients on a day hospital noticeboard and from talking to other service users). He was 29 years old, was employed as an internet web-page designer, and had a diagnosis of bipolar disorder (although he met DSM-IV criteria for schizophrenia at this time). He had a five-year history of such mental health problems, having experienced five manic episodes and three depressive episodes in this period. He often experienced positive psychotic symptoms during his manic episodes, and had recently had one such episode. He was currently prescribed lithium, carbamazepine, haloperidol, and depixol, and was compliant with all medication (medication was stable throughout intervention, with the exception of being taken off haloperidol at the patient's request). During the initial interview the PANSS (Kay, Fiszbein, & Opler, 1987) was administered by the therapist, as were the PSYRATS (Haddock, McCarron, Tarrier, & Faragher, 1999). The scores for each of these measures pre- and post-treatment can be seen in Table 8.1.

Table 8.1 Steven's PANSS and PSYRATS scores pre- and post-treatment

Measure	Pre-treatment	Post-treatment
PANSS: Total	66	41
PANSS: Positive	25	11
PANSS: Negative	10	9
PANSS: Global	31	21
PSYRATS: Delusions	15	0
PSYRATS: Hallucinations	25	17

Cognitive behavioural assessment, problem list, and goals

Steven identified his current concerns as hearing voices, believing that there was a conspiracy against him in which people were trying to cause him physical and mental harm, depression, an unsatisfactory social life, and sleeping too much. These were initially prioritised in the above order, and specific, measurable, proximal, and realistic goals were set in relation to each problem. For example, as regards voices the initial goals were set in relation to small (yet meaningful to him), measurable (using percentage ratings) changes in control over voices and distress caused by voices. The fact that changes in these dimensions may well correspond to changes in frequency was discussed. However, it was agreed that as changes in frequency may not be achievable they would be left off the goal list. Steven also agreed that if they were less distressing and he had more control over them then this would be a meaningful improvement, even if frequency was unaffected.

Initial formulations, persecutory beliefs, and selling the model

At the next session Steven identified the conspiracy as his target for the session in the agenda. Socratic questioning was used to develop a shared description of the recent specific incidents that had been disturbing him. A series of event–thought–feeling–behaviour cycles was collaboratively arrived at, and an example of one of the specific incidents summarised in this way is shown in Table 8.2. The therapist then used these to socialise Steven to the general cognitive model in relation to his fears about the conspiracy:

Therapist: So it sounds like your colleague at work coughs and you interpret this as meaning that he is involved in the conspiracy and is
criticising you for being lazy, which makes you feel upset and
become more alert to his behaviour. Is this correct?
Steven: Yes, that pretty much sums it up.
Therapist: If you wanted to change the way that you feel in this situation,
what would you have to do?
Steven: I could ignore him I suppose.
Therapist: Is there anything else that would make you less upset?

Table 8.2 Maintenance formulation for delusions

Event ⟶	Thought ⟶	Feeling ⟶	Behaviour
Man touched nose	He is angry He's going to damage my car	Frightened Panic	Get ready

Steven: If I knew he wasn't coughing about me.
Therapist: Are there any other possible reasons for him to be coughing?
Steven: Well he could have had a cold but I don't think so.
Therapist: Do you ever cough?
Steven: Yes.
Therapist: Why do you do it?
Steven: Sometimes I have a cold, sometimes it is a smokers' cough.
Therapist: Any other reasons why people might cough?
Steven: I guess some people might cough as a kind of nervous habit or to clear their throat.
Therapist: Could any of these things apply to your colleague.
Steven: I suppose so.
Therapist: Which seems most likely; one of these or them doing it to criticise you?
Steven: Probably some kind of habit.
Therapist: If, at the time, you were able to think through these different reasons and decide it was a habit, would you feel upset.
Steven: No.
Therapist: So what would you need to change in this cycle to affect how you feel—is it the event itself, how you interpret that event, or how you behave?
Steven: It is the interpretation of the event that has to change.

An examination of the specific incidents in relation to the conspiracy employing this framework was used over the course of three or four sessions to effectively decrease the frequency of his persecutory beliefs, the distress associated with these beliefs, and how much he believed them to be true. This was done partly because he had reprioritised the conspiracy as his main problem, partly because there were some small elements of risk associated with these beliefs (he had been involved in a fight as a result of this in the past and was a very highly skilled martial artiste), and partly because they seemed most likely to demonstrate quick success (and therefore contribute to engagement) and most amenable to instilling the process of cognitive therapy in him. These were used to show the usefulness of examining the evidence for interpretations of events, generating alternative explanations for events, and investigating such possibilities using behavioural experiments. An example of a behavioural experiment used in relation to the above situation was that Steven decided that he could investigate the situation further by keeping a record of how often his colleague coughed when he was working, when he was pretending to be working, and when he wasn't working. His prediction was that his colleague would cough most in the latter case, but he actually observed that the colleague coughed an approximately equal number of times in each condition. This resulted in a reduction of conviction from 70% to 5%. Similarly, the discussion of such specific incidents within sessions

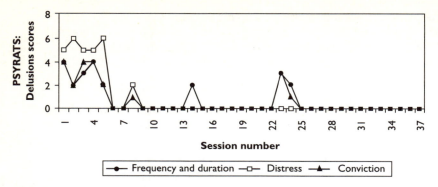

Figure 8.1 Steven's PSYRATS delusions scores.

usually resulted in a dramatic decrease in belief ratings and distress ratings. Changes over time for the PSYRATS ratings for beliefs in the conspiracy can be seen in Fig. 8.1.

Voices

Following the successful reduction of concerns about the conspiracy, Steven reprioritised the voices as his primary concern. Investigation of his voices began by analysing recent episodes of voice-hearing using the event–thought–feeling–behaviour framework which he had found useful in dealing with the ideas about a conspiracy. This same format was employed because he had agreed that this might be useful, and in order to help to instil a process of how to deal with distressing concerns and to aid generalisation. An example of such an analysis of a recent episode is given in Table 8.3.

Some discussion of these situations and the thoughts in relation to the voices enabled Steven to see that his interpretations of the voices were what caused the majority of the distress, rather than the voices themselves. The examination of such episodes was initially undertaken collaboratively within sessions, but soon was done as part of homework by filling in a modified dysfunctional thought record (DTR). The similarity of these analyses to those in relation to the conspiracy made the usefulness of examining the evidence for interpretations of voices, generating alternative explanations for

Table 8.3 Maintenance formulation for voices

Event ⟶	Thought ⟶	Feeling ⟶	Behaviour
Voice says: "Leave party or else"	I might do something foolish I won't be able to talk to anyone	Anxiety Tension	Go home Stop talking

voices, and investigating possible explanations of voices using behavioural experiments readily apparent.

Triggers and modulators

An examination of several weeks' worth of diaries (the modified DTRs) revealed a number of common themes in the internal and external events that preceded voice activity. These were social situations (particularly small enclosed spaces with lots of people present), use of cannabis, use of alcohol, anxiety, and paranoid thoughts. Factors that appeared to make the voices worse included the above potential triggers, as well as paying attention to the voices, resisting what they suggested doing, and driving a car. Factors that appeared to make the voices easier to deal with included going to bed, sometimes having an alcoholic drink, and obeying the voices. This information was used in collaborative discussions about the possible explanations of the voices, considering how each of these could be used as evidence for or against particular interpretations on the basis of whether they were compatible or not.

Interpretations of voices

Over a number of weeks several possible explanations of the voices were generated; this was done by starting with the most readily accessible interpretation, discussing what was consistent with this, and highlighting any discrepancies. Problem-solving techniques such as brainstorming were employed to generate other interpretations along with consideration of any that other people had suggested in the past. The explanations that were rated as being possibilities could be summarised as being related to three themes: the voices being a higher power; the voices being a form of mental illness; or the voices being an unusual thought process. The first of these was the interpretation that Steven started with.

He believed that the voices were a higher power for a number of reasons. They appeared to know personal information about him that other people would not (this is what Chadwick and Birchwood describe as the omniscience of voices). He also described physical sensations in which he felt that the voices were trying to compel him to say inappropriate things in social settings (sometimes successfully). Another factor that caused him to interpret his voices in this way was the visual imagery that occurred concurrently with the experience; he had images of the spirits of a number of people (friends and relatives) surrounding his head, and viewed this as indicative of some spiritual presence.

The possibility that his voices were a symptom of mental illness had been repeatedly presented to Steven as a fact by his psychiatrists. He saw several factors as being relevant to this: he had had several admissions to psychiatric hospitals; he had been given a diagnosis of bipolar disorder; he was taking several medications; and he had definitely experienced periods of excessively high mood in the past which had had difficult consequences. However, he was very sceptical of this possibility as the medication did not appear to help, the voices occurred independently of high mood, and he cited the fact that in many cultures voice-hearing is viewed as a sign of spirituality.

The possibility that the voices were an unusual thought process was arrived at slowly. Initially, Steven was given a lot of information regarding how common it is to hear voices. This included working out how many people in the UK would hear voices on the basis of epidemiology studies elsewhere and some discussion of more frequent hallucinatory experiences such as hypnogogic and hypnopompic phenomena. He was also given information about the fact that speech musculature has been found to move when people hear voices and that subvocalisation often inhibits voices. Analysis of the content of the voices from within session episode analyses and diaries highlighted the fact that the voices often spoke about things that were of high personal salience to him (girlfriends, behaving foolishly, fighting). This, in combination with some discussion about unwanted intrusive thoughts, allowed him to conclude that there may be some link between his thoughts and his voices. He summarised this possibility as the voices being a product of his own mind that was different to most other people's thoughts but not necessarily wrong or abnormal. However, he pointed out that he could distinguish between his thoughts and voices and that the following factors appeared to be involved: lack of deliberateness; no control over stopping them; the urges to say things; and reason becoming impossible. Discussion of these illustrated that they were not necessarily specific to voices, but were certainly most commonly associated with them. Some may argue that it is risky to consider the possibility that voices are related to thoughts with someone who hears voices telling them to do things (or command hallucinations in psychiatric jargon). However, by examining metacognitive beliefs (thoughts about thoughts) it can be very clear to people that having a thought does not mean that you will do it, that you are responsible for causing it, or that you are a bad person. It would seem likely that a voice perceived as a higher power (and therefore disobedience may be punished) is more likely to be obeyed than a thought, particularly when cognitive therapy has been shown to be very effective in dealing with unwanted thoughts (both in general and in relation to the prior concerns of this patient).

These three interpretations were considered in great detail. Analysis of how compatible the triggers and modulators were with each of them was undertaken, and any additional evidence for and against each that had naturalistically occurred throughout the week or been specifically gathered using behavioural experiments was integrated. An example of a typical session's evidence is shown in Table 8.4.

Table 8.4 Evidential analysis for interpretations of voices

Interpretation	Evidence for	Evidence against
A higher power	• The voice can predict unlikely things happening • Imagery of higher power • Physical feeling—it feels very convincing	• It could be coincidence • A lot of what they predict does not occur
A sign of illness	• It can be associated with high mood • Can be triggered by paranoia	• It doesn't seem to happen at work • It is different to high mood
An unusual thought process	• It could be a stress response • It can be triggered by cannabis • What they talk about is similar to things I think about	• It feels real

Content of voices

The content of voices was commonly used as evidence for or against the different interpretations of the voices. However, if there was distress that appeared to be related directly to the content of the voices, then this was challenged using the standard verbal reattribution techniques. One such example was when the voices told Steven he would never get a girlfriend. A quick examination of the evidence for and against this revealed that this was extremely unlikely to be true. He also felt that when the voices called him names that this may reflect low self-esteem, so work aimed at improving sense of self-worth was agreed upon (see later for details).

Attention

Selective attention also appeared to be implicated in the maintenance of his voices. Some discussion of how attention works in general, and how we selectively attend to personally salient information (using examples such as noticing other cars of the same type or colour as yours), was conducted. The role of attention in relation to the voices was investigated using within session analysis of recent situations in which the voices had been problematic and between session behavioural experiments to examine predictions. From his descriptions of the situations (particularly social situations—this is important to note because of the proposed role of self-focused attention in social phobia; cf. Clark & Wells, 1995), it seemed that Steven was engaging in high levels of self-focused attention. He reported monitoring his thoughts in such situations and "becoming more sensitive" to the possibility of hearing voices. This hypervigilance towards his thinking processes extended to monitoring physical sensations—he described a "ripple feeling" as preceding the voices. Using behavioural experiments Steven found that by focusing on his surroundings (very similar to the interrogation of the environment recommended to socially anxious individuals; Clark & Wells, 1995) he could ameliorate and sometimes prevent the voices from occurring.

Positive beliefs about voices

In dealing with the voices it also became apparent that there were a number of positive beliefs about the voices that were preventing intervention from being maximally effective and may have contributed to their maintenance (this issue is highlighted by Morrison, Wells, & Nothard, 2000). Steven perceived his voices as creating a fantasy world in which things appeared more vivid and in which he felt much more important, singled out, and like he had a destiny. He felt that they added excitement to his life and provided entertainment, and that without them life could be boring. The talk about fighting was particularly exciting, and gave him a sense of living on the edge that he described as like being on a roller coaster. These beliefs were examined in detail, because if it was thought that the advantages of voice-hearing outweighed the disadvantages intervention would have ceased to target them. However, it was collaboratively decided that if alternative sources of entertainment and ways of reducing boredom could be achieved then intervention should proceed (details of these aspects of intervention are given later).

This decision was not made definitively until after a relapse. Steven had become bored again and had decided to smoke some cannabis while away on a residential course. This had resulted in an initial period of excitement associated with the voice-hearing. However, this was shortly followed by terror and paranoia in association with voices that were very unpleasant in content. This culminated in some very socially inappropriate behaviour, a physical assault, the involvement of the police, and a hospital admission following an overdose. This situation appeared to remove any remaining ambivalence about the relative advantages and disadvantages of voice-hearing.

Final formulation

Towards the later stages of therapy a more detailed formulation in relation to the voices was collaboratively developed. This incorporated the most problematic interpretations, cognitive, behavioural, physical, and emotional

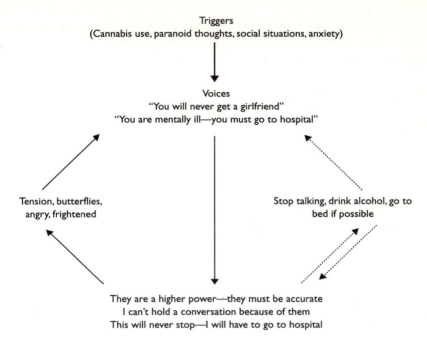

Triggers
(Cannabis use, paranoid thoughts, social situations, anxiety)

Voices
"You will never get a girlfriend"
"You are mentally ill—you must go to hospital"

Tension, butterflies,
angry, frightened

Stop talking, drink alcohol, go to
bed if possible

They are a higher power—they must be accurate
I can't hold a conversation because of them
This will never stop—I will have to go to hospital

Figure 8.2 Formulation for voices.

responses, as well as triggers, voice content, and the reciprocal relationships between these factors. An example of this is shown in Fig. 8.2.

Mood, social life and self-worth

Low mood, sleep, social life, establishing a daily routine and concerns about his job were all also identified on Steven's problem list. Some of these were prioritised because of their relation to the content of his voices or the necessity of providing alternative ways of gaining some of the benefits he identified in relation to the voices. These interventions were again formulation-driven, commonly drawing from techniques used in cognitive therapy for depression. These included activity scheduling, sleep hygiene, reviewing medication dosages and side effects in consultation with the psychiatrist, behavioural graded task assignments, and problem solving. In addition, schema-based interventions were employed to improve sense of self-worth; these included examining evidence for and against the belief "I am worthless" and positive data logs for activities deemed to be worthwhile.

Relapse prevention

The following blueprint or summary of what had been found to be useful and what could be done to minimise chances of relapse was collaboratively generated in the final session:

- Identifying triggers for episodes
- Event–Thought–Feeling–Behaviour
- Identify cycle
- Look for what to change
- Change thoughts:

    — Examining the evidence
    — What would you say to a friend? etc.
    — Are there different ways to interpret the event
    — Change interpretation of events—balanced thinking

- Making decisions:

    — Look at advantages and disadvantages

- Change behaviour:

    — Start a conversation
    — "Displacement activity"—reading, TV, etc.
    — Making social contact
    — Relaxation
    — Giving up cannabis
    — Look for interesting things to do

Outcome

The changes in the main voice-related outcome measure are shown in Fig. 8.3.

CONCLUSIONS

It appears that cognitive therapy based on the principles outlined by Beck (1976) can be effectively applied to the distress that is commonly experienced by people who hear voices. The cognitive models of auditory hallucinations appear to translate readily into formulation-driven interventions that can be applied collaboratively using the structure of cognitive therapy.

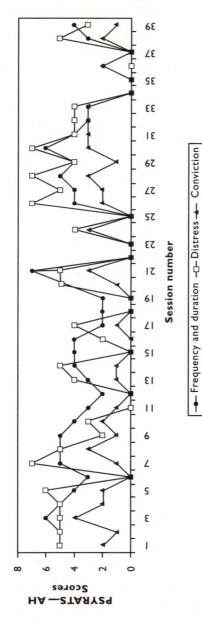

Figure 8.3 Steven's PSYRATS hallucinations scores.

REFERENCES

American Psychiatric Association (1994). *Diagnostic and statistical manual of mental disorders* (4th edn). Washington, DC: APA.

Baker, C., & Morrison, A.P. (1998). Metacognition, intrusive thoughts, and auditory hallucinations. *Psychological Medicine, 28*, 1199–1208.

Beck, A.T. (1976). *Cognitive therapy and the emotional disorders.* New York: International Universities Press.

Bentall, R.P. (1990). The syndromes and symptoms of psychosis: Or why you can't play twenty questions with the concept of schizophrenia and hope to win. In R.P. Bentall (Ed.), *Reconstructing schizophrenia* (pp. 23–60). London: Routledge.

Bentall, R.P., Baker, G., & Havers, S. (1991). Reality-monitoring and psychotic hallucinations. *British Journal of Clinical Psychology, 30*, 213–222.

Bentall, R.P., & Slade, P.D. (1985). Reality-testing and auditory hallucinations: A signal detection analysis. *British Journal of Clinical Psychology, 24*, 159–169.

Chadwick, P., & Birchwood, M. (1994). The omnipotence of voices. A cognitive approach to auditory hallucinations. *British Journal of Psychiatry, 164*, 190–201.

Chadwick, P.D., & Birchwood, M. (1995). The omnipotence of voices II: The Beliefs About Voices Questionnaire (BAVQ). *British Journal of Psychiatry, 166*, 773–776.

Clark, D.M., & Wells, A. (1995). A cognitive model of social phobia. In R. Heimberg, M. Leibowitz, D.A. Hope, & F.R. Schneier (Eds.), *Social phobia: Diagnosis, assessment, and treatment* (pp. 69–93). New York: Guilford Press.

Drury, V., Birchwood, M., & Cochrane, R. (1996). Cognitive therapy and recovery from acute psychosis: A controlled trial I: Impact on psychotic symptoms. *British Journal of Psychiatry, 169*, 593–601.

Frith, C.D. (1979). Consciousness, information processing, and schizophrenia. *British Journal of Psychiatry, 134*, 225–235.

Garety, P.A., Kuipers, L., Fowler, D., Chamberlain, F., & Dunn, G. (1994). Cognitive behavioural therapy for drug-resistant psychosis. *British Journal of Medical Psychology, 67*, 259–271.

Gould, L.N. (1950). Verbal hallucinations as automatic speech. *American Journal of Psychiatry, 107*, 110–119.

Haddock, G., McCarron, J., Tarrier, N., & Faragher, E.B. (1999). Scales to measure dimensions of hallucinations and delusions: The psychotic symptom rating scales (PSYRATS). *Psychological Medicine, 29*, 879–889.

Haddock, G., Slade, P.D., Bentall, R.P., Reid, D., & Faragher, B.F. (1998). A comparison of the long-term effectiveness of distraction and focusing in the treatment of auditory hallucinations. *British Journal of Medical Psychology, 71*, 339–349.

Hansson, L., Bjorkman, T., & Svensson, B. (1995). The assessment of needs in psychiatric patients. *Acta Psychiatrica Scandinavica, 92*, 285–293.

Heilbrun, A.R. (1980). Impaired recognition of self-expressed thought in patients with auditory hallucinations. *Journal of Abnormal Psychology, 89*, 728–736.

Kay, S.R., Fiszbein, A., & Opler, L.A. (1987). The Positive and Negative Syndrome Scale (PANSS) for schizophrenia. *Schizophrenia Bulletin, 13*, 261–276.

Kingdon, D.G., & Turkington, D. (1991). The use of cognitive behaviour therapy with a normalising rationale in schizophrenia. *Journal of Nervous and Mental Disease, 179*, 207–211.

Kingdon, D.G., & Turkington, D. (1993). *Cognitive behavioural therapy of schizophrenia*. New York: Guilford.

Kuipers, E., Fowler, D., Garety, P., Chisholm, D., Freeman, D., Dunn, G., Bebbington, P., & Hadley, C. (1998). London-East Anglia randomised controlled trial of cognitive behaviour therapy for psychosis III: Follow-up and economic evaluation at 18 months. *British Journal of Psychiatry, 173*, 61–68.

Kuipers, E., Garety, P., Fowler, D., Dunn, G., Bebbington, P., Freeman, D., & Hadley, C. (1997). The London-East Anglia randomised controlled trial of cognitive behavioural therapy for psychosis I: Effects of the treatment phase. *British Journal of Psychiatry, 171*, 319–327.

Margo, A., Hemsley, D.R., & Slade, P.D. (1981). The effects of varying auditory input on schizophrenic hallucinations. *British Journal of Psychiatry, 139*, 122–127.

Morrison, A.P. (1998). A cognitive analysis of auditory hallucinations: Are voices to schizophrenia what bodily sensations are to panic? *Behavioural and Cognitive Psychotherapy, 26*, 289–302.

Morrison, A.P., & Haddock, G. (1997a). Cognitive factors in source monitoring and auditory hallucinations. *Psychological Medicine, 27*, 669–679.

Morrison, A.P., & Haddock, G. (1997b). Self-focused attention in schizophrenic patients and normal subjects: A comparative study. *Personality and Individual Differences, 23*, 937–941.

Morrison, A.P., Haddock, G., & Tarrier, N. (1995). Intrusive thoughts and auditory hallucinations: A cognitive approach. *Behavioural and Cognitive Psychotherapy, 23*, 265–280.

Morrison, A.P., Wells, A., & Nothard, S. (2000). Cognitive factors in predisposition to auditory and visual hallucinations. *British Journal of Clinical Psychology, 39*, 67–78.

Slade, P.D., & Bentall, R.P. (1988). *Sensory deception: A scientific analysis of hallucination*. London: Croom Helm.

Tarrier, N. (1999). Specific effect of cognitive behaviour therapy for schizophrenia is not proved: Author's reply. *British Medical Journal, 318*, 331.

Tarrier, N., Beckett, R., Harwood, S., Baker, A., Yusupoff, L., & Ugarteburu, I. (1993). A trial of two cognitive behavioural methods of treating drug-resistant psychotic symptoms in schizophrenic patients: Outcome. *British Journal of Psychiatry, 162*, 524–532.

Tarrier, N., Yusupoff, L., Kinney, C., McCarthy, E., Gledhill, A., Haddock, G., & Morris, J. (1998). Randomised controlled trial of intensive cognitive behaviour therapy for patients with chronic schizophrenia. *British Medical Journal, 317*, 303–307.

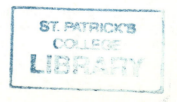

Chapter 9

Anxiety, associated physiological sensations, and *delusional* catastrophic misinterpretation: Variations on a theme?

Steven Williams

INTRODUCTION

In this chapter the psychological treatment of a young woman with a diagnosis of schizophrenia who had experienced just one episode of psychosis will be described. The cognitive model of panic disorder (Clark, 1986) will be used as a template to consider this young woman's psychotic experiences, in some ways developing the analogy between auditory hallucinations and panic disorder recently advanced (Morrison, 1998a) and in the context of some types of delusional beliefs, especially those involving the catastrophic and atypical misinterpretation of the physiological sensations associated with anxiety. It is not suggested that such a model would be helpful for all individuals experiencing psychosis, but that for a sub-group of people who *delusionally* misinterpret such sensations in a catastrophic manner (as distinct from individuals who misinterpret such sensations catastrophically in socially "acceptable" ways and are understood to suffer from panic disorder) such models may be helpful to consider as a guide to formulation for the therapist, and a route towards developing a potentially convincing alternative explanatory model for the affected person (as suggested by Morrison 1998b).

This approach to understanding and treating psychosis acknowledges the problematic nature of retaining one unifying concept (schizophrenia) to explain all apparently related phenomena, and suggests that explanatory psychological models of psychosis are constructed around the actual experience of symptoms rather than a "syndrome" that has been shown to be problematic in the scientific sense (Boyle, 1990) and in terms of its clinical utility (Bentall, 1990). It is consistent with the assertion (Clark, 1997) that the most effective psychological treatments have been constructed by building a model that seeks to explain what keeps the "problem" going (maintenance level model), if possible, what factors were involved in the development of the "problem", (longitudinal/aetiological level model), and with this understanding seek to treat the central pathology and disrupt and break the maintenance cycle. It is also of course an inherently empowering method of trying to understand and treat apparently "ununderstandable" (Jaspers, 1963) psychotic phenomena, in the sense that it emphasises collaboration and empiricism with the affected person as the basic ingredients of active therapy. Schema-level interventions, based on the longitudinal formulation collaboratively arrived at, to reduce this person's future vulnerability to similar difficulties will be described. A detailed case study will illustrate the development of the therapeutic procedures in this particular example. A discussion of the implications of such an approach to the treatment of individuals with similar difficulties will be conducted at the end of the chapter.

THEORETICAL BACKGROUND

A professional consensus has emerged in recent years with regard to an explanatory model of schizophrenia. This consensus has gathered around models of understanding schizophrenia (Nuechterlein & Dawson, 1984; Zubin & Spring, 1977), which are collectively known as the stress vulnerability hypothesis. Such models have been crucial in developing an understanding of schizophrenia that emphasises that this disorder in functioning is characterised by genetic predisposition mediated by stress. In some senses this type of model applies to many disorders including those of a physical nature such as diabetes.

This model, crude as its first articulation was in many ways, was a breakthrough in that it allowed for psycho-social interventions, especially with regard to the idiosyncratic experience of stress, irrespective of the actual or hypothesised genetic vulnerability that an individual had to contend with. In some respects the actual *relative* contributions of genetic vulnerability and stressful life events to the development of psychosis in an individual was irrelevant because it could be argued that we all have a genetic vulnerability to, for example, death, but this fact does not prevent most individuals trying to lead a fulfilled life of one kind or another! That we did not have to wait to weigh the relative contributions of genetics and stressful life events to the development and maintenance of psychosis in a particular individual was beneficial given that, despite a century of research into the genetic nature of schizophrenia, nothing could be demonstrated for certain despite the repeated claims of breakthrough (Bentall, 1990).

Following the failure of psychoanalytically orientated therapy to contribute to the effective treatment of people with diagnoses of schizophrenia, psychological intervention in such disorders was a fairly rare activity until these models began to be articulated. When interventions were attempted from a psychological perspective, they tended to follow the Zeitgeist and be concerned initially in *managing* the behavioural consequences of psychotic experiences, as often as not from the perspective of the institution that many people inhabited who were affected by psychosis during the 1960s and 1970s. Such models of intervention, heavily influenced by the successes of experimental behaviour therapy, tried to treat the behavioural manifestations of psychosis (and sometimes of institutionally generated behaviours often misunderstood as resulting from psychosis) by means of operant conditioning principles. These attempts at psychological intervention tried to apply universal learning theory principles to the complex problem of psychosis. They were characterised not by careful study of the nature of an individual's psychotic experiences but by the transfer to the business of helping people with distress associated with psychosis the principles and procedures that had been found helpful to other people experiencing different types of distress.

The results of such attempts at intervention were mixed, and specific models of understanding and treating people with psychosis were not particularly advanced in this respect. Other treatment approaches such as social skills training and life skills training were also used to help people with schizophrenia overcome some of the problems they encountered as a result of their "core" psychotic symptoms, and possibly therefore attempting to prevent the secondary disabilities associated with this disorder (interpersonal difficulties and reduction in social contacts) acting as a further stressor in people already vulnerable to psychotic breakdown. However, it was not until fairly recently that treatment approaches that involve affected people as full partners in therapy have been developed and evaluated.

An important study in this regard was Chadwick and Lowe's 1990 paper on belief modification (the language of operant conditioning still clearly retained here), which demonstrated that seemingly intransigent delusional beliefs were able to be influenced by the sorts of techniques that were involved in helping anyone (psychotic or not) fully review and consider the evidence for their beliefs (this seminal paper will be reviewed more thoroughly in the next section on supportive empirical studies).

While the stress vulnerability models outlined earlier were helpful in allowing both for a genetic predisposition and the influence of stress in schizophrenia, we are still not clear about the relative contributions of each side of the model in schizophrenic illness in general, and with regard to an affected person in particular. Given the wide ranging variability in presentation, course, and outcome in schizophrenia, the current lack of a conclusive genetic explanation for schizophrenia, and the apparent existence of psychotic phenomena in the general non-clinical population, allied to the evidence that the core symptoms of schizophrenia (hallucinations and, in terms of the person discussed here, particularly delusions) are subject to the same change processes as is the case for normal individuals, it is contended that for at least a significant sub-group of people so diagnosed the therapist can approach the treatment of the core symptoms as he or she would with a non-psychotic person with troublesome beliefs.

EVIDENCE SUPPORTING THEORY

It has been argued that it would be appropriate to approach the treatment of an individual suffering from schizophrenia on an individual basis, or at the very least on the basis that the affected person's experiences may be understood as a syndrome of schizophrenia rather than the inevitable playing out of a unifying disease process. Is there supportive scientific evidence to commend this position? This is the question that is often asked of therapists and researchers who articulate a person level or even (putative) syndrome level approach to the treatment of people with psychotic experiences, and yet this question compounds the earliest scientific errors in the history of the schizophrenia concept. It is a back-to-front argument to suggest that unless it can be demonstrated that a person's experiences can be proven *not* to be accounted for by a disease process, therapists should approach the treatment of that individual as if their experiences were disease driven. The appropriate hierarchical sequence is that those that maintain that individual experiences can be accounted for by a disease process must demonstrate this scientifically in order to require others to abandon a person level approach to the "treatment" of such experiences.

It is very clear that schizophrenia cannot yet be demonstrated to be a disease in any truly rigorous scientific sense (Boyle, 1990) and yet all too often therapists and researchers are asked to operate as though it has been, with possible deleterious consequences for the individual (inappropriate treatment regimes). One of the main principles of medicine is that of parsimony—the notion that we do the least invasive treatment possible and intervene only when there is compelling evidence that requires us to do so. Such a principle should not be abandoned in the treatment of people affected by psychotic experiences, and such experiences should be approached, at least initially, at the level of the person, rather than at the syndrome or disease level. It is clear to anyone who works with people with schizophrenia that the variability in presentation of people attracting this diagnosis is more evident than their similarities. This has been acknowledged even by traditionally orientated psychiatrists and researchers (Crow, 1980) who have suggested that perhaps there are three separate syndromes accounting for what we currently group together as schizophrenia. Of course, variability in presentation could still be possible even within a disease process.

There is also good evidence suggesting that the prevalence of schizophrenia is remarkably stable across differing cultures (World Health Organisation, 1979), yet even such observations of human behaviour and experiences utilising tight criteria to arrive at diagnosis do not prove the existence of a disease process. The same study also demonstrated the divergence of outcome in schizophrenia, with people in developing countries doing much better in terms of recovery than people living in developed industrialised nations. This divergence at least suggests that outcome in schizophrenia can be influenced by environment, a finding inconsistent with a rigid disease view. Other studies employing retrospective analysis of the records of public institutions appear to demonstrate that the course of schizophrenic illness is influenced by the slumps and booms characteristic of capitalist societies (Warner, 1994). Such evidence is advanced not in order to claim that schizophrenia does not exist—though some influential opinion now claims not to believe in it as a concept (Bentall, 1990)—but in order to claim the space in which therapists can work at a person level of understanding psychotic experiences with affected people.

While claims about the genetic nature of schizophrenic illness are widespread, the actual evidence seems more circumspect. Problems abound with the methodology, aims, and statistical manoeuvres employed by researchers who all too often have approached the issue as if the research question was "how do we demonstrate that schizophrenia is a genetic disease?" rather than "does genetic predisposition explain schizophrenia and to what extent?" (Marshall, 1990). Such unscientific a priori assumptions led to procedures including the determination of zygosity in twins by simple observation by the leading researcher, the same person already having also determined diagnosis, and yet the data that was obtained is routinely aggregated into the analysis demonstrating the genetic basis of schizophrenia. Even if schizophrenia does have a wholly genetic basis, we cannot conclude that interventions at the level of the person rather than the disease are irrelevant, because; "Just as drugs change behaviour, so will altered behaviour imposed by talking therapies change brains" (Rose, Kamin, & Lewontin, 1984, p. 228).

Perhaps the most compelling reason why therapists and researchers should approach work with people affected by psychotic symptoms at the person level is the evidence that phenomena that are routinely used to establish diagnostic criteria for schizophrenia appear to be prevalent in the non-clinical population, especially auditory hallucinations. Delusional beliefs, still considered as key phenomena in arriving at a diagnosis of schizophrenia and schizophrenia spectrum disorders, have been demonstrated to be phenomena present amongst the non-clinical population to a suprisingly large extent (Peters, Joseph, & Garety, 1999). Firm evidence is also now being reported (Raune, Kuipers, & Bebbington, 1999) that demonstrates that psycho-social stress is indicative not only of psychotic experiences in general, but quite possibly linked strongly to the *specific themes* that emerge in a person's symptoms, whether hallucinatory or delusional in nature, and that this may be especially the case in first or early episode patients. This (admittedly early) evidence, supporting earlier therapeutic "intuition" in this area, argues convincingly against the notion that psychotic experiences are "ununderstandable" phenomena (Jaspers, 1963), and can be seen to be consistent with the notion of approaching even seemingly bizarre phenomena at the level of the person rather than a disease or even syndromal level.

An attempt has been made to explain why it is important that therapists approach the treatment of people with psychotic symptoms as they would approach the treatment of any person presenting for help with distressing experiences, and do not make a priori assumptions about the treatability or otherwise of these phenomena. An important question that remains to be examined is whether or not such experiences are amenable to the same change processes as non-psychotic experiences are or not. Chadwick and Lowe's 1990 paper looked at the possibility of trying to treat people with strongly held delusional beliefs in a broadly standard psychological manner. Six people were included in this early study, with five of the six reporting 100% conviction in their delusional beliefs at base line and the other person's delusional belief conviction being more variable but never falling below 90%. They tried to ensure that they did not risk hardening conviction (if that was possible, given baseline scores!) by adopting four principles (Watts, Powell, & Austin, 1973) to minimise "psychological reactance":

1 Begin by considering beliefs that are problematic for the person but least strongly held.
2 Clients are asked not to adopt an alternative belief but to *consider* it.
3 The evidence rather than the belief is challenged.
4 Finally, the client is asked to voice the argument against their belief.

During the active treatment stage of the study, a verbal challenge was made to the client about the delusional belief. Clients were asked not to abandon their belief in its entirety, but to view it as only one possible explanation of the evidence. The belief itself was then challenged by pointing out any inconsistency, showing an alternative, and finally arguing that the alternative made more sense. This simple procedure led to one client entirely rejecting their belief and maintaining this at follow-up, a reduction in belief conviction from 100% to 40% for a second client, again maintained at follow-up, with a third client's belief conviction vacillating at around 40%, with similar results again at follow-up. A fourth client's belief remained at 100% throughout the study, although he claimed his concerns were now centred on what had happened rather than what was still happening. Verbal challenge alone had no impact on two clients. These two clients were then treated by means of "reality-testing", which involved the therapist and client collaborating to design a simple test of the delusional belief—e.g. one client believed he knew what was going to happen before it happened, and the test for this belief was to tape record a television news programme which the client did not watch, stop the tape at random points, and ask the client to predict what will happen next. This procedure proved to be completely effective in one case with conviction in the delusional belief falling from 100% to 0%, maintained at follow-up, and moderately effective with the other person with conviction falling from 100% to between 20% and 40% during treatment, and stabilising at around 40% conviction at follow-up. These impressive results do suggest that it is possible to modify delusional beliefs simply by careful and diplomatic challenges to such beliefs.

Although Chadwick and Lowe did utilise Watts et al.'s (1973) principles to avoid the risk of psychological reactance, in a sense this procedure could be equally applied to the treatment of many psychological disorders such as health anxiety. Indeed, the issue of engagement in health anxious patients is handled in a similar way (Salkovskis, 1996). More recently, Kingdon and Turkington (1994) have suggested that when examining delusional beliefs with affected people the therapist should use a "peripheral questioning" approach, where the evidence supporting the delusional belief is challenged or examined before the belief itself is. This is a very similar approach to that suggested by Chadwick and Lowe. It appears that providing the therapist is sensitive to the importance of the belief for the affected person, and approaches the treatment of such problematic beliefs in a sensitive and empathic way, that such difficulties may be amenable to intervention, and through the same mechanisms that therapists would use to help anyone review and consider beliefs that may be the source of some difficulties. The beliefs of ordinary people are often formed and maintained with little apparent regard to evidence: indeed only a minority of the population form their beliefs, even concerning issues of great importance to themselves and their families, in a way consistent with the logical rules of reasoning. In this sense, holding beliefs with little regard to the evidence is a normal occurrence. The aim of therapy with people affected by delusional beliefs is to subject such beliefs to some "scientific" enquiry where they cause distress to the person, in the same way that thinking errors are identified and discussed with people presenting with other types of psychological distress.

The cognitive model of panic (Clark, 1986) suggests that the main psychological process that underlies panic disorder is the misinterpretation of the normal physiological signs asociated with anxiety in a catastrophic way. Once this misinterpretation has occurred, the level of anxiety the affected person is experiencing becomes heightened, and the associated physiological sensations become more intense, leading to further catastrophic thinking and so on, thus creating the vicious cycle so familiar to most cognitive therapists. It will become evident why this is considered to be an appropriate template for developing a formulation of the person's difficulties about to be described in some detail.

CASE STUDY

Assessment

June (pseudonym) is a 32-year-old lady who lives in rented accommodation with her husband and her two young children. She had first presented to psychiatric services complaining of depression in the context of marital stress. A year later she had a "psychotic episode" and was admitted to hospital convinced that her husband was trying to kill her, despite a lack of "objective" evidence. She improved on antipsychotic medication, but still had times when she felt very strongly convinced that she was in great danger, and she was reluctant to continue with the medication on a long-term basis. The medical staff treating June's illness had diagnosed her as suffering from schizophrenia, and she had been referred to psychological therapy as an adjunct to the routine treatment she was receiving (antipsychotic medication, mental state monitoring in outpatients, and occasional visits by a CPN).

Prior to commencing therapy June was assessed with the PANSS (Kay, Fiszbein, & Opler, 1987) to establish a baseline of her positive and negative symptoms (if any) and general psychopathology. Other assessments used included the Social Functioning Scale (Birchwood, Smith, Cochrane, Wetton, & Copestake, 1990), Beck's Depression Inventory (Beck & Greer, 1987) and the delusions subscale of the PSYRATS (Haddock, McCarron, Tarrier, & Faragher, 1999). These assessments showed that while June had moderately distressing delusional beliefs, there was little evidence of any other psychotic phenomena; indeed her positive symptom subscale of the PANSS suggested no other clinical evidence of psychotic features. She was not depressed and her social functioning was very good as measured against norms for people with schizophrenia. Her delusional beliefs, while rated as "moderate" according to the PANSS, actually looked much more problematic when the parameters of this phenomena were more carefully assessed using the delusions subscale of the PSYRATS. This phenomena, where global measures of psychopathology are frequently quite poor measures of the full impact of delusional beliefs on the person, should be noted. The PSYRATS measure indicated that June thought about her beliefs very frequently (at least once an hour or so), found that once she started to think about her beliefs she would think about them sometimes for hours at a time, and while she had only a low level of conviction in the beliefs (less than 10%) she always experienced the beliefs as extremely distressing and markedly disruptive to her life (for example, she found it difficult to attend family events especially away from home, where she could just go to bed if her worries were bothering her too much). The delusions subscale of the PSYRATS rates delusional beliefs on six parameters using a five-point scale with zero being absent and four meaning severe. June's scores pre-treatment, post-treatment, and at one-year follow-up are presented towards the end of this chapter.

This assessment clearly suggested that a target for intervention could well be June's delusional beliefs and in particular the amount of time she spent thinking about these beliefs, getting distressed by them, and being unable to get on with her life properly as a consequence. As these measures were administered by an assessor who was not the treating therapist (because of the research design used in the service), it was clear that these were important areas to discuss at our first treatment session.

Treatment sessions

Session one

At the first treatment session it also became evident that the PSYRATS scores obtained by the assessing therapist did not tell the full story of June's delusional beliefs and her conviction in them. June explained that although her conviction in the delusional belief that we identified as being "The 'pulsing' sensation I experience means that someone, probably my husband, is trying to kill me" was currently only perhaps 1%, when the phenomena occurred it was 100%. She also rated her general level of distress as 20% and the frequency of the belief occurring as about 30%. We did similar ratings at sessions two and three, before much active treatment had started, and obtained the results detailed in Table 9.1.

Table 9.1 June's ratings for weeks one, two, and three

	Week 1	Week 2	Week 3
Belief now	1%	1%	2%
Belief when phenomena occurs	100%	65%	60%
Distress now	20%	1%	30%
Distress when phenomena occurs	—	90%	70%
Frequency of phenomena over last week	30%	5%	5%

During this first session, June stated that she had been admitted to hospital about a year ago after becoming convinced that her husband and/or others were trying to harm or possibly kill her by sending "pulses" through her body. She was discharged from hospital four months later having been prescribed and having taken an antipsychotic oral medication. By this time the pulsing had stopped, although June was not at all convinced that she had been suffering from an illness that had now improved as the explanation for these events; she considered it just as likely an explanation that her husband or whoever it was that had been trying to harm her had simply stopped doing so because the authorities were involved, and it was therefore more dangerous for them to continue. Despite these concerns, June tried to continue with her life as best as she could; she stopped taking her medication and several months later the pulsing phenomena returned.

June described the phenomena as being like an actual pulse in her fingertips and toes, then spreading across her chest. When she experienced this phenomena, June had associated thoughts such as "Here we go again" and worried about what might happen if the pulsing did not stop. To try to regain some control, June would sometimes try reasoning with herself, entertaining thoughts such as "Its got to be me", but this left her feeling quite sad as it implied to June that she might therefore be admitted to hospital again. Active coping was attempted by June, such as moving round the house to distract herself from the phenomena, but she did this only resentfully, entertaining thoughts such as "If it's him (her husband) that is doing it, why should I have to move around the house?"

June was also experiencing other odd phenomena such as seeing letters or numbers in ash in an ashtray or seemingly imprinted in bread, but she did not find this distressing, although offered no explanation whatsoever for the experiences. These experiences were not to become the source of much active intervention, though they were periodically monitored for any changes to associated frequency or distress ratings.

During this first session June was given a rationale for cognitive therapy which she appeared to find acceptable. Finally, an attempt was made to establish with June a simple understanding of her experiences based on the five systems model (Greenberger & Padesky 1995) and this early maintenance level formulation is included later in this chapter as Fig. 9.1.

Homework was set and involved considering the formulation as a basis for informing and developing our therapy work together. An initial therapy contract of six sessions prior to a review was agreed upon.

Session two

This session was concerned with developing our understanding of any connections between thoughts, feelings, behaviour, and physical sensations, and how these factors taken together could help us to understand what was happening to June and develop ideas for treatment/intervention.

The environment in which a person finds themselves is an important context for cognitive therapists, if often overlooked, and this was acknowledged and the contributions that June's particular circumstances could be playing in the genesis and/or maintenance of her problem was assessed. In particular, it was important to take full account of June's history of marital disharmony (the multi-disciplinary notes made reference to her stormy relationship with her husband). A more detailed account of a recent occasion in which the phenomena had occurred was attempted. On the Monday evening prior to the second therapy session, June had put the children to bed and sat down quietly for the first time all day at about 8pm. She was feeling tired, and she was sitting in the living room with her husband David when she became aware of the pulsing phenomena in her back. She described it as "a bit like if you stop the blood supply to your finger for a few seconds and it starts to really throb", but this sensation was described as going right through her body. At the time it occurred, she had just watched a few minutes of TV, which was on quietly more or less in the background. Possible explanations for the phenomena were brainstormed and the following list developed:

a   The house is "bugged".
b   June's teeth fillings are leaking.
c   The electricity supply in the house is faulty.
d   It is June's imagination.
e   It is the symptoms of anxiety/worry.
f   Static electricity.
g   It is connected to June's menstrual cycle.
h   Some physical cause.

When following this procedure it is important not to close the list down too quickly. It is extremely useful to the therapy process if the therapist can become aware of all possible reasons for the phenomena/experience that the client is considering in order to fully review evidence, design behavioural experiments, etc. Time given to this process also allows the therapist to gain awareness of the person's thinking processes for later intervention. People also often find their idiosyncratic or delusional explanations difficult to voice as an awareness of how odd such ideas can sound to others is sometimes maintained even when the belief is personally held with complete conviction. For all these reasons therapists should proceed within an appropriate time frame, as the generation of a possible hypothesis is an early step in "scientific" thinking, and taking time to signpost it as such may pay dividends later in empowering people to change thinking/reasoning styles rather than simply changing an opinion about a particular event or phenomena.

Following compilation of this list (which was compiled in true brainstorming style, with no censoring of possible explanations allowed), June ruled out explanations b, c, d and h immediately on the grounds of information she already had established. Her dentist had explained to her that leaking fillings could not cause this phenomena and she accepted this explanation. The explanation that the electrics were faulty was dismissed because the phenomena continued to occur in places other than at home, notably during her time in hospital, and other people had not complained of the phenomena. June did experience the pulsing phenomena and she was unwilling to accept that it could be explained entirely by imagination, given the very real physical sensations that occurred within her. Agreement was reached that, whatever the explanation, something was certainly going on, so putting it all down to imagination did not seem helpful. While an in-patient on the psychiatric unit, the medical staff had taken blood and other tests to rule out any possible physical cause, and these procedures had left June satisfied that this particular explanation could be discounted.

This left as possible explanations that the house was bugged, the symptoms of anxiety or worry, static electricity, or the menstrual cycle. June rated her belief in the house being bugged as only 1% during the session but as high as 65% during an episode. It was agreed that all the other contending explanations needed more information before their validity or otherwise could be decided. In order to aid this process, it was agreed that collecting information about the phenomena more systematically would be helpful, and accordingly homework was agreed upon that involved June keeping a diary of the occurrence of the pulsing, listing the situation or circumstances, the event (pulsing), and associated thoughts, feelings, and behaviours.

Sessions three to six

Session three was delayed several weeks due to June being physically unwell and the therapist's annual leave commitments, but when it did take place it was immediately apparent that June had not managed to complete the homework assignment as she found that when the phenomena did occur she was unable to do more than attend to it. However, the frequency of the phenomena had fallen, and over a four-week period it had occurred on only two occasions. The frequency rating June recorded over this period was therefore down to 5% from a therapy baseline of 30%, while conviction in the original belief had fallen to 60% at the time of the pulsing sensation (down from 100%), although the in-session rating had risen from 1% at baseline to 2% now. June did appear to be more distressed by the phenomena with a "distress now" rating of 30% and distress during an episode rating of 70%, compared to a distress rating at therapy baseline of 20% (only distress now rating provided). These rather puzzling ratings (particularly for distress) were discussed, and June explained that thinking about the phenomena rather than simply pushing it to the back of her mind as she had previously been doing may have accounted for this. This short-term consequence of cognitive therapy, observed by other therapists treating people with other conditions, is a predictable side effect and in retrospect should have been discussed with June before therapy commenced. June also explained that she thought she may be pregnant again, and she was worried about this for a number of reasons.

In this session a detailed review of a recent episode was again conducted given June's non-completion of homework, and then we went on to gather some of the additional information required regarding possible explanations for her experiences. In particular, information was given by the therapist concerning the physiological sensations associated with anxiety, and a Socratic questioning style was used to help the client consider any similarity with her own experiences. Homework was agreed upon to include consideration of the physiological sensations associated with anxiety as a possible explanation for June's experiences, and consideration of the benefits and costs of keeping a concurrent record of thoughts/feelings/behaviour associated with the pulsing phenomena following discussion in session along these lines.

Session four required a diversion from the original therapy plan because June revealed she was indeed pregnant, and became quite distressed in the session when discussing this fact. This allowed the therapist to opportunistically demonstrate the utility of the cognitive model with June by identifying via the "downward arrow technique" what it was about being pregnant that she found so distressing. A hot thought concerning being pregnant was identified, which was "I will have to stop medication because I am pregnant, therefore I will get ill again, end up back in hospital and possibly lose my kids". After having established the hot thought in this manner, the dysfunctional thought record was then used to arrive at a more balanced and less distressing thought, namely: "Even if I do get ill and have to go back into hospital, I would have to spend some time away from my children, which is upsetting, but I would not lose them just because I was ill". June rated her belief in this thought as 75% and there was a big reduction in associated distress.

This impromptu demonstration of the utility of the cognitive model was helpful in legitimising this approach to June's distressing delusional beliefs. While some authorities have counselled against working with emotionally aroused clients with psychotic disorders (Fowler, Garety, & Kuipers, 1995) and inexperienced therapists can panic and diverge from a cognitive model when distress is high, such circumstances actually present therapeutic opportunity if handled well.

During session four we also discussed whether or not stress was a useful explanation for June's experiences of pulsing, and she stated that it might be the explanation. Homework was agreed on and involved June canvassing trusted family members to see if they had any experiences similar to her pulsing phenomena. Where "hot thoughts" occurred that distressed June, particularly in relation to the target delusional belief, she agreed to try and use the thought record to help us to be clear about the thoughts that were triggering her distress.

At session five, June had not completed the homework because she had not had any occasions when she had become very distressed concerning her beliefs. Her ratings were as follows: belief now 0%; belief when phenomena occurs 1% at last occurrence; distress now 5%; distress when phenomena occurs 2%; frequency of phenomena over last week 8–10%. There had been only one occasion over the week where June had noticed the phenomena, but on this occasion she attributed it to having just eaten ice-cream, perhaps too quickly, and we acknowledged how this attribution, rather than her usual catastrophic one, prevented the vicious circle commencing and escalating. Despite the fact that June had had a week in which the phenomena was not very pronounced, our initial formulation was developed a little to take into account the circumstances in which the pulsing appeared to occur. It was agreed that what could account for the fact that the phenomena appeared to occur when June had sat down perhaps for the first time in the day, was that the trigger was probably hypervigilance leading to the awareness of her own pulse, which sometimes leads, through a process of catastrophic thinking and associated heightened sensory acuity "magnifying" the sensation 10-fold, to the shuddering pulsing sensations and symptoms of anxiety/panic that she was so familiar with. Homework to test out this hypothesis was suggested by June and involved trying to relax/feel calm at her mother's in the middle of the day to enhance awareness of her own heartbeat in an attempt to induce the sensations she normally associated with the catastrophic thought that someone was trying to harm or kill her. It was acknowledged that this could take several sessions to achieve, and June confirmed that if she did get the phenomena at her mother's in the middle of the day, it would not lead her to draw the conclusion that her mother was involved in such a plan, but rather that the phenomena she had been calling pulsing was probably completely normal.

In session six there were more examples of June reattributing the physical sensations that she had labelled "pulsing" to ordinary, non-catastrophic explanations. For example, on the previous Friday night she had gone to bed alone as her husband was having a night out, and although she felt nervous being alone in bed in the house and she did become aware of her heartbeat and some of the pulsing phenomena through her body, she explained it away as the consequence of arousal/anxiety and did not begin to think that it meant someone was trying to harm her. Another possible explanation she had begun to consider to account for awareness of her heartbeat was her pregnant state: she reasoned that given her pregnancy-related weight gain, it might be quite normal to become more aware of her heartbeat as her heart had to work a little harder than before she was pregnant.

Sessions seven to twelve

At the end of session six it was agreed that the initial therapy contract of six sessions would be extended by another six sessions. The areas addressed in sessions seven to twelve were further information gathering and experiments concerning the possible explanations for June's pulsing phenomena, the attempted elimination of safety behaviours, and the beginnings of a longitudinal formulation in response to June's question "why did this happen to me?"

At session seven the impact of how June was thinking on her actual physical experiences was demonstrated by showing how June's thought of "I've eaten ice-cream too quickly" effectively meant that her anxiety levels did not escalate and the pulsing phenomena did not therefore occur. This was established by asking June to recall the event and in particular the physical sensation she first experienced, and then, using the five-systems model, to schematically represent the different effects of thinking "I've eaten ice-cream too quickly" and "someone is trying to harm or possibly kill me" on the actual physical sensations themselves. While this may seem to have been repetitive, it was considered helpful in preparing the ground for an important behavioural experiment in June's treatment, which was the induction of the pulsing phenomena in session. The confidence that June was beginning to gain in the hypothesis that the strength of the pulsing phenomena was related to how anxious she was, which in itself was largely mediated by how she was thinking, was crucial in persuading June to try out the induction of the pulsing phenomena in session. In this sense it is again clearly analogous to the psychological treatment of panic disorder, which does require therapists to help sufferers gain some confidence in the new psychologically orientated hypothesis before they can be persuaded to try out panic induction exercises that attempt to demonstrate that the phenomena that is being misattributed as harmful is in fact harmless (Clark, 1996).

The induction of the pulsing phenomena was attempted in session eight using the following procedure. June was asked first to simply focus her attention on her pulse by holding her fingertips together firmly. She was then asked to become vigilant to any signs of the pulsing phenomena in the rest of her body. Once she had located such phenomena, she was then asked to read a sentence written down from her thought records that suggested that this phenomena was evidence of people attempting to harm her. Finally, to de-escalate June was told by the therapist that the pulsing she had noticed was a normal phenomena, that it was intensified by anxious thoughts, and it would be more accurate to consider the phenomena of pulsing as simply her body working normally and responding to worries and perceptions of threat in a normal way. Using guided discovery to help June take account of the whole experience, we concluded the following:

1   By focusing her attention on her pulse, June became much more conscious of it.
2   The suggestion (from the thought record) that the pulsing phenomena indicated she was in some personal danger led to certain physiological changes in June; in particular her breathing became more shallow and rapid, her chest felt tight, and she began to sweat more.
3   When it was suggested by the therapist that the phenomena of pulsing demonstrated no more than June's body working normally and that she was not in any personal danger, her chest felt less tight, she cooled down (that is she felt less hot), the pulsing receded to just her fingertips, and eventually after two to three minutes her breathing returned to normal.

In summary, June concluded that worrying thoughts lead to a spiralling of the anxiety/pulsing phenomena, and in contrast, thoughts that what is happening is a normal physiological process lead to the spiralling of the pulsing phenomena not occurring or subsiding. June also identified that at the stage in the cycle when her chest becomes tight she often smokes a cigarette to help her feel less anxious, and we discussed the likely physio-logical effects of this and how it could actually enhance the pulsing phenomena because of smoking's action in narrowing capillaries.

It became evident during this cycle of sessions that June had a number of safety behaviours that she engaged in as part of an attempt to cope with her distress due to her thoughts and worries about the pulsing phenomena. Safety behaviours can be understood as being behaviours engaged in by a person to prevent a feared catastrophy occurring, but which actually may prevent disconfirmation of the catastrophic cognition (Salkovskis, 1991): for example, in panic disorder the person with palpitations who misinterprets this normal phenomena as a warning sign of an imminent heart attack and therefore immediately sits down and stops all physically exerting behaviour. In addition to smoking a cigarette when she had noticed the early signs of the phenomena, June also engaged in mock humour with her partner, attempting to laugh off "what he might be up to". She also tried to reassure herself by saying things to herself such as "whatever he is up to I will find out sooner or later so there's no point in worrying about it now". We discussed safety behaviours in session and identified how such behaviours, while understand-able as an attempt to cope with distressing experiences, actually potentially prevented June from discovering that the phenomena of pulsing was normal and not in any way dangerous, and that worrying thoughts about the experi-ence actually exaggerated it greatly. She agreed to try and drop these safety behaviours given their counter-productive nature, and to replace the use of these strategies with the "challenging" strategies concerning the normality of the phenomena and the understanding of how worrying thoughts drive the spiral of worry/sensation/worry. The following section of dialogue may help to illustrate this:

Therapist: How do you think "jokingly" dealing with your worries about the pulsing influences what your beliefs about the pulsing are?

June: I'm not sure how it influences my beliefs but it helps me cope with the worries by having a joke about them.

Therapist: It sounds like you use humour to help you deal with the worries you have about what might be happening: does this help you establish whether your worries are accurate or not?

June: No, not really. Dealing with the worries in this way sort of pushes them to the back of my mind for a while, that's all.

Therapist: Do you find that is an effective way of dealing with this worry on a once and for all basis?

June: Well the worry always comes back so I suppose this method just puts it off really.

Therapist: I wondered whether it also prevents you honestly looking at the evidence about your worries, thinking it through in the way we have discussed, and trying not to jump to any conclusions.

June: Laughing it off is an alternative to thinking it through really—it prevents me thinking through the evidence in the way we talked about.

Therapist: So it's possible that although laughing it off is done as an attempt to feel better in the short term, it may actually prevent you from working through your worries and perhaps concluding that the sensations or the pulsing are normal and not harmful?

June: Yes, it's possible that dealing with the worry in this way is actually not really helpful.

Therapist: Given what we have said, do you think you will deal with the worry any differently next time?

June: I think it would be better to use the thought challenge technique to deal with it directly rather than just trying to laugh it off.

June was clearly getting benefit from the sessions in terms of preventing the vicious cycle of sensation/worrying thoughts/sensations/worrying thoughts occurring. There was reduction in the frequency of the pulsing phenomena, the duration of the phenomena when it did occur, and the degree of distress experienced. On occasions there were still problems and, in particular, on a long trip to a family wedding that necessitated an overnight stay, June had a difficult time with the pulsing phenomena occurring and finding it difficult to challenge the catastrophic cognitions concerning this. We agreed that a lapse was different to a relapse, and tried to identify any special indications about the trip that made June particularly vulnerable to the phenomena occurring and difficulty with the thought challenge technique, for future reference and perhaps to include in a relapse prevention blueprint later in therapy.

During therapy sessions we had identified basic or dysfunctional assumptions underlying June's negative automatic thoughts by use of the "downward arrow technique" (Burns, 1980). This technique allows the therapist and patient to establish potentially problematic beliefs by accepting the validity of distressing thoughts at face value *temporarily*, and asking "supposing that were true, what would that mean?" until a general assumption or dysfunctional belief operating in multiple situations is established. This process highlighted a belief that "I cannot trust anyone", and this belief hinted at a longitudinal formulation that helped us to consider an important question therapeutically that June raised in session, namely "Why did this happen to me?" It was towards the end of this tranche of therapy sessions that June first articulated this question, which neatly allowed us to consider a longitudinal formulation in an attempt to possibly reduce future vulnerabilities to similar schema-driven misattributions.

Sessions thirteen to eighteen

These sessions were characterised by attempts to identify and expose to critical scrutiny, in an atmosphere of collaborative empiricism, deeper level beliefs that may have made June vulnerable to developing the worries she did under the specific circumstances that held at the time (see the section entitled "A note on formulation"). We also continued to carry out further behavioural experiments away from the session to increase June's belief in the psychological explanation for her experiences that we had together been developing.

An example of a session from this end section of treatment is session seventeen. The notes from this session list agenda items including current perceptions and beliefs, and an historical formulation section. The current perceptions and beliefs section allowed us to cover possible explanations for the last pieces of evidence supporting June's original delusional beliefs regarding her partner's attempts to harm her. In particular, we focused on the perception that June had, that her husband made odd movements and had odd mannerisms. She had sometimes regarded this as further evidence that he may be "up to something", and following a discussion about selective attention in the session, and how such attention is often driven by existing beliefs in a self-fulfilling prophecy manner, June agreed to put this as a possible psychological explanation for her experiences to the test by deliberately manipulating her attention while with her mother to see if she could also generate signs of similar odd behaviour or mannerisms that could also be interpreted in a sinister way. We chose June's mother as the focus for this experiment as June had assured me that there were no circumstances under which she would really believe that her mother was trying to harm her, therefore, if this worked with her mother, it really would show that selective attention could account for this piece of evidence, and it could then be dismissed.

In terms of work at a more schematic level, we identified that June had a belief that she should never really relax or let her guard down, even with family or close friends. We examined this belief and identified that it was based on beliefs about herself, the world, and other people that may have left June vulnerable to the development of psychotic symptoms. For example, June's core or basic beliefs about others was that other people should not be trusted, and the connection of this to her beliefs and worries about her partner was evident. We had already identified experiences in June's early life that led her to this conclusion about others, in particular sexual abuse at the hands of an adult, and failure of a parent to respond adequately to June's contemporaneous disclosure of this event. In order to create the space to examine and possibly amend core beliefs and therefore reduce possible future vulnerability, a rationale must be shared with the patient. The method used to do so with June was to agree that, given what had happened to her, the belief about other people was an understandable conclusion to draw at the time and possibly important in maintaining her safety given the circumstances of what occurred, but that such a strong belief with its obvious and possibly deleterious consequences should at least be re-examined to check for current validity and to ensure that no thinking errors were occurring that "confirmed" the belief even with possibly ambiguous evidence. Schema modification procedures used with June along these lines included a "life events review" to ensure that existing beliefs were not selectively influencing what was noted about others, and use of a positive data log to collect evidence supporting a slightly modified and less global core belief (Greenberger & Padesky, 1995). The results of therapy (using the delusions subscale of the PSYRATS) can be seen in Table 9.2.

Booster sessions

Three sessions were offered to June as boosters to cover the following:

- A fully integrated formulation emphasising how early experiences led to the formation of basic or core beliefs about the world, self, and others, and then the formation of dysfunctional assumptions, which under certain circumstances led to the appearance of the distressing symptoms of psychosis. Once these symptoms had occurred, a vicious cycle developed, including worrying thoughts and the related appearance of physical symptoms of anxiety, which were in turn misinterpreted and exacerbated the symptoms associated with anxiety.
- Identification of thinking errors that maintained the problem once it had started, and putting in place a plan to monitor the existence of such thinking errors as a relapse prevention plan.
- Agreeing steps June could continue to take to help her newly modified core beliefs take hold and flourish.

Table 9.2 June's PSYRATS delusions scores

Variable	Pre-treatment	Post-treatment	One-year follow-up
Amount of pre-occupation	4	0	0
Duration of pre-occupation	4	4	2
Conviction	1	2	1
Amount of distress	4	1	4
Intensity of distress	4	2	3
Disruption	3	0	0

A note on formulation

The therapist worked with June to develop a possible understanding of her experiences from a psychological perspective. Although this is probably always the aim for psychological therapists, the manner in which it is done needs careful attention and consideration so as not to risk problems with engagement, which is described as a rate-limiting step by Kingdon (1998), and the approach adopted to this has been described throughout this case study. As discussed earlier, the formulation was developed with June from the present and then back to the past to identify and modify possible vulnerabilities to future problems/difficulties. Developing a symptom formulation is crucial to the development of a plan, collaboratively arrived at with the affected person, to try and reduce the distress associated with the symptoms. While it is crucial it is not always possible, and it is perhaps unfortunate that the ethos of our professional backgrounds mitigates against publication of studies where therapists may have not got this far in therapy with affected people. Therapists working as part of the Socrates trial (a multi-site randomised controlled trial of cognitive behavioural therapy for early, acute psychosis) have conceptualised the different stages of therapy reached with people with psychosis (Everett et al., 1999) and this is a useful model for honestly evaluating the success of programmes of care, and enabling therapists to feel that they have achieved something, even if "only" engagement, thus perhaps maintaining the motivation of the therapist(s).

Symptom level formulation

Our understanding of what was happening for June when the phenomena occurred focused on her appraisal of threat in relation to the bodily sensations she had become aware of, and how such an appraisal would intensify the sensations she erroneously believed to indicate she was in some danger, which of course would keep the worry that she was in danger going, and so on (see Fig. 9.1). We had not identified a clear trigger to these experiences, but it became apparent from monitoring homework June completed that most occurrences happened in the evening when it was peaceful and she was not busy with the children. Clearly the trigger was self-monitoring for any signs that she was being harmed, which led to awareness of sensations, and started the vicious cycle.

Longitudinal formulation

The identification of June's tendency to monitor for signs that she was in any danger, while perhaps easy enough to understand once the belief had occurred to her that she was in danger, left us with the question of where this tendency to self-monitor for signs of danger had come from. June also proved herself to be quite psychologically minded, and once we had reduced her current levels of belief in her delusion, even under conditions where the pulsing occurred and she was aware of it, she directly asked a question that facilitated discussion of a longitudinal formulation (and subsequent modification of vulnerability factors emanating from this), which was "but why did this happen to me?"

It can be seen from the schematic representation of June's longitudinal formulation (see Fig. 9.2) that early experiences in which in particular she had been sexually abused by an adult, and then not fully supported by a parent after disclosing this information, left her to draw conclusions about herself, the world, and other people, that while perhaps understandable (and possibly accurate) at the time, needed reconsideration as an adult in the light of *all* her experiences. Certainly, it does appear reasonable that the assumption(s) that she used as her way of managing in the world, given her early formed beliefs about it and her degree of vulnerability in it, left her open to potential psychological disturbance at some future point. The assumption that she should never fully drop her guard/relax in any situation is a particularly hard

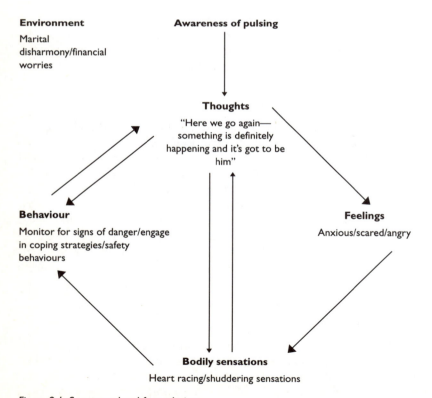

Figure 9.1 Symptom level formulation.

Early experiences

Parents divorced, abused by parental "friend", parent
unsupportive regarding this disclosure. Oldest sibling—took care
of sister

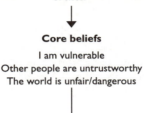

Core beliefs

I am vulnerable
Other people are untrustworthy
The world is unfair/dangerous

Basic assumptions

Unless I know for *sure* about other people I should keep my guard up
Unless I keep my guard up other people will take advantage of me

Critical incidents

Having children, moving house, living with partner who was older and had
previously been married

Negative automatic thoughts

Alan is up to something/trying to harm me

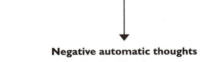

Behaviour

Monitor for signs of danger
Engage in coping strategies/safety
behaviours

Feelings

Anxious/scared/angry

Bodily sensations

Heart racing/shuddering sensations

Figure 9.2 Longitudinal formulation.

taskmaster and perhaps designed to create the conditions for psychological difficulties.

DISCUSSION AND CONCLUSIONS

It is contended that the case study presented in this chapter demonstrates that an approach to the psychological treatment of people suffering with psychosis can be adopted that addresses the particular symptoms in a similar way to how therapists would approach the treatment of other distressing symptoms and experiences such as panic disorder. Schizophrenia and panic disorder may be considered at opposite ends of the spectrum in terms of the development of psychological methods of treatment of proven effectiveness in some respects, and yet certain cases currently understood to fall under the schizophrenia umbrella may have much in common with typical presentations of panic disorder, apart from the socially unacceptable nature of the catastrophic misinterpretation (Morrison, 1998b)—e.g. "someone is trying to kill me" rather than "I am having a heart attack". The nature of the catastrophic misinterpretation *is* clearly of significance and cannot just be dismissed as unimportant, but we must also take note of how standard methods of psychological treatment utilised with people with "mild to moderate" disorders can be of benefit to people with severe mental illness such as schizophrenia, perhaps especially early on in the development of the illness when the secondary disabilities so often associated with this disorder have not yet taken effect. Once the presenting symptom level disorder can be treated using standard psychological methods, attempts can also be made to reduce future vulnerabilities by addressing dysfunctional assumptions and schema level beliefs.

Such an approach will not be effective in all cases, and specific symptom or syndrome level research will be necessary to identify which types of symptoms affecting which types of people, currently grouped together under the unifying (but perhaps scientifically unhelpful) schizophrenia diagnosis, can be aided most effectively by such psychological approaches. Research to identify and understand the underlying and different psychological processes that may account for some of the presentations currently grouped together as schizophrenia is clearly indicated in order to follow Clark's assertion (Clark, 1997) of how progress has been made historically with the psychological understanding and treatment of disorders at a symptom level. This position—that continuing to try to research the schizophrenia concept as if it was a demonstrably proven disease entity may be counter-productive to the business of unravelling the disorders grouped together *currently* as schizophrenia—has been articulated for at least a decade (Bentall, 1990) and in its place a symptom or at the most syndromal level of enquiry commended. In order to have protocol-driven, person level psychological treatments in place for people experiencing psychotic phenomena, such research is clearly indicated and must be conducted.

Therapeutic pessimism abounds in the field of the treatment of people with schizophrenia. Professionals too often have catastrophic cognitions themselves about outcome—cognitions that are often transmitted to the sufferer and family members with unhelpful results. Such pessimism is not always empirically valid: outcome in schizophrenia is more variable and frequently more favourable than many treating professionals realise. The treatment of people with schizophrenia can be approached with some hope that the tools used to help people with less severe problems may be of benefit here too.

REFERENCES

Beck, A.T., & Greer, R. (1987). *Beck Depression Inventory scoring manual.* New York: Psychological Corporation.

Bentall, R.P. (1990). (Ed.). *Reconstructing schizophrenia.* London: Routledge.

Birchwood, M., Smith, J., Cochrane, R., Wetton, S., & Copestake, S. (1990). The Social Functioning Scale: The development and validation of a scale of social adjustment for use in family intervention programmes with schizophrenic patients. *British Journal of Psychiatry, 157,* 853–859.

Boyle, M. (1990). *Schizophrenia: A scientific delusion?* London: Routledge.

Burns, D.D. (1980). *Feeling good.* New York: New American Library.

Chadwick, P.D.J., & Lowe, C.F. (1990). Measurement and modification of delusional beliefs. *British Journal of Psychiatry, 162,* 524–532.

Clark, D.M. (1986). A cognitive approach to panic disorder. *Behaviour Research and Therapy, 24,* 461–470.

Clark, D.M. (1996). Panic disorder: From theory to therapy. In P.M. Salkovskis (Ed.), *Frontiers of Cognitive Therapy* (pp. 318–344). New York: Guilford Press.

Clark, D.M. (1997). Panic disorder and social phobia. In D.M. Clark, & C.G. Fairburn. (Eds.), *Science and practice of cognitive behaviour therapy.* Oxford: Oxford University Press.

Crow, T.J. (1980). Molecular pathology of schizophrenia: More than one disease process? *British Medical Journal, 280,* 66–68.

Everett, J., Ledley, K., Grazebrook, K., Benn, A., Siddle, R., & the Socrates Group (1999). *The Socrates study: The process of cognitive behaviour therapy for acute, early schizophrenia.* Paper presented at the third international conference on psychological treatments for schizophrenia, Oxford, England.

Fowler, D., Garety, P., & Kuipers, E. (1995). *Cognitive behaviour therapy for psychosis: Theory and practice.* Chichester: Wiley.

Greenberger, D., & Padesky, C.A. (1995). *Mind over mood.* New York: Guilford Press.

Haddock, G., McCarron, J., Tarrier, N., & Faragher, E.B. (1999). Scales to measure dimensions of hallucinations and delusions: The psychotic symptom rating scales. *Psychological Medicine, 29,* 879–889.

Jaspers, K. (1963). *General psychopathology.* Manchester: Manchester University Press.

Kay, S., Fiszbein, A., & Opler, L. (1987). The Positive and Negative Syndrome Scale (PANSS) for schizophrenia. *Schizophrenia Bulletin, 13*, 261–275.

Kingdon, D.G. (1998). Cognitive behaviour therapy for psychotic symptoms in schizophrenia. In N. Tarrier, A. Wells, & G. Haddock, (Eds.), *Treating Complex Cases*. Chichester: Wiley.

Kingdon, D.G., & Turkington, D. (1994). *Cognitive behaviour therapy of schizophrenia*. New York: Guilford Press.

Marshall, R. (1990). The genetics of schizophrenia: Axiom or hypothesis? In R.P. Bentall (Ed.), *Reconstructing schizophrenia*. London: Routledge.

Morrison, A.P. (1998a). Cognitive analysis of the maintenance of auditory hallucinations: Are voices to schizophrenia what bodily sensations are to panic? *Behavioural and Cognitive Psychotherapy, 26*, 289–302.

Morrison, A.P. (1998b). Cognitive behaviour therapy for psychotic symptoms in schizophrenia. In N. Tarrier, A. Wells, & G. Haddock (Eds.), *Treating Complex Cases* (pp. 195–216). Chichester: Wiley.

Nuechterlein, K.H., & Dawson, M.E. (1984). A heuristic vulnerability-stress model of schizophrenic episodes. *Schizophrenia Bulletin, 10*, 300–312.

Peters, E.R., Joseph, S.A., & Garety, P.A. (1999). Measurement of delusional ideation in the normal population: Introducing the PDI. *Schizophrenia Bulletin, 25, 3*, 553–576.

Raune, D., Kuipers, E., & Bebbington, P. (1999). *Psycho-social stress and delusional and verbal auditory hallucination themes in first episode psychosis: Implications for early intervention*. Paper presented at the third international conference on psychological treatments for schizophrenia, Oxford, England.

Rose, S., Kamin, L.T., & Lewontin, R.C. (1984). *Not in our genes*. London: Penguin.

Salkovskis, P.M. (1991). The importance of behaviour in the maintenance of anxiety and panic: A cognitive account. *Behavioural Psychotherapy, 19*, 6–19.

Salkovskis, P.M. (1996). The cognitive approach to anxiety: Threat beliefs, safety-seeking behaviour, and the special case of health anxiety and obsessions. In P.M. Salkovskis (Ed.), *Frontiers of cognitive therapy* (pp. 48–74). New York: Guilford Press.

Warner, R. (1994). *Recovery from schizophrenia: Psychiatry and political economy.* New York: Routledge.

Watts, F.N., Powell, G.E., & Austin, S.V. (1973). The modification of abnormal beliefs. *British Journal of Medical Psychology, 46*, 359–363.

World Health Organisation (1979). *An international follow-up study*. Chichester, England: WHO.

Zubin, J., & Spring, B. (1977). A new view of schizophrenia. *Journal of Abnormal Psychology, 86*, 103–126.

Chapter 10

Cognitive therapy for an individual with a long-standing persecutory delusion

Incorporating emotional processes into a multi-factorial perspective on delusional beliefs

Daniel Freeman and Philippa A. Garety

INTRODUCTION

Cognitive interventions are driven by formulations, tailored for each individual, of the factors maintaining disorder. In the case of anxiety, detailed frameworks have been developed to guide treatment of each type of anxiety disorder, such as panic disorder (Clark, 1986), obsessive-compulsive disorder (Salkovskis, 1985), and generalised anxiety disorder (Wells, 1994). In this way, therapeutic practice has been linked to theoretical developments. Cognitive therapy for psychosis is no different, with therapy being guided by formulations developed in the initial appointments (e.g. Chadwick, Birchwood, & Trower, 1996; Fowler, Garety, & Kuipers, 1995; Kingdon & Turkington, 1994). However, both the therapeutic practice and the psychological understanding of symptoms in this area are in their infancy in comparison with cognitive therapy for non-psychotic disorders (neurosis). As a consequence, the intervention frameworks for psychotic symptoms are less well developed. Therefore, discussion and sharing by clinicians of formulations used in interventions for individuals with psychosis is valuable.

In describing our theory and practice of cognitive therapy for psychosis, we aim to make further connections between the psychological understandings of psychosis and neurosis. Each has been studied and treated separately as a result of a classificatory divide that systematised the view that psychosis, in contrast to neurosis, was "ununderstandable" in terms of normal psychological processes, and, furthermore, that it "trumped" neurosis. This led to the neglect of the study of the influence of emotional processes on the development and maintenance of symptoms of psychosis, such as delusional beliefs. However, recent theoretical developments in anxiety and depression research have great promise for the development of cognitive behaviour therapy for psychosis. To illustrate this potential, we describe in this chapter a cognitive intervention for an individual with a persecutory delusion. This intervention was based upon a multi-factorial formulation that incorporated both processes associated with psychosis and processes traditionally associated with neurosis.

CONTEMPORARY THEORIES OF PERSECUTORY DELUSIONS

Since the late 1980s the individual symptoms of psychosis have become recognised as important phenomena in their own right, leading to a marked increase in the study of delusional beliefs, and our cognitive therapy formulations draw upon this recent literature. Three main theoretical accounts of (persecutory) delusions have received the most attention: this is the work concerning reasoning biases, theory of mind difficulties, and attributional defences. Therefore, we will briefly summarise these approaches (for a detailed review of the empirical literature see Garety & Freeman (1999)).

Reasoning biases

The idea that delusions are continuous rather than discontinuous with normal beliefs has led to the proposal that the "confirmation bias" (Wason, 1960), a tendency only to look for evidence consistent with beliefs, will maintain and enhance delusions (e.g. Maher, 1974). Chadwick (1993) notes such a reasoning bias in his first-hand account of an episode of psychosis ("Everything that verified my ongoing thoughts and ideas I voraciously used and remembered"). Chadwick also describes how his "criterion for the acceptance of 'reasonable quality data' started to plummet", which is somewhat similar to the "jumping to conclusions" reasoning style found in studies by Garety and colleagues (e.g. Garety, Hemsley, & Wessely, 1991). Dudley, John, Young, and Over (1997) and Garety and Freeman (1999) argue that the experimental data, considered as a whole, indicate that "jumping to conclusions" by individuals with delusions may reflect a data gathering bias—that is, a tendency to seek less information in order to reach a decision—and that such a bias may contribute to delusion formation and maintenance.

Theory of mind difficulties

Drawing upon research into children's understanding of "folk psychology", Frith (1992) proposes that schizophrenic symptoms develop from newly acquired deficits in a person's metarepresentational ability or "theory of mind" (ToM) (Premack & Woodruff, 1978). ToM refers to the ability to understand mental states (beliefs, desires, feelings, and intentions) in the self or others. Frith argues that delusions of persecution and reference arise from the person with schizophrenia knowing that people have mental states that cannot be directly viewed, but making invalid attempts at inferring them (i.e. there is a dysfunction in the representation of the mental states of others). According to Frith, delusions of reference occur because a person with schizophrenia mistakenly labels an action as having an intention behind it. Persecutory delusions arise because the person notices that other people's actions have become opaque and surmises that a conspiracy exists. From the experimental evidence (e.g. Corcoran, Mercer, & Frith, 1995) it can be concluded that theory of mind difficulties are particularly associated with negative symptoms, but that such difficulties are also present in some individuals with persecutory delusions. This suggests that, while ToM difficulties may plausibly contribute to some persecutory delusions, Frith's theory does not fully account for such delusions.

Attributional defences

Bentall and colleagues have recently reframed and re-examined the idea that persecutory delusions result from defensive processes. For instance, Bentall (1994) argues that individuals with persecutory delusions have underlying low self-esteem, and that in order to prevent the low self-esteem thoughts reaching consciousness, causes of negative events are attributed to external factors. The delusion is thought to reflect this externalising bias. More recently, it has been further suggested that the attributional defence involves blaming negative events on other people, rather than situations or the self (Kinderman & Bentall, 1997). The experimental findings indicate that many individuals with persecutory delusions do have an externalising bias for negative events (e.g. Kaney & Bentall, 1989), but the evidence is less clear that this functions as a defence against the intrusion into consciousness of underlying low self-esteem or self-concept discrepancy (Garety & Freeman, 1999).

Overview: The multi-factorial perspective

In sum, contemporary accounts of delusions have focused upon reasoning (Garety & Hemsley, 1994), representational ability (Frith, 1992), and attributional defences (Bentall, 1994). Elements of all these theories have received support although, to date, little research attention has been given to alternative explanations of the findings. The majority of the participants in the experimental studies have had current delusional beliefs, and therefore the evidence is stronger for the idea that these factors *maintain* delusions rather than contribute to formation. It is also apparent that each account of delusions is unlikely to stand alone. We argue that the heterogeneity found both in the experimental research and clinical presentations indicates that a multi-factorial perspective on delusion formation and maintenance is appropriate (e.g. Garety & Hemsley, 1994): delusional beliefs are unlikely to share a common cause.

More broadly, the multi-factorial approach to delusions can be allied with a stress vulnerability conceptualisation of psychotic disorder. The picture of heterogeneity in the development of delusional beliefs is mirrored by heterogeneity in researchers' views of schizophrenia. But there is wide agreement on the heuristic value of stress vulnerability conceptualisations of the development of schizophrenia, and these models prove useful frameworks for understanding delusion theories within. Stress vulnerability models (e.g. Zubin & Spring, 1977) integrate variables known to have an association with illness, and contain the idea that the emergence of symptoms depends upon an interaction between vulnerability (e.g. from genetic, biological, psychological, and social factors) and stress (e.g. from the occurrence of life events). Therefore, with regard to the psychological theories of delusions, it is plausible to view delusional beliefs as forming at times of stress and high emotion, when reasoning biases, attributional biases, and theory of mind dysfunction are likely to be exaggerated.

INCORPORATING THEORETICAL IDEAS FROM NEUROSIS

A multi-factorial perspective on the formation and maintenance of delusional beliefs allows the integration of ideas from research into emotional disorders. Despite past interest from theoreticians (e.g. McReynolds, 1960; Mednick, 1958), consideration of direct roles for emotional processes in delusion formation and maintenance has, until recently (e.g. note Morrison, 1998), been strikingly absent from the renewed interest in delusional beliefs. Therefore, we will consider the issue in some depth, but will confine our discussion to potential roles of processes associated with anxiety and depression, where there is a (small) literature of interest.

Anxiety

Processes associated with anxiety may be especially important in the formation and maintenance of persecutory delusions, because anxiety and persecutory beliefs share a common theme of the "anticipation of danger". Similar cognitive processes are therefore likely to be operative in both disorders. What roles could anxiety processes play in symptom development? Three such processes may be of particular importance: information processing biases, safety behaviours, and metacognitive beliefs.

Anxiety is associated (in individuals with high trait anxiety or who have clinical disorder) with biases in information processing (Williams, Watts, Macleod, & Mathews, 1988). Examples of such biases include the interpretation of ambiguous situations as threatening (e.g. Mathews, Richards, & Eysenck, 1989) and the preferential processing of threat (see Williams,

Mathews, & Macleod, 1996). Anxiety may, therefore, trigger processes that provide evidence or substantiation for persecutory beliefs. Consistent with this idea, individuals with persecutory delusions have been found to demonstrate preferential processing of threat words in the emotional Stroop task (e.g. Bentall & Kaney, 1989). Such processing biases are likely to be related to, or at least to be enhanced by, a self-focused cognitive style—which may also be associated with both emotional disorder (Ingram, 1990) and paranoia (Freeman, Garety, & Phillips, 2000; Smári, Stefánsson, & Thorgilsson, 1994).

The second anxiety process of relevance to persecutory delusions is that of safety behaviours. Recently, it has been suggested that the use of "safety behaviours" contributes to the maintenance of individuals' conviction in persecutory delusions (Freeman, 1998; Morrison, 1998). There has been no data on this issue beyond clinical description (but see Freeman, Garety, & Kuipers, in press). However, the concept is of potential theoretical and clinical importance, and therefore a detailed consideration is valuable.

Safety behaviours have been defined by Salkovskis (1991) as responses to threat that are believed by the individual to prevent the feared consequences from happening, but which actually contribute to the maintenance of anxious fears by preventing disconfirmation. Thus, episodes that should have provided evidence against the threat occurring are turned, instead, into "near misses" by the use of safety behaviours. Salkovskis (1996) outlines three main categories of safety behaviours by anxious individuals: (1) avoidance of situations that the person thinks are threatening; (2) escape from a situation that is believed to be threatening; and (3) within-situation behaviours that are carried out when the individual believes they are in a position of potential danger. These categories are likely to prove useful in understanding the safety behaviours of individuals with persecutory delusions.

In psychosis, our experience suggests that many individuals with persecutory delusions display avoidance behaviours. For example, some individuals with persecutory delusions avoid particular places (e.g. local shops, the pub) in order to minimise the likelihood of harm, and, at levels seen in agoraphobia, this may extend to avoiding leaving the home. Escape behaviours are often reported by individuals with persecutory delusions. For example, an individual may cut short a shopping trip and rush home after believing that people in the street were looking towards him or her in a prelude to an attack. Little has been documented about the subtle within-situation safety behaviours that individuals with persecutory delusions may use. Examples of within-situation safety behaviours from our clinical work include individuals with persecutory delusions ensuring that they had the company of a friend when entering threatening situations, and other individuals not answering the front door and keeping the curtains drawn when they felt vulnerable to attack in their own home.

Some safety behaviours may be particularly relevant for persecutory delusions. For example, to reduce the chances of threat occurring, individuals may comply with, or give in to, the demands or wishes of the persecutor. Individuals with delusions may also be more likely to try to get the help of others in reducing the threat, for example by asking friends to help or contacting the police or solicitors. Some individuals with persecutory delusions may confront, or go up to, the person who is thought to be trying to harm them, and this is perhaps also best conceptualised as a safety behaviour. Lastly, it is worth remembering that for some individuals the persecution is happening (for example, they feel that the persecutors have spread rumours around the neighbourhood, or are hitting them, or driving them crazy), and therefore when assessing safety behaviours in these cases there needs to be enquiry about attempts to minimise the level of harm.

Finally in our discussion of processes generally associated with anxiety, Freeman and Garety (1999) have reported preliminary evidence that meta-cognitive processes associated with generalised anxiety disorder contribute to the clinically important dimension of delusional distress: in individuals with persecutory delusions, metaworry concerning the control of delusion-relevant thoughts was found to be associated with higher levels of delusional distress. That is, individuals may become most distressed when they worry that they cannot control their thoughts about persecution as well as they would like. This indicates the importance of considering individuals' appraisals of their delusional beliefs.

Depression

Bentall and colleagues' defence account of persecutory delusions postulates an indirect role for processes associated with depression, examining the hypothesis that the *avoidance* of negative emotion is the motivation for delusion formation. However, there may also be direct roles for depression in delusion formation and maintenance. For example, although Trower and Chadwick (1995) believe that the majority of persecutory delusions can be explained by a delusion-as-defence hypothesis, they also suggest that a specific second type exists in which very low self-esteem and depression are prominent and readily acknowledged by the individual. It is postulated that the person with "bad-me" paranoia has extremely negative self-evaluative thoughts and believes that the persecution is deserved punishment for his or her badness. Chadwick, Birchwood, and Trower (1996) describe how a person who had sexually molested a young girl therefore viewed himself as totally bad and perverted, believed that other people knew about this by reading his mind, and were consequently punishing him. Low self-esteem associated with depression may also have other direct roles (Freeman et al., 1998). For instance, it may give the individual a feeling of social exclusion and therefore a sense of being a target for others. Low self-esteem could also contribute to symptom development by leading individuals to believe that other people view them as inferior and therefore targets for persecution (although the individual does not believe that this is justified). In essence, schemas may be important; as for auditory hallucinations (Close & Garety, 1998), the use of thought chaining from the delusion to beliefs about the self may be clinically useful.

FROM THEORY TO THERAPY

Thus, in order to construct a formulation to guide the subsequent intervention, the assessment phase of cognitive therapy for psychosis should try to determine which of the psychological factors (reasoning biases, ToM difficulties, attributional biases, emotional processes) are involved in the formation and maintenance of an individual's delusional belief. To understand the aetiology of the delusion, the psychological processes are placed within a general diathesis stress model. The individual's own stresses and illness vulnerabilities are assessed, drawing upon the wider schizophrenia literature (see Fowler et al., 1995) and, in this way, important social and biological factors are not overlooked.

Each of the theoretical ideas presented in this chapter may help in understanding symptom formation and maintenance. Conceptually, however, it is helpful for the therapist to separate the formation from the maintenance of the symptom, and sometimes also to distinguish the reaction to or appraisal of the symptom. The reason for this is simple: factors involved in formation may not be involved in maintenance and vice versa. For example, the belief confirmation bias will only operate once a delusional idea is formed. The potential usefulness for the therapist in distinguishing the factors that determine individuals' appraisals of their symptoms stems from the likelihood that it is the reaction to a symptom, rather than simply its presence, which determines whether clients come to the attention of services (Freeman & Garety, 1999).

A theory-led approach, based upon careful assessment, has been emphasised. However, the importance of core therapeutic skills should not be underestimated in working with people with psychosis (see Rothwell & Duffy, 1999 and Fowler et al. 1995). One of the findings to emerge from the recent randomised controlled trials of cognitive-behaviour therapy for psychosis (e.g. Tarrier et al., 1998) is that the non-cognitive behaviour therapy control conditions (e.g. supportive counselling) lead to some improvement in symptoms, suggesting that simply providing a safe environment in which the person with psychosis can discuss their problems can be beneficial.

Clearly we advocate an individualised approach, but our multi-factorial perspective has a common thread: delusions are viewed as *explanations of experience; as attempts to make sense of events*. In therapy, therefore, the aim is to provide the client with an alternative, plausible, and less distressing explanation of their experiences. If a client finds that he or she cannot accept an alternative explanation, then the aim of therapy must be for the client to be less distressed and disrupted by their established belief.

CASE EXAMPLE: MRS GREEN

Mrs Green (a pseudonym) was 60 years old, had 2 children, and was in part-time employment. Certain details in this case example have been changed in order to protect client anonymity.

Presenting problems

Mrs Green said that she believed that practically all the local children, particularly teenagers, were deliberately trying to annoy her. She was absolutely certain that this was happening (100% sure), and did not think that she could be mistaken. She said that she thought about the belief all the time, found it difficult to control the thoughts, and found the belief extremely distressing. Her husband and family had not witnessed any incidents supportive of the belief, and did not think that it was correct.

It was believed by Mrs Green that the local children tried to annoy her by laughing, shouting, whistling, or bumping into her. For instance, she would hear laughter while sitting on a bus, and conclude that it was aimed at her. Such events were reported by Mrs Green as occurring about fortnightly, but she thought that they would occur much more frequently if she left the house more often. On occasions, Mrs Green had shouted at the children whom she believed to be laughing at her, and this had resulted in the children shouting back in rather nasty exchanges. Detailed questioning indicated that the laughing and shouting heard by Mrs Green were not auditory hallucinations.

Mrs Green believed that she was the only person the children targeted. She was not sure why she was persecuted, although she thought that she was a "soft target". She wondered whether a curse had been put on her. She also wondered whether she was being punished for having been outspoken when she was an adolescent, although she did not believe that her behaviour at that time merited such a response.

A further belief was that the next-door neighbours had installed equipment in order to watch her in the home, and that this was also done to annoy. However, this persecutory belief was held with low degrees of preoccupation and distress.

The belief that children were deliberately trying to annoy her had made Mrs Green very anxious and miserable. She had become fearful of leaving the home, and had therefore reduced the number of times she did so. If children were seen in the street by Mrs Green, she would not go outside. However, she believed that the risk of threat was diminished when in the company of another person, such as her husband. Mrs Green acknowledged that she often spent time worrying, even about issues not directly related to the delusion. She reported feeling sad all of the time. Self-esteem was low, and she described herself as "not good enough, not intelligent enough, bit of a bore". Thoughts of suicide were present, although she said that she would not carry them out. On the Beck Depression Inventory Mrs Green scored 46, indicating severe depression. On the Beck Anxiety Inventory Mrs Green scored 18, indicating mild–moderate anxiety.

Mrs Green described her life as "boring", and felt that this gave her time to think about the persecution. Apart from her part-time work, Mrs Green engaged in no other activities outside of the home. She said that she had no friends, had never made friends, and believed that she would not be socially accepted. However, Mrs Green did have friendly interactions with work colleagues and with people in the local neighbourhood, where she had lived for many years. She also enjoyed a good relationship with her daughter-in-law. At interview, Mrs Green was initially shy, but she soon began to speak thoughtfully, established a good rapport with the therapist, and was able to insert humour into the conversation. Indications of high expressed emotion in the family were not apparent. The family were supportive of Mrs Green's wish to have psychological therapy.

History

Mrs Green's biological mother was unmarried, which led to Mrs Green being raised by foster parents from a very early age. From the age of five, Mrs Green spent ten years in a residential home for children (an orphanage). She described the conditions in the residential home as good, and said that she had no complaints except that, like the other children, she received only limited attention from the (small number of) adults. Mrs Green had been the subject of some verbal teasing, although she recalled no particularly distressing incidents. Contact with her biological mother was renewed when Mrs Green was older. Mrs Green had been employed in a number of posts including, for example, that of a domestic cleaner in a hospital.

Mrs Green's belief concerning persecution had lasted approximately 30 years. In the year prior to the onset of the belief, she had given birth to her first son, and had then become increasingly isolated, unsupported, and depressed. Her husband was working nights and was also spending time drinking in the pub. It was at this time that she first heard children laughing and concluded that she was the subject of the laughter, and that the aim was to annoy. Mrs Green did not have a good recall of the events at this time. No grandiose delusions, hallucinations, subjective thought disorder, or replacement of will experiences were reported as ever having occurred.

Soon after the development of the delusion, Mrs Green had a three-month psychiatric admission; she described having been given medication there, but receiving no help for her persecutory thoughts. One further admission took place a few years later. Since that time, Mrs Green had received a regular low dose of conventional neuroleptic medication, and, more recently, had tried risperidone, but the ideas of persecution had persisted, and they had become more intrusive over the last four years, since her second son had left home. She described having close relationships with her children, while her relationship with her husband had greatly improved. Her sons had not exhibited behavioural difficulties during childhood. Mrs Green reported a history of mental illness in current and older generations of her family, including her biological mother. The referral for psychological therapy arose out of Mrs Green's gradual increase in distress and a change in her psychiatrist, who asked for advice at a community mental health team meeting at which the therapist (DF) was present.

Formulation

In summary, Mrs Green had distressing and preoccupying delusions of reference and persecution, and met diagnostic criteria for delusional disorder, persecutory type (DSM-IV; American Psychiatric Association, 1994). She had co-morbid depression and symptoms of anxiety. The delusions had developed at a time of stress: when she was looking after her baby, was isolated, and began to feel vulnerable and depressed. It was hypothesised that this mood state, allied to a "jumping to conclusions" reasoning style and a poor understanding of the intentions of others (the latter a consequence perhaps of the lengthy period in the residential home), may have resulted in the creation of the delusion, especially given the previous experiences of being teased. On the basis of her family history of mental illness, a genetic vulnerability to reasoning biases was also incorporated into this stress vulnerability conceptualisation of the onset of delusional ideas.

A detailed model of the maintenance of the delusion was constructed. It incorporated a number of factors, and this is displayed in Fig. 10.1. Anxiety was viewed as playing a key role in embedding the belief. For example, safety behaviours were apparent. Mrs Green reacted to her threat belief by avoiding contact with children, which meant that the belief had not been fully tested, and that disconfirmatory evidence had not been received. Similarly, Mrs Green endeavoured to have another person present in situations that she perceived as threatening, and reasoned that this accounted for the absence of persecution on those occasions. Mrs Green also preferentially processed perceived threat in the environment (e.g. laughter, shouting), and adopted threatening interpretations of ambiguous situations (e.g. laughter on a bus), both of which provided a continuing stream of evidence supportive of the threat belief. With regard to the presence of depression, it was postulated that low self-esteem had a direct influence on symptom development by making her feel vulnerable to attack ("a soft target"). It was also apparent that Mrs

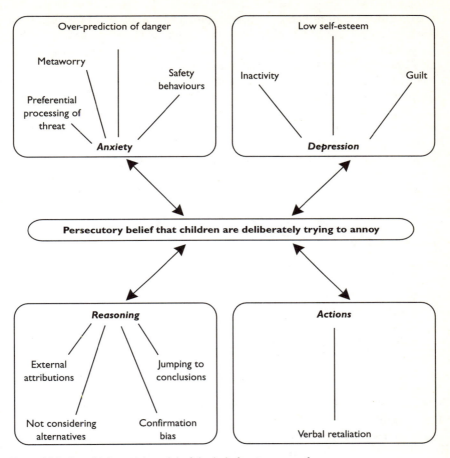

Figure 10.1 A multi-factorial model of the belief maintenance factors.

Green's inactivity had left her with considerable time to think about the persecution.

Reasoning biases were also identified, and these may have overlapped with the processing biases associated with anxiety and depression. Mrs Green clearly had difficulty in thinking of alternative explanations for events and showed a rapid acceptance of threatening ideas (i.e. "jumping to conclusions"). It was also hypothesised that she tended to search for excessively external causes for her feelings of anxiety and guilt. In the construction of the formulation, it was acknowledged that children may have directed their attention at Mrs Green on occasions (although there was nothing especially distinctive in her appearance), but that she interpreted their behaviour as personal to her, rather than more simply as examples of typical youthful exuberance. Mrs Green's verbal retaliation was thought to exacerbate the situation. Although difficulties understanding the intentions of others were identified as present at the time of onset of the belief, it was less clear that this was an ongoing general difficulty, and theory of mind dysfunction was therefore not included in the model of maintenance.

During the development of the formulation with Mrs Green, the reciprocal nature of the relationships between the maintaining factors and the persecutory belief were readily apparent (i.e. "vicious cycles"). For example, anxiety processes appeared to lead to a strengthening of the belief, which would then make Mrs Green feel more anxious, and so on. These reciprocal relationships, together with the consequent reduction in support, reassurance, and activities caused by Mrs Green's second son leaving home (to live with his wife), were hypothesised to have been factors in the increase in distress in recent years.

Intervention

There were four main components to the intervention:

- building a therapeutic alliance;
- constructing a (non-delusional) explanation of the client's experiences;
- verbally evaluating the persecutory belief; and
- reducing the influence of hypothesised maintaining factors.

This division of therapy into components provided a simple overall framework to guide the intervention. However, the components should not be viewed as discrete stages that followed one after the other; there was overlap. For example, the formulation could not be devised without an initial joint evaluation of the persecutory thoughts, behaviours, and events, and there could not be more rigorous evaluation without the formulation.

The first component of therapy was building and maintaining a trusting therapeutic alliance, which formed a basis for the subsequent elements of therapy. The therapist needed to demonstrate an uncritical and empathic attitude; this was of particular importance in the case of Mrs Green, who worried that her beliefs could be construed as "mad" or "crazy" by other people and felt embarrassed and a little ashamed. Therefore, in the first meeting the therapist used a number of standard cognitive therapy techniques to help develop trust. Active listening and communication skills were employed. The therapist empathised with the client by the use of phrases that made the link between thoughts and feelings (e.g. "I can see that you would have been very anxious if you thought that . . ."), but which did not imply that the therapist viewed the thoughts as accurate. To alleviate obvious anxieties about therapy, there was rapid agreement to the request from Mrs Green that her daughter-in-law be present at the first appointment. Mrs Green then felt able to attend subsequent sessions on her own. At the end of the first meeting, which was spent eliciting information, the goals of therapy were agreed, conveying the message that Mrs Green had control over the progress of therapy. The goals were:

- to develop an understanding of the development of the threat beliefs;
- to devise ways of helping Mrs Green to cope with them;
- to reduce the distress and anxiety that they caused; and
- to increase the number of her positive activities and to improve her mood.

(It is of note that a reduction in the conviction with which the belief was held was not a principal aim of therapy.) Another means of reducing client concerns about therapy is to provide information on the process and general techniques of therapy. Thus, Mrs Green was told that the therapist and client would work collaboratively, and that therapy would proceed by exploring and evaluating worrying thoughts; examining the links between events, thoughts, and feelings; and by using between-session tasks. Mrs Green also found it helpful to know that the therapist had met and helped other people distressed by persecutory beliefs. It was agreed to meet for six sessions, and then to review progress.

The second component of therapy was the development with Mrs Green of a shared understanding of the formation and maintenance of the persecutory belief, and this model evolved over the course of therapy (see the preceding "Formulation" section). Elements of the formulation were introduced from the second appointment onwards, with the role of avoidance being discussed first:

Therapist: What do you think is the consequence of avoiding all children?
Mrs Green: Well, I won't get harmed by them.
Therapist: Sure. Other than children being nasty to you, how else could they *possibly* act?
Mrs Green: They might ignore me, or smile at me, be okay.
Therapist: That's true. So, the children might be nasty, indifferent, or kind, although you're fairly sure that they would be nasty. If you avoid children then, what will be the consequence?
Mrs Green: I won't find out what they will do.
Therapist: I think that's right. What could you do instead then?
Mrs Green: I could be around children and find out.
Therapist: Yes, the trouble with avoidance is that you don't get a chance to check out or test your fears, and, therefore, the fears will remain whether they are true or not. The alternative is to check them out, test them. This seems a particularly good idea for thoughts that are distressing.

Each part of the formulation was discussed prior to the whole being presented, in order to ensure that there would be a large degree of agreement at that stage. At the fifth session the formulation was written down and both the therapist and Mrs Green kept copies. A simple verbal summary by the therapist was as follows:

> It seems that your belief developed at a time when you were quite stressed, and isolated, perhaps couldn't think too straight. As you felt vulnerable, and some of your family members have had times of upset too, it's not so surprising that when you heard children laughing you felt that they were getting at you. And once an important emotional belief is formed, it is very difficult to change. People "run" with their beliefs: they look for evidence consistent with their belief, interpret events as supporting the belief (forget ones that don't). And by avoiding situations, they don't fully test their fears. So, I don't think that it's surprising that your belief has lasted such a long time. As you said, you became very "sensitive to children". Does this make sense?

The presentation of the formulation included a strong element of normalisation. This is achieved, first, by explaining the belief in terms of psychological processes (making experiences understandable) and, secondly, by recognising that these are common processes used by others (an analogy with political beliefs and other strongly held beliefs is useful to discuss with the client).

The third strand of therapy involved verbal discussion of the evidence for and against the (delusional) belief. In keeping with basic cognitive therapy techniques, the aim was for the client to generate the evidence and form her own conclusions. (For this reason, the persecutory belief was not referred to as a delusion, although in a later session the use of this term by others was discussed.) The therapist's role during this stage was merely to prompt. For instance, if Mrs Green was having difficulties generating evidence inconsistent with the belief, then the therapist might suggest to her that she imagine that she was another person viewing the situation or that someone had come to her with a similar account of events. Mrs Green was also encouraged to think about what her life would be like if all the children were against her (it was agreed that they would probably smash her windows and her flower-pots, spray graffiti on her walls, and they would call out her name) and to consider the degree to which it fitted with her experiences (none of the suggested events had occurred). Mrs Green was given a diary sheet to complete between (a number of) therapy sessions. The sheet comprised columns for Mrs Green to record and evaluate weekly events viewed as *consistent* with the belief, and a second sheet was given to record events *inconsistent* with the belief. It should also be noted that there was discussion of the consequences of Mrs Green's persecutory belief being found to be incorrect. As she mostly saw benefits to this outcome the discussion was brief, but in some cases this can be a lengthy and important topic.

The fourth component of therapy was the reduction of the influence of the hypothesised maintaining factors. Once the formulation had been presented, it was possible to be quite specific with the client about the aims and predictions of this stage of therapy: if the hypotheses were correct, then a maintaining factor could be changed and the strength of the belief would alter.

For instance, safety behaviours, particularly avoidance, were discouraged. Instead, it was suggested that the persecutory belief could be tested by going outside alone. This discouragement of the use of safety behaviours can be seen as a gentle manoeuvre to encourage the client to begin to empirically test and question the threat belief. Two of the therapy sessions comprised the therapist accompanying Mrs Green in activities that she had avoided, in order to help initiate this strategy. Homework exercises were then set along such lines: for example, Mrs Green was encouraged to visit the local park and to walk past local schools. When devising such tasks with Mrs Green, particular attention was given to precluding the use of subtle within-situation safety behaviours. Before and after such activity, Mrs Green was asked to rate both the expectation of threat and level of anxiety on Subjective Units of Distress scales (SUDs). The ratings served as a method of assessing the test of the threat belief and could illustrate a tendency to over-predict the likelihood of danger. The dropping of safety behaviours provided ample opportunity for empirical testing of Mrs Green's beliefs, but it should be noted that for some delusional beliefs more elaborate tests may need to be devised.

Processes associated with depression were targeted by a small number of simple techniques: discussing causes of the mood state; encouraging the engagement in more activities (e.g. voluntary work); and by providing reading material about challenging negative thoughts.

Reasoning biases were addressed by discussing alternative interpretations of ambiguous situations that the client had taken as evidence for the belief, work which tied in with the diary sheets, and by noting the influence of information processing biases. The ambiguous situations were discussed in detail using an A–B–C framework. To facilitate the client's understanding of this process, the classic cognitive therapy "noise-in-the-night" illustration of how an event can be interpreted and experienced differently was introduced early in therapy. An example from near the start of therapy is presented:

Therapist: So, as you walked down the street you heard children were laughing and you knew that they were laughing at you.

Mrs Green: Yes, there were two of them, and they ran past me, laughing at me.

Therapist: Okay, so you saw the children laughing and had the thought that they were laughing at you.

Mrs Green: No, I didn't see them laughing at me. I was trying not to look at them, I just heard the laughter when they went past.

Therapist: Oh, how did you know that they were laughing at you?

Mrs Green: I knew it.

Therapist: Do you remember when we talked about the "noise in the night", and how you came up with several explanations for the noise? Thinking about it now, are there any other potential explanations for the children laughing?

Mrs Green: They might have been playing a game I suppose. Or just laughing as children do.

Therapist: Is that possible?

Mrs Green: Yes, it is. I was convinced at the time that they were laughing at me, but I'm less sure of that now. They didn't bump into me when they could have.

As Mrs Green often did not think of alternative explanations to the delusion when in anxious situations, a flashcard was developed to assist her ("Think of an alternative. Think more about it. Am I jumping to conclusions? Maybe it has nothing to do with me").

Finally, another method used to reduce the influence of the maintaining factors was to discuss different ways for Mrs Green to act when she felt that people were trying to annoy her, with an emphasis on how retaliation could be counter-productive.

It can be seen from this section that the therapist took care to ensure that methods were devised to help Mrs Green to retain and implement the lessons learned in the therapy sessions. These included the setting of homework tasks, the writing down of ideas, the provision of reading material, and frequent revision of key points. Follow-up appointments were scheduled to help consolidate progress. Additional techniques that could be used are encouraging the client to keep their own notes during therapy sessions, or audiotaping the appointments and providing the client with a copy of the recording.

Measures

At the beginning of therapy, the presence of positive symptoms was assessed using PSE-10 (Schedules for Clinical Assessment in Neuropsychiatry; World Health Organisation, 1992). Personal questionnaires were then used in each therapy session to assess the degree of conviction, preoccupation, and distress in the main persecutory belief (Brett-Jones, Garety, & Hemsley, 1987). Delusional conviction was also measured by obtaining a percentage rating of the strength of the belief. For the second (less distressing and preoccupying) belief, conviction and distress were measured at the beginning and end of therapy. Levels of depression and anxiety were measured at regular intervals by the Beck Depression Inventory (Beck et al., 1961) and the Beck Anxiety Inventory (Beck et al., 1988) respectively.

Outcome

Therapy lasted for eleven one-hour sessions, which spanned three months. There were a further two appointments, one and two months after the end of the main sessions.

There was rapid progress, coinciding with the beginning of active therapy in the second appointment. Mrs Green began to accept a non-delusional explanation of her experiences in terms of the model described above. The conviction in the persecutory belief fell from 100% to 10%, and this was maintained at follow-up (Fig. 10.2). Both the preoccupation and, importantly, the distress associated with the belief also fell considerably (Fig. 10.3). The ratings of distress fell from "more than extremely distressing" to "more than a little distressing but less than moderately distressing". The improvements in the delusional belief were mirrored by improvements in levels of depression and anxiety (Fig. 10.4). By the final follow-up appointment, levels of depression and anxiety were in the non-clinical range. It is also of interest that the conviction and distress associated with the second persecutory belief, concerning the neighbours annoying Mrs Green, had decreased slightly by the time of the final follow-up appointment, even though this belief had not been targeted in therapy.

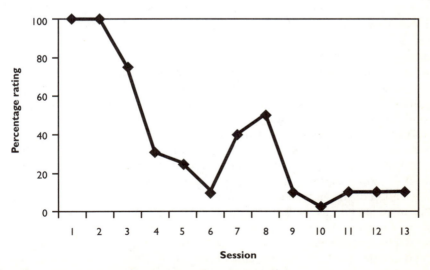

Figure 10.2 Percentage ratings of delusional conviction.

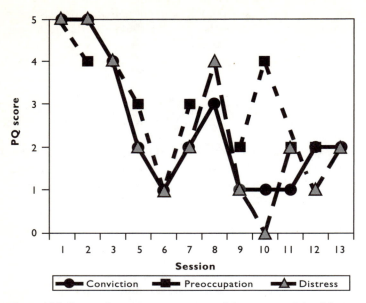

Figure 10.3 Personal questionnaire ratings of dimensions of the delusion.

As regards changes in behaviour, Mrs Green's avoidance had been reduced (e.g. she could now leave her home at around the time of the end of the school day); she now thought that it was best to ignore, rather than retaliate, when she suspected that people were trying to annoy; and there had also been a modest increase in activity (e.g. use of the local library). In terms of cognitive techniques, Mrs Green had learned the value of "checking out" anxious thoughts, rather than trying to avoid threat. But it was evident, from the temporary increases in belief conviction associated with the occurrence of ambiguous events (see Fig. 10.2, sessions 7 and 8), that she was still developing the skill of generating alternative explanations. Mrs Green was resistant to prompts to increase social activities further, and it seemed apparent that she still held some beliefs about herself that prevented her from becoming more engaged in activities in the community. Finally, Mrs Green said that she had found therapy extremely useful, and rated herself as "very satisfied" on a form administered at a later date, while her psychiatrist also provided confirmation of the improvement in mental state.

As an addendum to the formal outcome data, news was received concerning Mrs Green's longer-term progress: eight months after the final appointment she was considered well enough to be discharged from the community mental health team back into the care of her GP. At this time her psychiatrist wrote: "She remains quite well, although describes some general anxiety. She

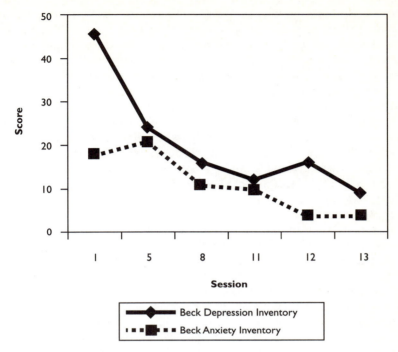

Figure 10.4 Depression and anxiety scores.

continues to work, and function quite well outside of work. She did not appear overtly paranoid".

DISCUSSION

In recent years a number of randomised controlled evaluations of cognitive behaviour therapy for psychosis have been reported (Drury et al., 1996; Kuipers et al., 1998; Tarrier et al., 1998), and together these have provided demonstrations of the effectiveness of this approach. However, at least as regards those with medication-resistant symptoms, a proportion of individuals (30–50%) do not make clinically significant improvements, while only a small minority are symptom-free after therapy (Kuipers et al., 1997, 1998). Therefore, innovations in the practice of cognitive therapy for psychosis, derived from the growing understanding of the mechanisms underlying symptoms, should be encouraged. This is a complex and challenging task, because symptoms of psychosis, such as delusions, may need to be understood from a multi-factorial perspective, with the recognition that differences in causal processes may exist even between delusions of the same content.

Consistent with the therapeutic promise of cognitive therapy for the difficulties of psychosis, we have described in this chapter how a long-standing delusional belief was reduced in a three-month period using an intervention that built upon previously developed methods by including techniques from work with emotional disorders. Encouragingly, a multi-dimensional assessment of the client's delusion showed significant reductions in delusional conviction, preoccupation, and distress. This resulted from Mrs Green accepting an alternative explanation of her experiences in terms of the formulation. Establishing a plausible alternative explanation is essential. Simply setting out to disprove a delusional belief is likely to be fruitless; typically, clients are then left with a choice between their delusional explanation and their only other salient, alternative explanation—that they are "mad". Despite the presentation of an alternative model in psychological terms, the rapid progress achieved was nevertheless unexpected, because the client initially showed little cognitive flexibility concerning her belief (see Garety et al., 1997): at the start of the intervention she did not think that she could be mistaken. While this absence of cognitive flexibility may have made the intervention more difficult because she presented at first as unwilling to consider an alternative explanation, it is possible that the absence of ongoing anomalous experiences (e.g. auditory hallucinations) may have made the intervention less difficult. In our experience, anomalous experiences are frequently taken as powerful evidence for delusional beliefs.

The intervention also succeeded in significantly reducing levels of anxiety and depression, even though emotional distress was not directly targeted except where it was thought to influence the persistence of the delusion. This is consistent with a hypothesis contained within the formulation that there were reciprocal relationships between the maintaining factors and the delusion. Although a single case cannot be taken to be representative, the client's presenting levels of anxiety and depression were not uncommon for an individual with a medication-resistant persecutory delusion (Freeman et al., 1998). In short, an intervention that promoted evaluation of the evidence for a delusional belief, while reducing the influence of a number of postulated maintaining factors, succeeded in reducing delusional conviction, delusional distress, and mood disturbance.

It could be expected, however, that the client will lapse back into old modes of thinking, since the delusion had been firmly held for 30 years. For instance, Mrs Green will still be very vulnerable to misinterpreting situations in line with the delusion. Therefore, additional "booster" sessions, perhaps implemented by a key-worker, would be beneficial to consolidate the progress made. It is expected that further improvements in symptoms would be brought about by additional long-term work that aimed, for example, to improve Mrs Green's levels of self-esteem, activities, and resources for dealing with anxiety. Addressing Mrs Green's tendency to worry may help prevent a subsequent elevation in the persecutory belief. She described herself as a "worrier", and it is of note that metaworry concerning the control of delusion-relevant worries was reported (see Freeman & Garety, 1999), indicating that exploration of beliefs about worry and the use of thought control strategies would be appropriate.

The formulation can therefore provide a continuing guide to intervention, though which factors exert the greatest influence may of course change with time. The formulation can also be expanded. In this relatively brief intervention the focus was the *maintenance* of the delusional belief. However, discussion of aetiological factors are important in therapy. Models of symptom formation provide a means for the individual to understand his or her difficulties, and they may also have a normalising benefit, because the development of a delusion is described in terms of the operation of normal psychological processes (albeit biased). In the present case, additional sessions would allow the client's personality and prior learning and experiences, including her childhood, to be discussed in greater detail. However, the aetiological factors may of course be distinct from the maintaining factors, and cannot be determined with any certainty because, unlike the maintaining factors, they cannot be directly changed during therapy.

Finally, the description of therapy has highlighted how ideas from research into neurosis informed the intervention. In this respect, therapeutic practice is ahead of theoretical development. While the literature indicates that emotional processes are plausible factors in delusion formation and maintenance, little experimental work examining the direct influence of such processes on psychosis has, as yet, been carried out. In this chapter, we have hypothesised in particular that interpretative biases and safety-seeking behaviours associated with anxiety and depression contribute to the maintenance of delusional beliefs. Whether such processes are tied exclusively to the emotional disorders, or whether, as is likely, they are mechanisms also important in the maintenance of psychotic disorders, is an empirical question. We also envisage that in the future we may develop our understanding of the role of anger in the maintenance of persecutory delusions, because central to anger are judgements of blame and attributions of intent: processes that are of obvious relevance to persecutory delusions. From a multi-factorial viewpoint, which specific emotion is influential in each individual delusion will differ. Determining if there are phenomenological characteristics of the delusion that allow clinicians to identify more readily the key emotional processes operating would be valuable. We would also highlight the possibility that psychotic and neurotic processes will interact. For example, a data-gathering reasoning bias would be exacerbated by dichotomous thinking and internal attentional self-focus. Clearly, examining the relationship between emotional processes and positive symptoms of psychosis is a future area of both clinical practice and research that is likely to provide clinically worthwhile and theoretically interesting results—and illustration of the interplay between therapeutic practice and theoretical development.

REFERENCES

American Psychiatric Association (1994). *Diagnostic and statistical manual of mental disorders, Fourth Edition.* Washington, DC: American Psychiatric Association.

Beck, A.T., Epstein, N., Brown, G., & Steer, R. (1988). An inventory for measuring clinical anxiety: psychometric properties. *Journal of Consulting and Clinical Psychology, 56,* 893–897.

Beck, A.T., Ward, C.H., Mendelson, M., Mock, J., & Erbaugh, J. (1961). An inventory for measuring depression. *Archives of General Psychiatry, 4,* 561–571.

Bentall, R.P. (1994). Cognitive biases and abnormal beliefs: Towards a model of persecutory delusions. In A.S. David & J. Cutting (Eds.), *The Neuropsychology of Schizophrenia* (pp.337–360). Hove, UK: Lawrence Erlbaum & Associates Ltd.

Bentall, R.P., & Kaney, S. (1989). Content specific processing and persecutory delusions: an investigation using the emotional Stroop test. *British Journal of Medical Psychology, 62,* 355–364.

Brett-Jones, J., Garety, P., & Hemsley, D. (1987). Measuring delusional experiences: A method and its application. *British Journal of Clinical Psychology, 26,* 257–265.

Chadwick, P. (1993). The stepladder to the impossible: A first hand phenomenological account of a schizoaffective psychotic crisis. *Journal of Mental Health, 2,* 239–250.

Chadwick, P.D.J., Birchwood, M.J., & Trower, P. (1996). *Cognitive therapy for delusions, voices and paranoia.* Chichester: Wiley.

Clark, D.M. (1986). A cognitive model of panic. *Behaviour Research and Therapy, 24,* 461–470.

Close, H., & Garety, P.A. (1998). Cognitive assessment of voices: Further developments in understanding the emotional impact of voices. *British Journal of Clinical Psychology, 37,* 173–188.

Corcoran, R., Mercer, G., & Frith, C.D. (1995). Schizophrenia, symptomatology and social inference: Investigating "theory of mind" in people with schizophrenia. *Schizophrenia Research, 17,* 5–13.

Drury, V., Birchwood, M., Cochrane, R., & MacMillan, F. (1996). Cognitive therapy and recovery from acute psychosis: A controlled trial, I: Impact on psychotic symptoms. *British Journal of Psychiatry, 169,* 593–601.

Dudley, R.E.J., John, C.H., Young, A.W., & Over, D.E. (1997). Normal and abnormal reasoning in people with delusions. *British Journal of Clinical Psychology, 36,* 243–258.

Fowler, D., Garety, P.A., & Kuipers, L. (1995). *Cognitive behaviour therapy for psychosis: Theory and practice.* Chichester: Wiley.

Freeman, D. (1998). *Neurosis and psychosis.* Unpublished Ph.D. thesis. University of London.

Freeman, D., & Garety, P.A. (1999). Worry, worry processes, and dimensions of delusions: An exploratory investigation of a role for anxiety processes in the maintenance of delusional distress. *Behavioural and Cognitive Psychotherapy, 27,* 47–62.

Freeman, D., Garety, P., Fowler, D., Kuipers, E., Dunn, G., Bebbington, P., & Hadley, C. (1998). The London-East Anglia randomised controlled trial of cognitive behaviour therapy for psychosis, IV: Self-esteem and persecutory delusions. *British Journal of Clinical Psychology, 37,* 415–430.

Freeman, D., Garety, P.A., & Kuipers, E. (in press). Persecutory delusions: Developing the understanding of belief maintenance and emotional distress. *Psychological Medicine*.

Freeman, D., Garety, P.A., & Phillips, M.L. (2000). An examination of hypervigilance for external threat in individuals with generalised anxiety disorder and individuals with persecutory delusions using visual scan paths. *Quarterly Journal of Experimental Psychology*, *53A*, 549–567.

Frith, C.D. (1992). *The cognitive neuropsychology of schizophrenia*. Hove, UK: Lawrence Erlbaum & Associates Ltd.

Garety, P.A., Fowler, D., Kuipers, E., Freeman, D., Dunn, G., Bebbington, P.E., Hadley, C., & Jones, S. (1997). The London-East Anglia randomised controlled trial of cognitive behaviour therapy for psychosis, II: Predictors of outcome. *British Journal of Psychiatry*, *171*, 420–426.

Garety, P.A., & Freeman, D. (1999). Cognitive approaches to delusions: A critical review of theories and evidence. *British Journal of Clinical Psychology*, *38*, 113–154.

Garety, P.A., & Hemsley, D.R. (1994). *Delusions: Investigations into the psychology of delusional reasoning*. Oxford: Oxford University Press.

Garety, P.A., Hemsley, D.R., & Wessely, S. (1991). Reasoning in deluded schizophrenic and paranoid patients: Biases in performance on a probabilistic inference task. *Journal of Nervous and Mental Disorder*, *179*, 194–201.

Ingram, R.E. (1990). Self-focused attention in clinical disorders: Review and a conceptual model. *Psychological Bulletin*, *107*, 156–176.

Kaney, S., & Bentall, R.P. (1989). Persecutory delusions and attributional style. *British Journal of Medical Psychology*, *62*, 191–198.

Kinderman, P., & Bentall, R.P. (1997). Causal attributions in paranoia and depression: Internal, personal, and situational attributions for negative events. *Journal of Abnormal Psychology*, *106*, 341–345.

Kingdon, D.G., & Turkington, D. (1994). *Cognitive behaviour therapy of schizophrenia*. Hove, UK: Lawrence Erlbaum & Associates Ltd.

Kuipers, E., Fowler, D., Garety, P.A., Chisholm, D., Freeman, D., Dunn, G., Bebbington, P.E., & Hadley, C. (1998). The London-East Anglia randomised controlled trial of cognitive behaviour therapy for psychosis, III: Follow-up and economic evaluation at 18 months. *The British Journal of Psychiatry*, *173*, 61–68.

Kuipers, E., Garety, P.A., Fowler, D., Dunn, G., Bebbington, P.E., Freeman, D., & Hadley, C. (1997). The London-East Anglia randomised controlled trial of cognitive behaviour therapy for psychosis, I: Effects of the treatment phase. *British Journal of Psychiatry*, *171*, 319–327.

Maher, B.A. (1974). Delusional thinking and perceptual disorder. *Journal of Individual Psychology*, *30*, 98–113.

Mathews, A., Richards, A., & Eysenck, M.W. (1989). The interpretation of homophones related to threat in anxiety states. *Journal of Abnormal Psychology*, *98*, 31–34.

McReynolds, P. (1960). Anxiety, perception, and schizophrenia. In D.D. Jackson (Ed.), *The etiology of schizophrenia* (pp.248–292). New York: Basic Books.

Mednick, S.A. (1958). A learning theory approach to research in schizophrenia. *Psychological Bulletin*, *55*, 316–327.

Morrison, A.P. (1998). Cognitive behaviour therapy for psychotic symptoms in schizophrenia. In N. Tarrier, A. Wells, & G. Haddock (Eds.), *Treating complex cases: The cognitive behavioural therapy approach* (pp.195–216). Chichester: Wiley.

Premack, D., & Woodruff, G. (1978). Does the chimpanzee have a theory of mind? *Behavioural and Brain Sciences, 4,* 515–526.

Rothwell, N., & Duffy, L. (1999). Towards an integrated psychotherapeutic approach in psychosis: Three case studies. *Clinical Psychology and Psychotherapy, 6,* 227–235.

Salkovskis, P.M. (1985). Obsessional-compulsive problems: A cognitive-behavioural analysis. *Behaviour Research and Therapy, 25,* 571–583.

Salkovskis, P.M. (1991). The importance of behaviour in the maintenance of anxiety and panic: A cognitive account. *Behavioural Psychotherapy, 19,* 6–19.

Salkovskis, P.M. (1996). The cognitive approach to anxiety: Threat beliefs, safety-seeking behaviours, and the special case of health anxiety and obsessions. In P.M. Salkovskis (Ed.), *Frontiers of cognitive therapy* (pp.48–74). New York: Guilford Press.

Smári, J., Stefánsson, S., & Thorgilsson, H. (1994). Paranoia, self-consciousness, and social cognition in schizophrenics. *Cognitive Therapy and Research, 18,* 387–399.

Tarrier, N., Yusupoff, L., Kinney, C., McCarthy, E., Gledhill, A., Haddock, G., & Morris, J. (1998). Randomised controlled trial of intensive cognitive behavioural therapy for patients with chronic schizophrenia. *British Medical Journal, 317,* 303–307.

Trower, P., & Chadwick, P. (1995). Pathways to defense of the self: A theory of two types of paranoia. *Clinical Psychology: Science and Practice, 2,* 263–278.

Wason, P.C. (1960). On the failure to eliminate hypotheses in a conceptual task. *Quarterly Journal of Experimental Psychology, 12,* 129–140.

Wells, A. (1994). Attention and the control of worry. In G. Davey & F. Tallis (Eds.), *Worrying: Perspectives on theory, assessment and treatment* (pp. 91–114). Chichester: Wiley.

Williams, J.M.G., Mathews, A., & MacLeod, C. (1996). The emotional Stroop task and psychopathology. *Psychological Bulletin, 120,* 3–24.

Williams, J.M.G., Watts, F.N., Macleod, C., & Mathews, A. (1988). *Cognitive psychology and emotional disorders.* Chichester: Wiley.

World Health Organisation (1992). *SCAN: Schedules for Clinical Assessment in Neuropsychiatry.* Geneva: WHO.

Zubin, J., & Spring, B. (1977). Vulnerability: A new view of schizophrenia. *Journal of Abnormal Psychology, 86,* 260–266.

Chapter 11

Attributional therapy: A case of paranoia and hallucinations

Peter Kinderman and Andy Benn

INTRODUCTION

This chapter outlines recent theoretical and empirical developments in the understanding of causal attributions in paranoia and persecutory delusions, and illustrates novel clinical approaches to therapeutic intervention targeted at changing causal attribution within a course of treatment using cognitive behavioural therapy.

The study of individual symptoms of psychosis (Bentall, Jackson, & Pilgrim, 1988; Persons, 1986) rather than of broadly defined syndromes such as schizophrenia has led to theoretical advances in our understanding of paranoia, paranoid ideation, and persecutory delusions. Using the theoretical framework offered by attribution theory Bentall, Kinderman, and colleagues (Bentall & Kinderman, 1999; Bentall, Kinderman, & Kaney, 1994) have proposed and developed a model of paranoid ideation based upon attributional abnormalities, attentional bias, self-discrepancies, negative self-representations, and theory of mind (ToM) deficits.

The attributional model of paranoia (illustrated in Fig. 11.1) proposes that people with paranoid delusions show an attentional bias towards material that is both threat-related (Bentall & Kaney, 1989) and related to negative self-representations (Kinderman, 1994). People experiencing persecutory delusions make abnormally internal attributions for positive events and abnormally external attributions for negative events (Candido & Romney, 1990; Fear, Sharpe, & Healy, 1996; Kaney & Bentall, 1989, 1992; Sharp, Fear, & Healy, 1997). It is suggested that this pattern—which is only evident on explicit as opposed to implicit measures (Lyon, Kaney, & Bentall, 1994)—serves as a mechanism to maintain a positive self-image in the face of threats resultant from the attentional bias.

The choice of attribution employed also appears significant. Kinderman and Bentall (1996) identified three loci of attributions; internal, external-personal, and external-situational. Kinderman and Bentall (1997b) found that paranoid individuals demonstrated not only an externalising bias (attributing more positive events than negative events to internal loci) but

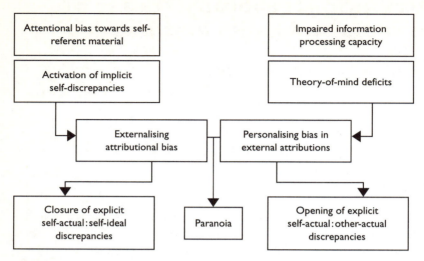

Figure 11.1 A diagrammatic representation of the attributional model of paranoia.

also a personalising bias (allocating the majority of their external attributions to personal as opposed to situational loci).

Bentall and Kinderman (1999; also Kinderman, Dunbar, & Bentall, 1999) have suggested that this pattern of attributional abnormalities might, in part, be a consequence of failure of cognitive systems associated with social cognition. Because psychotic episodes are associated with dysfunctions of information processing capacity (Green, 1992), and ToM tasks appear to make considerable demands on cognitive resources, it is possible that the ToM deficits and attributional abnormalities experienced by paranoid patients reflect these more general psychological impairments.

SEARCH AND TERMINATION STRATEGIES IN CAUSAL ATTRIBUTION

Research in social psychology has suggested that the process of causal attribution can usefully be thought of in terms of two relatively independent processes. People make effortful searches for possible explanations for social events. In addition, people employ heuristic and idiosyncratic rules for terminating this search.

Gilbert and colleagues (Gilbert, 1989; Gilbert, McNulty, Giuliano, & Benson, 1992) have suggested that social attributions for the actions of other people involve an active search for situational factors. This search is effortful and easily disrupted. Thus, when participants in research experiments were required to make judgements about an actor while performing an additional cognitive task, they tended to make more dispositional attributions for behaviour than under no additional load (Gilbert, Krull, & Pelham, 1988). This mirrors the personalising attributional bias observed in paranoid individuals (Kinderman & Bentall, 1997b) and the tendency to underestimate the situational causes of behaviour referred to as the "fundamental attribution error". This has strong similarities with the tendency to "jump to conclusions" reported by other researchers of delusional reasoning (Huq, Garety, & Hemsley, 1988), where people with paranoid delusions tend to guess at the answers to questions without much information, rather than narrow down the field of possible answers.

It seems clear that people pursue a strategic search for material pertinent to making causal attributions. It also seems clear that, in keeping with the links between the attributional model of paranoia (Bentall & Kinderman, 1999) and theory of mind difficulties, the search for situational attributions may place a particular strain on this strategy. Fatigue, stress, depression, anxiety, and the presence of general or specific deficits in social cognition might limit the search strategy. The search strategy might also be biased as a result of affect mediated motivational stances. It may also be influenced by experience. So far this framework has not been widely used to understand causal attributions, but we may speculate that all of these factors will influence attributional search strategies.

Social psychologists have suggested that there exists a strong requirement for people to develop interpretative frameworks of their social world that satisfy a motivational need for "structure" or "closure" (DeGrada, Kruglanski, Mannetti, & Pierro, 1999; Dijksterhuis, van Knippenberg, Kruglanski, & Schaper, 1996). This research implies that people possess idiosyncratic rules for the closure or termination of search strategies for causal attributions. That is, people seem to search for possible explanations for social events, choosing from the possible explanations generated. This search appears to terminate when an account is generated that is psychologically satisfactory. Satisfactory explanations may of course include the matching of current explanations with prior explanations or beliefs, bringing the problem of circular reasoning into play. Causal attributions are extremely important in determining emotional and behavioural reactions to personally salient events (Buchanan & Seligman, 1995; Heider, 1958; Weiner, Russell, & Lerman, 1978). Termination rules for attributional search strategies are unlikely therefore to be limited to "closure" but will involve other motivational goals, including maintenance of affect and self-concept.

Clearly therapeutic strategies aimed at altering maladaptive attributional styles must address both the search for possible explanations and the choice of an appropriate conclusion. In the last few years cognitive behavioural interventions have also been shown to be effective in patients suffering from delusions (Chadwick & Birchwood, 1994; Garety et al., 1997; Kuipers et al., 1997; Tarrier et al., 1993). The strategies developed by cognitive behaviour therapists working with psychotic patients involve explicit attempts to modify patients' explanations for events, together with attempts to address problems of self-esteem and hopelessness (Fowler, Garety, & Kuipers, 1995).

Kinderman and Bentall (1997a) reported a single case study of cognitive behavioural therapy directed at modifying maladaptive attributions driving persecutory delusions. In that case, a man suffering from persecutory delusions was helped to reattribute negative life experiences to situational causes rather than to a conspiracy directed towards himself. A reduction in paranoid ideation, which was maintained at follow-up, was accompanied by changes on formal measures of attributions. That study illustrated the potential applicability of cognitive therapy specifically targeted at altering patterns of causal attributions.

Given the attributional abnormalities seen in schizophrenia, it would seem appropriate to conclude that a therapeutic approach using cognitive behavioural therapy is warranted. Future research into the cognitive abnormalities underlying psychotic symptomatology is likely to lead to increases in the effectiveness of this kind of treatment. Kinderman (2001) used the two-phase model of causal attribution to develop potential strategies for altering paranoid explanations. Because paranoid causal attributions are conceptualised as arising from both a truncated search and an idiosyncratic set of termination rules, both of these processes can be targeted. The case described in the next section is an example of such a therapeutic strategy.

CASE DESCRIPTION: MR RATTIGAN

The following case study concerns a patient recruited into the Socrates study (a multi-site randomised controlled trial of cognitive behavioural therapy for early, acute psychosis). This case has been selected for the purposes of highlighting the concepts and therapeutic concepts under consideration here, rather than for its representativeness of patients in the Socrates study. The approach to therapy in the Socrates study was compiled from contemporary clinical and research interventions in the treatment of individual psychotic symptoms field (Bentall, Haddock, & Slade, 1994; Chadwick & Lowe, 1990; Haddock, Bentall, & Slade, 1993; Kingdon & Turkington, 1994).

Initial clinical assessment

Mr Rattigan was a 28-year-old white single male. He was admitted to an acute psychiatric ward under Section 3 of the 1983 Mental Health Act following an assessment by his GP and an approved social worker. He had one previous voluntary admission nine months before his current admission—his parents had encouraged him to seek help when they noticed his self-care had deteriorated, he seemed continually anxious, was not sleeping, and was avoiding social contact. This admission had lasted 10 days during which time he was treated for and received a discharge diagnosis of depression. His current admission had been prompted by a similar presentation of deterioration of self-care, avoidance of social contact, loss of sleep, second and third person auditory hallucinations, and persecutory delusions together with the use of neologisms. He was given a provisional diagnosis of schizophrenia and treated with Sulpiride 400mg in the morning and 400mg at night, with 20mg of Procyclidine daily.

Mr Rattigan had been unemployed for approximately five years. His mother and father were still alive but divorced. He did not have much contact with his father, although his father had visited him twice since he was admitted to hospital. His mother had remarried during his late teens and he saw his mother and stepfather weekly. Mr Rattigan stated that, when well, most of his time was spent shopping, visiting friends, looking for work, learning the guitar, going out for drinks with friends, and reading, with a particular interest in the occult.

He was recruited to the Socrates project by the project psychiatrist two days after his admission to the ward. He met the study admission criteria in the following ways:

- he was aged between 18 and 65;
- it was his second admission, but his first admission was less than two years ago;
- his symptoms included auditory hallucinations and delusions and he had received a provisional diagnosis of schizophrenia;
- illegal drugs were not thought to be the primary cause of his symptoms;
- he had no history of head injury or evidence of organic brain damage; and
- he gave informed consent for taking part in the study.

He was randomised into treatment using cognitive behavioural therapy and both the project psychiatrist and the ward clinical team were blind to this randomisation.

Mr Rattigan was seen for a total of 13 sessions of cognitive behavioural therapy including 4 post-discharge sessions. Mr Rattigan had been hospitalised 13 days and started on antipsychotic medication following assessment by his admission team prior to the first contact with the therapist. The first two to three sessions of therapy were mainly focused on assessment. Mr Rattigan reported that he had been stressed in his personal relationships over the past year and, in particular, stressed as a result of a relationship with a woman. He said he kept hearing voices of "chatter about myself" from air conditioning fans, washing machines, vacuum cleaners, and occasionally cars. The initial assessment also revealed that Mr Rattigan was fully convinced at that time that he had been subjected to the malign influence of "black magic" causing him to hear these voices. He had previously taken the voices to be benign, as they appeared to give advice about how and when to carry out everyday tasks, and how to avoid a group of people he feared. These voices had encouraged him to shoplift and after he had been caught shoplifting Mr Rattigan concluded that whoever was behind the "black magic" was evidently part of a wider plot to have him dehumanised. He believed that because of his shoplifting offence he would be killed, perhaps in prison, then he would be secretly taken out of the prison, sold on the black market, his body dried and turned into a waste basket. These beliefs had been a feature of Mr Rattigan's life for four months prior to his admission to hospital and during those four months he had avoided almost all social contact and taken to travelling at night, staying out of view of people and sometimes crawling along hedgerows.

During the initial assessment phase Mr Rattigan denied the use of illicit drugs excepting the occasional use of cannabis. However, he later told the therapist that he had been using amphetamine sulphate for the previous four and a half years up until two months prior to his admission to the hospital.

Formal assessment

As part of the Socrates study, Mr Rattigan's mental health and psychological functioning was regularly assessed by a research psychiatrist independent of the therapist, independent of the clinical team, and blind to his allocation to cognitive behavioural therapy. Mr Rattigan's symptoms were assessed using the Positive and Negative Syndrome Scale (PANSS; Kay & Opler, 1987)—a 30-item rating scale composed of a "positive" symptom subscale (7 items), a "negative" symptom subscale (7 items), and a 16-item "general" psychopathology subscale. The Auditory Hallucinations Rating Scale (AHRS) and Delusions Rating Scale (DRS), now known as the Psychotic Symptom Rating Scale (PSYRATS, Haddock, McCarron, Tarrier, & Faragher, 1999), were used to assess the severity of a number of dimensions for each scale. The results of these assessments are presented in Table 11.1, and confirm the clinical picture of anxiety, auditory hallucinations, and persecutory delusions.

Unfortunately, it was not possible for Mr Rattigan to complete a formal measure of attributional style at the beginning of therapy. However, research evidence (outlined earlier) has been very clear about the abnormally defensive and personalising attributions accompanying paranoid delusions. It must also be noted that all formal assessments, including assessments of attributional style, were made blind to therapy. Nevertheless, Mr Rattigan's paranoid delusions and associated abnormal causal attributions were jointly agreed as therapeutic targets by the client and therapist in line with the Socrates study intervention protocol. Table 11.2 presents data related to measures of self-esteem (the Rosenberg Self-Esteem Inventory; Rosenberg,

Table 11.1 Formal symptomatic assessment using the PANSS and PSYRATS

| Date of assessment (post-admission) | PANSS | | | | | | | | |
| | PANSS subscales | | | | Individual PANSS items | | | PSYRATS | |
	Positive	Negative	General	Total	Delusions	Hallucinations	Suspiciousness	AHRS	DRS
13 days	24	26	33	93	5	4	4	30	18
28 days	20	21	42	83	4	3	3	24	13
34 days	18	18	38	74	4	3	2	20	10
42 days	12	16	29	57	3	2	1	13	7
48 days	9	11	16	46	2	1	1	11	5
Discharged from hospital after 61 days									
97 days	10	11	26	47	1	1	2	0	0
265 days	13	12	37	62	3	2	3	12	10
512 days	16	12	26	54	1	2	3	0	0

Notes: This table presents the scores on the PANSS for Mr Rattigan on the specified assessment dates. Data presented are the individual subscale scores as well as the individual scores for Mr Rattigan's key problems. Also presented are the corresponding scores on the PSYRATS subscales, the AHRS (Auditory Hallucinations Rating Scale) and DRS (Delusions Rating Scale).

Table 11.2 Psychological assessments

Date	Rosenberg Self-Esteem Inventory	Internal, Personal, and Situational Attributions Questionnaire								
		Number of attributions to individual loci						Derived scores	
		Positive items			Negative items			Externalising bias	Personalising bias
		a+	b+	c+	a–	b–	c–		
13 days	29								
28 days									
34 days									
42 days									
48 days	29								
Discharged from hospital after 61 days									
97 days	25	3	3	2	1	5	2	2	0.71
265 days									
512 days	29	4	4	0	0	4	4	4	0.50

Notes: This table presents the scores on the Rosenberg Self-Esteem Inventory and the IPSAQ (Internal, Personal, and Situational Attributions Questionnaire). IPSAQ data presented are the number of attributions made to each attributional locus for both positive and negative items, as well as the derivative scores.

1965) and causal attributions (Internal, Personal, and Situational Attributions Questionnaire, IPSAQ; Kinderman & Bentall, 1996).

As can be seen from Table 11.2, Mr Rattigan's self-esteem remained relatively constant over the course of therapy and during the follow-up period. This is consistent with two related processes. First, that his externalising and personalising attributional style served to maintain a positive global self-view, despite severe negative events in his life. Essentially these negative events were distressing and frightening, but they did not mean things were his fault, or that he was essentially a bad person. The fact that Mr Rattigan's self-esteem remained consistent while his symptoms (outlined in Table 11.1) changed dramatically partially supports this conclusion, but also suggests that his attributional style changed from a personalising, to a more situational one.

This is partially supported by the data from formal assessment of attributional style. Unfortunately, Mr Rattigan was only able to complete the IPSAQ following his discharge from hospital. Important data, concerning his pattern of explanations when very deluded and paranoid, are missing. Nevertheless, we can see that his pattern of attributions changes from predominantly personal (personalising bias of 0.71) to more situational (personalising bias of 0.50). This echoes the general continuation of positive improvement by Mr Rattigan post-discharge.

Qualitative analysis of the processes of attributional change in therapy

The processes of attributional change will be illustrated by highlighting case material from Mr Rattigan's therapy. As already mentioned, the strategy for the package of cognitive behavioural therapy offered to Mr Rattigan was based on a generic manual. However, within this model, active steps to address his dysfunctional causal attributions were attempted. This chapter focuses on these, and describes how relatively conventional cognitive behavioural therapy techniques can be used to widen truncated attributional search strategies, and challenge maladaptive attributional search termination rules.

Attributions about hospitalisation

Mr Rattigan perceived his admission to be a negative and undesirable event: he reported that his admission into hospital had been "a mistake". He said that his GP and a social worker had visited him, were concerned about him, and they had decided that he was experiencing mental health problems and required admission into hospital. Mr Rattigan disagreed that he was experiencing mental health problems. He said that what had actually happened was that he had been subjected to black magic that had caused him to hear voices.

This explanation for the distressing events that had been happening to him could be seen as consistent with a personalised and external set of attributions.

Mr Rattigan continued to hear voices occasionally within the hospital that seemed to him to be coming from the washing machines on the ward. A homework task was agreed with Mr Rattigan in order to help in the search for additional possible explanations for his voices. Over the weekend he agreed to think about possible links between the washing machines in the hospital, his voices, and the situations in which he heard voices while he was still living in his flat. On the first meeting after the weekend, Mr Rattigan reported that he had not experienced any voices when he was in the vicinity of the washing machines and had no further ideas about what may have caused him to hear voices other than black magic. In view of this potential impasse the therapist and Mr Rattigan agreed to look at the context in which he had initially begun to hear voices.

In terms of previous research on search strategies in attribution (Gilbert, 1989; Gilbert, McNulty, Guiliano, & Benson, 1992), this strategy can be seen to draw the client's attention to situational factors that may be relevant to the event. Therapeutic effort is directed first at expanding the attributional search (using "scientific" methods of experimentation and collection of evidence). In addition, however, it is clear that there is a subtle effect whereby the client's initial attribution of cause is not assumed to be the only valid conclusion. That is, the client's termination rules are gently massaged into more appropriate focus.

Explanations for voices

Mr Rattigan had first heard voices approximately six months before his admission to hospital. He had been sleeping little and had been almost constantly fearful of being killed. From where he lived he could hear the constant hum of the air-conditioning of a nearby shop. It was from this air-conditioning that he first heard the commentary on himself. In the few weeks after the onset of this symptom Mr Rattigan found that the voices were triggered by noises, such as vacuum cleaners, washing machines, and fan systems. Clinical assessment had highlighted that the voices involved a running commentary in the third person. Examples of the content of the hallucination included: "why doesn't he have a wash?" "why doesn't he watch the television?"; "lie down?"; "make a cup of coffee?" Given his previous account of how he had begun to neglect himself, the therapist enquired whether he himself had thought similar thoughts about himself and whether it was possible that the voices were his own thoughts. Mr Rattigan reported that "they are my thoughts, but they're not". Additional discussion took place using a normalising rationale (Kingdon & Turkington, 1994) concerning the role of sleep deprivation in causing some people to hallucinate.

Mr Rattigan accepted that it was possible that his fearfulness and loss of sleep may have contributed to him beginning to hear voices.

At this stage in therapy the therapist sought to reopen the search for an explanation for an event (hearing voices) for which Mr Rattigan appeared to have an entirely adequate subjective explanation (black magic causing him to hear voices). Several sessions later when Mr Rattigan related that he had taken amphetamine regularly for the past four and a half years, the question of the situational causes for his voices was raised again. The role of amphetamine in triggering symptoms like the ones he experienced, and the effect that taking amphetamine has on sleep were discussed. Within these discussions the therapist elicited attributions from Mr Rattigan that incorporated both of these additional possible causes of hearing voices and linked them with the results of the first search for alternative explanations for why he heard voices.

Occult beliefs and attributions

The assessment of the antecedents to the onset of Mr Rattigan's voices progressed to identifying the social circumstances in which he was living at the time. He had been part of a group of friends who took amphetamine. However, he found that over a period of time his positive experiences while taking the drug became less frequent while those of his friends appeared to become more frequent. He reported that he believed that they experienced a "better high" and were "receiving more minor damage" than himself. He began to suspect that some of the group were taking cocaine. He had stopped buying amphetamine some three months previously but by this time he believed that he was under their control through black magic influences.

At this point during therapy Mr Rattigan indicated that one of the main things about his voices was that they compounded his existing worries. His voices led to considerable paranoid anxiety, in part because a paranoid explanation was his solution to the experience of voices. He agreed to talk about his concerns, which involved "Wizz Religion". Mr Rattigan indicated that he was unsure where he had first come across this term and was unsure of its precise meaning, but that he believed himself to be a victim of this concept. He explained that a group of friends began taking amphetamine together but that one person ends up, inevitably, buying the amphetamine for the group. He believed that a black witch had orchestrated the situation around him. He also claimed that he had been "set up" for a minor crime and that this was associated with a plot in which he would be imprisoned, killed, and turned into an ornament. His fear had been compounded therefore by fears for losing his own life and being humiliated even in death by being transformed. He believed that the people who organised and orchestrated such things went to live in Switzerland and were able to afford anything. Because he thought their finances were virtually unlimited, he believed they were able to obtain anything they wanted and that an ornament that had been a human body was how he would end up.

Mr Rattigan said he had indeed shoplifted and that he would be prosecuted. He believed that he was acting under the control of others and therefore the shoplifting had not been intentional, but said he intended to plead guilty to the charge. Additionally, by being admitted to hospital he had breached his bail conditions and had not turned up for his trial, believing that he would be imprisoned for this breach.

In the next session Mr Rattigan explored the links between his voices and his beliefs about Wizz Religion. He reported that the voices had told him to dress up as a woman and that he would be able to evade detection by the people involved in Wizz Religion by this method. At the time this was happening, Mr Rattigan viewed the voices as benign and even helpful. It was only later after he had been arrested for shoplifting that he came to view the voices as being produced by the very people he believed were against him. Additionally in this session, he began to describe his relationship with a woman. About four years previously he had met a woman who had introduced him to a "crazy way of life which felt dangerous" but which felt exciting, rewarding, and vital to him. He also reported that this woman had been very supportive when he had split up from his previous relationship, he first began taking amphetamine in the company of this woman, and that she became part of his life. Approximately 18 months prior to his admission, Mr Rattigan suddenly lost contact with this woman. He told his therapist that he went round to her flat and found her gone, and continued trying to contact her but failed to do so. During a discussion of the effects of amphetamine use, Mr Rattigan was able to identify that the use of amphetamine had caused him to lose much sleep over quite a lengthy period and that he himself had known people who had strange experiences due to amphetamine.

Formulation

The clinical formulation is now described. A 28-year-old man, with a remote genetic predisposition to mental illness (maternal grandmother had a history of depression) loses inertia in his working life and becomes socially isolated. He meets interesting people and a woman he becomes fond of while taking stimulants. His consumption of stimulants increases but he finds that he is buying stimulants and sharing them while none of his co-consumers are reciprocating. As he is unemployed and has little money he stops seeing his associates and stops taking stimulants. He subsequently becomes depressed for a short period and is successfully treated for depression. His sleep pattern does not recover fully and he continues to sleep chaotically. A few months later he attempts to contact his former associates and finds they are no longer where they last lived. He begins hallucinating and at the same time begins attempting to account for this experience. His search is terminated rapidly when he concludes that his purchasing of amphetamine for his group of friends was deliberate. He came to believe he had been subjected to black magic and was afraid as he already had a belief in the possibility of genuine effects of black magic. He concluded that his friends wanted him dead and to sell him on as a "luxury" waste bin. He attributes the source of this black magic to the influence of the woman of whom he was so fond but who left without contacting him. He is hospitalised involuntarily but responds quickly to antipsychotic medication, and engages well with the therapist in the collaborative venture to reattribute the cause of his hallucination.

Overview of attributional interventions

As therapy progressed, particular focus was applied to Mr Rattigan's causal attributions. The therapist attempted to help him develop fuller attributional frameworks, and to challenge his inappropriate conclusions to the search for explanations. This process took place over several sessions during the intervention period. First was the recognition of delusional beliefs. Second, how Mr Rattigan had developed the beliefs was ascertained, with particular attention played to the use of causal attributions within his description of his subjective experience. Next, discussion and clarification with Mr Rattigan led to a shared and agreed version of what he believed to be the case. This could be summarised as follows: "I know I'm being influenced by black magic because I took the advice of a voice I've been hearing from an air-vent"; "I subsequently stole some cosmetics from a shop so that I could escape with my life from some so-called friends who want to convert me into a waste bin"; "They are, themselves working with the black witch"; "This leads me to conclude that I was actually being 'other peopled'—made to act like a shop-lifter by remote influence of this black magic"; "I know this to be true, because these so-called friends lulled me into buying amphetamine and sharing it with them—a one-way sharing"; "And three months after I stopped buying it and seeing them they all disappear and it was just at that time that I started to hear the voice".

Thirdly, Mr Rattigan was invited within session and between the sessions (his inter-session task or "homework") to try and identify other things that may have caused the "voice" to occur. It was not explicitly stated to Mr Rattigan that he was wrong in his attribution of black magic causing the "voice" to occur. The therapist told him that his explanation appeared to be based on an interpretation of certain events. Often this may lead to the general query of "what other ways are there of looking at it then?" Even in the absence of this puzzlement or surprise at the possibility of other explanations being possible, the therapist's task is to be collaborative but secure agreement that the "search" for an alternative explanation for the experiences is warranted. Affirmation of Mr Rattigan's efficacy at working out the best possible explanation of experiences was made. The affirmation was couched in a temporal sequence that helps the client locate the formation of their beliefs in time and place distinct from the hospital setting, and helps establish that the current endeavour of searching for an alternative explanation gives an opportunity for re-interpretation.

Fourthly, when Mr Rattigan did not identify other possible causes of his "voice" the therapist reminded him of other setting events that were identified during the assessment. Thus Mr Rattigan's prolonged use of amphetamine and his poor sleep were discussed as possible contributory factors, and the consequences for the formulation were discussed.

The main beneficial therapeutic factors appear to have been medication, respectful psycho-social assessment and formulation, cognitive behavioural therapy targeted at reopening the search for causal explanation, guiding the search, and terminating the search with a more comprehensive and reality based causal explanation.

This process is illustrated by two excepts from therapy. Again, these are not randomly selected excerpts, but are two particular sections of the taped transcript that illustrate the development of richer and more appropriate explanations for disturbing events during therapy.

Excerpt one: Session five

Therapist:	In the second or third session, we were looking at the voices you heard. And I don't know if you remember, but I said that there are a lot of situations that could cause people to hear voices. Do you remember me mentioning that?
Mr Rattigan:	Yes. I remember you mentioning it.
Therapist:	Because if you remember, you went into the washing room to see if the noise of the washing machine made it . . .
	. . .
Mr Rattigan:	It often struck me that if these were normal people, one thing that I always thought that if these were normal people that were creating the voices in my head, they must be able to stay awake an awful long time.
Therapist:	Right.
Mr Rattigan:	Because . . . (chuckles)
Therapist:	Right.
Mr Rattigan:	Because they do it in the middle of the night, and they do it in the day or whatever . . .
Therapist:	Right. It sounds a bit unusual doesn't it?
Mr Rattigan:	Yes, it means they are almost permanently awake.
Therapist:	Sure. That's quite difficult for someone to actually do.
Mr Rattigan:	And I'm wondering how they'd do it as well.
Therapist:	Yes. Have you any thoughts on that?

Mr Rattigan:	No, I really can't explain it. You know, the more you think about it, the more baffling it gets.
Therapist:	Yes.
Mr Rattigan:	So you think, what is it? Thought transference? What is it that's occurring—if it is—and what are these people doing?
Therapist:	Right. Is there any scientific evidence for things like that happening? Thought transference or telepathy?
Mr Rattigan:	Not that I know of, not that I'm aware of, no.
	. . .
Mr Rattigan:	Which makes me wonder who the hell's doing it, or how the heck they're doing it.
Therapist:	Or if there's a different explanation for it.
Mr Rattigan:	Maybe a different explanation for it. That's all it can be really. (30 seconds' pause)
Therapist:	Other sorts of situations that can cause people to hear voices are . . . You know, periods of stress . . . In the sense of people worrying about things too much or having more things on their plates than they can cope with . . . Periods of stress can cause people to hear voices. Um. Long periods of loss of sleep can also cause that. Those are some . . .
Mr Rattigan:	Which could be due to the amphetamines I'd been taking, then stopped taking.
Therapist:	Right. Yes. Yes.
Mr Rattigan:	Because I had long periods of no sleep at all.
Therapist:	Right.
Mr Rattigan:	And then suddenly I stopped taking altogether.
Therapist:	Right.
Mr Rattigan:	So maybe there's something that's compensating.
Therapist:	Sure. Yes. Yes.
Mr Rattigan:	Not compensating, but getting in there because . . . As it were . . .
Therapist:	Do you think that's likely to be possible?
Mr Rattigan:	I think it's a possibility.

Excerpt two: Session six

Mr Rattigan:	I hitched all the way to Lewisham, to try to get away from the voices. But it was still going on in Lewisham.
Therapist:	Right, so you were still having the voices, when you were in Lewisham?
Mr Rattigan:	Yes.
Therapist:	Right.
Mr Rattigan:	Oh yes, it didn't matter where I went. I could go to Notting Hill, I'd still be hearing the voices.

Therapist:	Right.
Mr Rattigan:	I'd be hearing them on the train to Notting Hill, I'd hear them in Notting Hill. If I went to Lewisham, I was hearing them when I was in Lewisham.
Therapist:	Yes. How could that possibly be done?
Mr Rattigan:	I don't know (sigh) I don't know. I had all kind of theories about what could possibly be going on. From whether it was something to do with (company name) laying cables everywhere to, like I say, just the influence of black magic being so massive, so great.
Therapist:	And, what about what we've discussed subsequently, that long periods of stress or loss of sleep . . .
Mr Rattigan:	I've been wondering this myself—if it is me that's wondering it—I've been wondering myself if it's emotional stress. I'm thinking that, it's something subconscious maybe that I didn't realise at the time.
Therapist:	Um.
Mr Rattigan:	Can that be a possibility? That it's some kind of emotional stress that I was under?
Therapist:	Oh sure.
Mr Rattigan:	That maybe I didn't realise, or didn't think I was under?
Therapist:	Right.
Mr Rattigan:	Was causing it—this . . .

These transcripts illustrate the two specific elements of the attributional intervention well. In both cases Mr Rattigan expresses some confusion or concern to explain the occurrence of his experiences. In both cases he appears to have difficulty explaining the events, but requires some assistance in searching for, and accepting, appropriate explanations. In both cases, the therapist gently explores Mr Rattigan's original views, and exposes some inconsistency. He develops, explicitly, the need for explanation, he does not accept maladaptive explanations, and assists Mr Rattigan in searching for more potential explanations. It is also worth noting that the therapist explicitly reinforces situational explanations for psychotic events—explanations in terms of environmental and personal stress.

Therapeutic outcome

Following the Socrates protocol for cognitive behavioural therapy in acute schizophrenia, therapy ended 35 days after it commenced. The therapeutic envelope ended four months from first contact. Mr Rattigan had attended nine sessions over the first thirty-five days, and one follow-up session at two weeks, four weeks, eight and twelve weeks after the thirty-fifth day. His "voices" had ceased approximately one week after therapy and his delusional beliefs by about the fourth week. At this time he was discharged from the hospital. At discharge, Mr Rattigan's causal explanation for his symptoms included: sleeplessness, caused by stress from the fears he had been holding and as an after effect of long-term amphetamine use; a pre-existing belief in the possibility of occult influence; misinterpreting the behaviour of friends and associates as malign; and the attribution of the occurrence of the "voice" as being caused by a woman he was fond of when she was imprisoned and went away without contacting him.

Follow-up sessions focused on the identification of warning signs of relapse and the development of an action plan to implement if symptoms begin to reappear (Birchwood, 1995; Birchwood, McGorry, & Jackson, 1997). Mr Rattigan remained well at the last follow-up session and continued to talk of his experiences in terms of the revised attributional formulation.

Clinical outcome

Mr Rattigan was discharged from the ward 61 days after admission. Clinically he had improved greatly. On the PANSS, his scores had dropped from 93 on admission to 46 (remembering that the PANSS does not have a lowest possible score of 0, but rather 30). Moreover, his scores on the key clinical symptoms of delusions, hallucinatory behaviour, and suspiciousness also dropped markedly. On the PSYRATS, he also showed marked clinical improvement. It is worth noting, however, that his scores did not drop to zero, symptom-free.

Following discharge, Mr Rattigan continued to show clinical improvement over the next 18 months. He appeared to have an improvement (with AHRS and DRS scores dropping to zero) at about three months' post-discharge, followed by a minor increase of symptomatology at nine months, followed by another clinical improvement. This pattern of continuing improvement over the course of 18 months following the delivery of cognitive behavioural therapy is consistent with previous research reports.

DISCUSSION

This chapter has described a relatively conventional case of cognitive behavioural therapy for psychotic delusions. Although the problems exhibited by Mr Rattigan were exotic, they were not unusual. In addition, the package of therapy employed was not only conventional, it was specifically designed to be a manual-based example of formulation-driven cognitive behavioural therapy. Nevertheless, the case serves to illustrate a specific pattern of intervention designed to address attributional abnormalities. This followed a formulation of the client's problems founded on research evidence.

The case illustrates well how a combination of a truncated search for plausible explanations for distressing or ambiguous events, coupled with a maladaptive set of termination rules can produce delusional beliefs and contribute to hallucinatory experiences. The therapy employed was designed to broaden Mr Rattigan's search for explanations and also to select, from a wider range of possible explanations, more appropriate conclusions. This strategy appeared to be successful in that Mr Rattigan altered his pattern of explanations for distressing events in his life, and experienced a reduction in the distressing symptoms. This benefit appeared to continue beyond the duration of therapy itself.

Of course, as with all single cases, many questions are left unanswered. Mr Rattigan received conventional medical interventions in addition to cognitive behavioural therapy. He also resided on a ward, unable to use street drugs. Both of these influences were presumably beneficial. To conclude that Mr Rattigan's clinical benefits were only due to cognitive behavioural therapy, and more specifically to the reattributional strategy described, would be unwise. Mr Rattigan was, however, a participant in a major, multi-centre randomised, controlled trial for cognitive behavioural therapy in early schizophrenia. It is to be hoped that trials such as these will provide evidence for the efficacy of cognitive behavioural therapy. Individual case studies such as this one allow the identification of the mechanisms and techniques that underpin this efficacy.

REFERENCES

Bentall, R.P., Haddock, G., & Slade, P.D. (1994). Cognitive behavior therapy for persistent auditory hallucinations: From theory to therapy. *Behavior Therapy*, *25*, 51–66.

Bentall, R.P., Jackson, H.F., & Pilgrim, D. (1988). Abandoning the concept of schizophrenia: Some implications of validity arguments for psychological research into psychotic phenomena. *British Journal of Clinical Psychology*, *27*, 303–324.

Bentall, R.P., & Kaney, S. (1989). Content-specific information processing and persecutory delusions: An investigation using the emotional Stroop test. *British Journal of Medical Psychology*, *62*, 355–364.

Bentall, R.P., & Kinderman, P. (1999). Self-regulation, affect and psychosis: The role of social cognition in paranoia and mania. In T. Dalgleish & M. Power (Eds.), *Handbook of Cognition and Emotion* (pp.351–381). Chichester: John Wiley.

Bentall, R.P., Kinderman, P., & Kaney, S. (1994). The self, attributional processes, and abnormal beliefs: Towards a model of persecutory delusions. *Behaviour Research and Therapy*, *32*, 331–341.

Birchwood, M. (1995). Early intervention into psychotic relapse: Cognitive approaches to detection and management. *Behaviour Change*, *12*, 2–19.

Birchwood, M., McGorry, P., & Jackson, H. (1997). Early intervention in schizophrenia. *British Journal of Psychiatry*, *170*, 2–5.

Buchanan, G.M., & Seligman, M.E.P. (Eds.) (1995). Explanatory style. Hillsdale, NJ: Lawrence Erlbaum Associates Inc.

Candido, C.L., & Romney, D.M. (1990). Attributional style in paranoid vs depressed patients. *British Journal of Medical Psychology*, *63*, 355–363.

Chadwick, P., & Birchwood, M. (1994). The omnipotence of voices: A cognitive approach to auditory hallucinations. *British Journal of Psychiatry*, *164*, 190–201.

Chadwick, P., & Lowe, C.F. (1990). The measurement and modification of delusional beliefs. *Journal of Consulting and Clinical Psychology*, *58*, 225–232.

DeGrada, E., Kruglanski, A.W., Mannetti, L., & Pierro, A. (1999). Motivated cognition and group interaction: Need for closure affects the contents and processes of collective negotiations. *Journal of Experimental Social Psychology*, *35(4)*, 346–365.

Dijksterhuis, A., van Knippenberg, A., Kruglanski, A.W., & Schaper, C. (1996). Motivated social cognition: Need for closure effects on memory and judgement. *Journal of Experimental Social Psychology*, *32(3)*, 254–270.

Fear, C.F., Sharpe, H., & Healy, D. (1996). Cognitive processes in delusional disorders. *British Journal of Psychiatry*, *168*, 61–67.

Fowler, D., Garety, P., & Kuipers, E. (1995). *Cognitive behaviour therapy for psychosis: Theory and practice*. Chichester: Wiley.

Garety, P.A., Fowler, D., Kuipers, E., Freeman, G., Dunn, G., Bebbington, P., Hadley, C., & Jones, S. (1997). London-East Anglia randomised controlled trial of cognitive behavioural therapy for psychosis, II: Predictors of outcome. *British Journal of Psychiatry*, *171*, 420–426.

Gilbert, D.T. (1989). Thinking lightly about others: Automatic components of the social inference process. In J.S. Uleman & J.A. Bargh (Eds.), *Unintended thought* (pp.189–211). New York: Guilford.

Gilbert, D.T., Krull, D.S., & Pelham, B.W. (1988). Of thoughts unspoken: Social inference and the self-regulation of behaviour. *Journal of Personality and Social Psychology*, *55*, 685–694.

Gilbert, D.T., McNulty, S.E., Giuliano, T.A., & Benson, J.E. (1992). Blurry words and fuzzy deeds: The attribution of obscure behavior. *Journal of Personality and Social Psychology*, *62(2)*, 18–25.

Green, M.F. (1992). Information processing in schizophrenia. In D.J. Kavanagh (Ed.), *Schizophrenia: An overview and practical handbook* (pp.45–58). London: Chapman and Hall.

Haddock, G., Bentall, R.P., & Slade, P.D. (1993). Psychological treatment of chronic auditory hallucinations: Two case studies. *Behavioural and Cognitive Psychotherapy*, *21*, 335–346.

Haddock, G., McCarron, J., Tarrier, N., & Faragher, E.B. (1999). Scales to measure dimensions of hallucinations and delusions: The psychotic symptom rating scales (PSYRATS). *Psychological Medicine*, *29*, 379–390.

Heider, F. (1958). *The psychology of interpersonal relations*. New York: Wiley.

Huq, S.F., Garety, P.A., & Hemsley, D.R. (1988). Probabilistic judgements in deluded and non-deluded subjects. *Quarterly Journal of Experimental Psychology*, *40A*, 801–812.

Kaney, S., & Bentall, R.P. (1989). Persecutory delusions and attributional style. *British Journal of Medical Psychology*, *62*, 191–198.

Kaney, S., & Bentall, R.P. (1992). Persecutory delusions and the self-serving bias. *Journal of Nervous and Mental Disease*, 180, 773–780.

Kay, S.R., & Opler, L.A. (1987). The Positive and Negative Syndrome Scale (PANSS) for schizophrenia. *Schizophrenia Bulletin*, *13*, 507–518.

Kinderman, P. (1994). Attentional bias, persecutory delusions, and the self concept. *British Journal of Medical Psychology*, *67*, 53–66.

Kinderman P. (2001). Changing causal attributions. In D. Penn & P. Corrigan (Eds.), *Social cognition of schizophrenia*. Chicago: American Psychological Association.

Kinderman, P., & Bentall, R.P. (1996). A new measure of causal locus: The Internal, Personal, and Situational Attributions Questionnaire. *Personality and Individual Differences*, *20(2)*, 261–264.

Kinderman, P., & Bentall, R.P. (1997a). Attributional therapy for paranoid delusions: A case study. *Behavioural and Cognitive Psychotherapy*, *25*, 269–280.

Kinderman, P., & Bentall, R.P. (1997b). Causal attributions in paranoia and depression: Internal, personal, and situational attributions for negative events. *Journal of Abnormal Psychology*, *106(2)*, 341–345.

Kinderman, P., Dunbar, R., & Bentall, R.P. (1999). Theory-of-mind deficits and causal attributions. *British Journal of Psychology*, *89*, 191–204.

Kingdon, D.G., & Turkington, D. (1994). Cognitive behavioural therapy of schizophrenia. Hove, UK: Lawrence Erlbaum Associates Ltd.

Kuipers, E., Garety, P., Fowler, D., Dunn, G., Bebbington, P., Freeman, D., & Hadley, C. (1997). The London-East Anglia randomised controlled trial of cognitive behavioural therapy for psychosis, I: Effects of the treatment phase. *British Journal of Psychiatry*, *171*, 319–327.

Lyon, H.M., Kaney, S., & Bentall, R.P. (1994). The defensive function of persecutory delusions: Evidence from attribution tasks. *British Journal of Psychiatry*, *164*, 637–646.

Persons, J. (1986). The advantages of studying psychological phenomena rather than psychiatric diagnoses. *American Psychologist*, *41*, 1252–1260.

Rosenberg, M. (1965). *The measurement of self-esteem*. Princeton: Princeton University Press.

Sharp, H.M., Fear, C.F., & Healy, D. (1997). Attributional style and delusions: An investigation based on delusional content. *European Psychiatry*, *12*, 1–7.

Tarrier, N., Beckett, R., Harwood, S., Baker, A., Yusupoff, L., & Ugarteburu, I. (1993). A trial of two cognitive behavioural methods of treating drug-resistant residual psychotic symptoms in schizophrenic patients, I: Outcome. *British Journal of Psychiatry*, *162*, 524–532.

Weiner, B., Russell, D., & Lerman, D. (1978). The cognition-emotion process in achievement-related contexts. *Journal of Personality and Social Psychology*, *37*, 1211–1220.

Part III

New developments in cognitive therapies for psychoses

Cognitive therapy for preventing transition to psychosis in high-risk individuals

A single case study

Paul French, Anthony P. Morrison, Lara Walford, Alice Knight, and Richard P. Bentall

INTRODUCTION

There is a growing body of evidence to suggest that it is possible to identify people who are at a high risk of developing a psychotic illness. Significantly, in the latest reforms to the British National Health Service there is an emphasis on the need to develop strategies and teams to deliver early interventions for psychosis.

The aetiology of schizophrenia and related psychotic disorders is at present unknown, but there exists a general consensus among researchers and clinicians that a stress vulnerability model best accounts for the available data (Gottesman, 1991; Gottesman, & Shields, 1982; Neuchterlein & Dawson, 1984; Zubin & Spring, 1977). This kind of model suggests that there exists some biological vulnerability to the disorder but that transition to psychotic illness is determined by exposure to environmental stressors. The first person to articulate this type of model was Paul Meehl (1962), who proposed the concept of "schizotaxia" to describe the neurointegrative deficit that he believed conferred vulnerability to schizophrenia. According to Meehl, most schizotaxic individuals will never go on to develop schizophrenia but instead will show schizotypal personality characteristics. However, a proportion who are exposed to appropriate stressors will "decomponsate" and become ill.

Biological factors that contribute to vulnerability to psychosis have attracted a great deal of attention from researchers since the publication of Meehl's seminal paper. For example, vulnerability has been attributed to genetic predisposition (Murray & McGuffin, 1993) and to events that might subtly damage the developing nervous system, such as foetal exposure to the influenza virus (McGrath & Murray, 1995). Theories of this sort aim to explain why some individuals appear to be at greater risk of developing psychotic symptoms in general compared with most people in the population. In contrast, psychological theorists have recently turned away from all-encompassing models of psychosis and have instead attempted to develop cognitive models of specific symptoms. For example, Morrison, Haddock, and Tarrier (1995) and Morrison (1998a) have generalised from some theories of anxiety in the attempt to explain some aspects of hallucinated voices, and Bentall, Kinderman, and Kaney (1994) have attempted to explain paranoid delusions using concepts borrowed from attribution theory. As some vulnerability factors may operate to create a non-specific increase in risk of serious mental disorder, whereas specific psychological processes may be implicated in specific symptoms, it may be possible to reconcile these two approaches and integrate them within a general framework.

WHY IDENTIFY PEOPLE AT RISK AND INTERVENE EARLY?

Clinical researchers have recently drawn attention to the likely benefits of providing interventions early in the course of a psychotic illness (McGlashen, 1996). There is now a growing body of evidence suggesting that there is often a considerable lapse of time between when a person first experiences psychotic symptoms and treatment, known as duration of untreated psychosis (DUP). Averages from four recent studies suggest that DUP in developed countries ranges between 52 weeks and 156 weeks, and that the mean duration of untreated illness (DUI, which includes the prodromal phase) can range between 112 and 239 weeks (Larsen, McGlashen, & Moe, 1996). Therefore, most people will be actually experiencing psychotic symptoms for around a year prior to treatment. Studies of the pathways to treatment confirm this general picture; for example, in the Northwick Park study (Johnstone et al., 1986) it was found that patients experienced an average of six helper contacts before adequate treatment was delivered. This observation suggests that people experiencing psychosis often present for assistance without their symptoms being picked up by professionals. This could be for a number of reasons. For example, patients may be reluctant to disclose their difficulties (Moller & Husby, 2000), professionals may be unable to recognise prodromal symptoms, and there may be a shared desire to minimise symptomatology for fear of labelling. However, recent studies have shown that the DUP is implicated in long-term outcome (Loebel et al., 1992; McGlashen & Johannessen, 1996) with lengthier periods without treatment associated with poorer outcome. Wyatt (1995) has therefore suggested that untreated psychosis may be biologically toxic. There would therefore seem to be a strong case for reducing DUP (Sullivan, 1927) and this might be achieved by effective monitoring of people at high risk of experiencing psychotic episodes.

So far, most interventions designed for this purpose have been directed towards secondary prevention, with the aim of reducing the risk of further episodes in people who have already been ill. Most strategies in this have focused on the ability of indicators to identify relapse patterns (Herz & Melville, 1980) and interventions have typically been pharmacological. More recently, however, the use of cognitive models to understand the process of relapse and to guide psychotherapeutic interventions has been explored (Gumley & Power, 2000).

Primary prevention interventions in mental health have been few and far between, although Mrazek and Haggerty (1994) have outlined three basic strategies that might be used for this purpose. These are universal (adopting strategies aimed at the whole population), selective (focusing on all those exposed to risk factors), and indicated (focusing on high-risk individuals with minimal but detectable signs). Of these, indicated prevention appears to be the most practical in terms of the resources required. The statistics relating to schizophrenia alone support this viewpoint. Although the lifetime risk of schizophrenia in the general population is about 1%, this increases as a function of genetic proximity to a relative with the disorder to around 45% for a child of two parents diagnosed with schizophrenia (Sham et al., 1994). This means that even if we target interventions at the selective group according to biological theories, the maximum transition to psychosis we could expect is 45%. We also need to consider that the majority of people who develop psychotic disorders have no familial history (Asarnow, 1988), which again tends to advocate against selective interventions. The universal strategy, in contrast, would require a great deal of resource provision. It would have to rely upon education, which is certainly an important factor in overall attempts at reducing stigma and increasing public knowledge about psychosis, although the efficacy of this approach to prevention is uncertain. Therefore, in terms of the most appropriate strategy available to be delivered in a pragmatic manner, indicated prevention seems to be the way forward.

CAN HIGH-RISK INDIVIDUALS BE IDENTIFIED?

There is emerging evidence that risk indicators can be used to predict psychotic episodes (Falloon et al., 1996; Olin & Mednick, 1996; Yung & McGorry, 1996; Yung et al., 1998); some combinations of indicators (both state and trait factors) can effectively identify a high-risk sample of whom 40% became psychotic after just 6 months (Yung & McGorry, 1996; Yung et al., 1998). One study suggests that primary care staff can be trained to identify risk indicators (Falloon, 1992) and other studies suggest that teachers' reports can be powerful predictors of later psychotic episodes (Olin et al., 1998). Other risk factors identified to date have included adolescent and childhood problems, schizotypal personality (Yung et al., 1998), schizotypal traits (Chapman et al., 1994), and a family history of schizophrenia spectrum disorders (Asarnow, 1988).

These studies have either used a prospective or retrospective design. The former include the genetic high-risk studies, which have identified children of parents with an existing disorder and followed them up over time, limiting the number of cases available for study and ignoring those people who have no family history. Although the retrospective design enables more people to be studied, research of this sort is reliant on the accuracy of memory or records.

A new approach was recently proposed by Yung et al. (1998). They embraced the prodromal approach, which has been utilised for some time in studies of the relapse prodrome in psychotic patients (Birchwood & Mac-Millan, 1993; Linszen et al., 1998; McGlashen, 1996). However, Yung et al.'s (1998) study attempted to identify people who were in the initial prodrome prior to developing psychotic symptoms. They describe how 40% of their sample made the transition to psychosis over a 12-month period. The criteria used by Yung et al. (1998) to define someone as being at incipient risk of psychosis produced two groups. Specific state risk factors operationally defined by the presence of either transient psychotic symptoms (brief limited intermittent psychotic symptoms, or BLIPS according to Yung et al.'s terminology) or attenuated psychotic symptoms (subclinical), both of which used duration and severity criteria (the latter based on BPRS cut-off scores), made up one group. Trait plus state risk factors operationally defined by the presence of an at risk mental state plus either a first degree relative with a history of any psychotic disorder or a diagnosis of schizotypal personality disorder in the individual accounted for the second group.

HOW TO INTERVENE?

The improved ability to accurately define high-risk groups achieved by the work of Yung and her colleagues has led researchers to attempt prevention with atypical neuroleptic medication (Miller & McGlashen, 2000). In this study an atypical neuroleptic (olanzapine) is compared with placebo medication. If someone does make the transition to psychosis then the blind is immediately broken and neuroleptics prescribed. However, the problem then arises that, although the onset of a psychotic illness may be prevented in up to 40% of the population identified, a further 60% of those identified will be treated aggressively with neuroleptic medication without good cause.

Given that the risks associated with using pharmacological interventions with false positive cases are considerable (Yung & McGorry, 1996), the logical alternative would seem to be the use of psycho-social interventions already proven in the treatment of psychotic disorders (Falloon, 1992). Cognitive behavioural therapy (CBT), perhaps the best researched and most widely recognised treatment of this sort, would pose little risk to the false positive group; indeed the problem-orientated nature of this intervention would mean that it may even be of benefit to these individuals.

An initial paper by Beck in 1952 examined the potential of cognitive interventions to challenge delusional beliefs. Subsequent to this, there were a number of small-scale studies (Chadwick & Lowe 1990; Watts, Powell, & Austin 1973) that served to maintain interest in the ability of cognitive and behavioural interventions to impact on the symptoms of psychosis. However, the past decade has seen a growing interest in CBT for psychotic symptoms and a number of carefully conducted randomised controlled trials have indicated the efficacy of this form of treatment (Drury et al., 1996; Kuipers et al., 1997; Sensky et al., 2000; Tarrier et al., 1998). In fact, on the basis of a meta-analysis of the data on the randomised controlled trials to date, it has been suggested that not to provide CBT for psychosis would be unethical (Beck & Rector, 2000). The success of cognitive therapy for both psychotic symptoms and mood-related symptoms (which are highly prevalent in psychotic prodromes; Birchwood et al., 1998) suggests that this approach may be uniquely suitable for preventing transition to psychosis.

Therefore, our strategy is to identify an indicated high-risk group and then offer a psychological intervention (CBT) with the aim of preventing the transition to psychosis. This chapter describes a single case from a randomised controlled trial that aims to evaluate the efficacy of this approach.

A SIMPLE HEURISTIC MODEL FOR UNDERSTANDING THE ONSET OF PSYCHOSIS

One of the fundamental principles of CBT is that therapy should be based on a cognitive model. There are several models that attempt to explain the maintenance of psychotic symptoms, such as the model for hallucinations proposed by Morrison (1998a) and the model of delusions proposed by Bentall, Kinderman, and Kaney (1994), but there has been less attention paid to the development of psychosis and the initial onset of symptoms. A simple heuristic model will be outlined here, followed by a case that illustrates it more fully.

The model, shown in Fig. 12.1, draws on the stress vulnerability literature (Neuchterlein & Dawson, 1984; Zubin & Spring, 1977); stress and vulnerability factors are presumed to interact to leave the person at a high risk for the subsequent development of symptoms. We assume that some individuals will experience triggering events, which can be external to the person (e.g. someone looking at them strangely) or internal (e.g. the experience of a very unusual thought), and that these events will therefore lead to unusual cognitive and perceptual experiences as explained by previous models of psychotic symptoms. In the model, the ability to generate and evaluate alternative explanations for these experiences is an important factor determining outcome, and this includes both external factors (e.g. having someone that the person can speak to in order to check things out) and cognitive abilities (e.g.

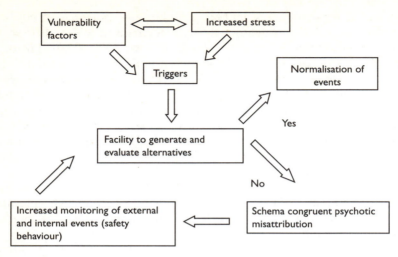

Figure 12.1 Model of development of early psychotic symptoms.

problem-solving and evaluation strategies). If this ability is impaired, it is possible that the stressed and vulnerable individual will start to make sense of the trigger in ways that are congruent with their dysfunctional schemas, possibly leading to a psychotic misattribution of the initial trigger. (Morrison (2001) has suggested that it is the cultural unacceptability of an interpretation that leads to it being regarded as psychotic; an impaired ability to generate alternative explanations is likely to result in an increase in culturally unacceptable interpretations because they are not subject to social validation or scrutiny.) This may then lead to an increase in self-monitoring behaviour, again directed at both external events (e.g. reading the papers more avidly to see if any news is personally-directed), and internal events (e.g. increased monitoring of unusual thoughts to see if they are repeated). This idea is similar to the concept of safety behaviours (strategies employed to avert feared catastrophes; see Salkovskis, 1991), which has recently been suggested to contribute to the maintenance of psychotic symptoms (Morrison, 1998b). Once further threatening events are detected because of increased self-monitoring, the person may again fail to generate and evaluate alternative explanations for these experiences, potentially creating a vicious cycle.

The exit from this cycle may be via the ability to generate and evaluate alternatives, which might be facilitated by a close friend, or a cognitive behaviour therapist who can help the individual to consider other ways of thinking, encourage better hypothesis testing strategies, and normalise the triggering events.

The model provides an account of psychosis that is acceptable to clients, is easily understood, and yet allows for a detailed cognitive exploration of symptom development. It suggests a possible explanation of why non-specific interventions such as befriending may reduce symptoms in the short term (Sensky et al., 2000), and is supported by the work of Moller and Husby (2000), who found that patients experiencing their first episode reported "reduced will" and a "reduced ability" to disclose their initial psychotic experiences. A case will shortly be described that highlights the various components of the model and their implications for treatment.

SPECIFICS OF THE THERAPY PROCESS: ENGAGEMENT

Engaging clients in this kind of work presents particular challenges. A flexible and collaborative approach is required in order to engage and subsequently maintain the client in therapy. The development of trust and rapport early on in the therapeutic relationship will play a key role in achieving this. Good engagement early in treatment may also lead to future benefits should the transition to psychosis occur, including improved adherence with a treatment programme and enhanced cooperation with the psychiatric team. This may lead to a reduced requirement for in-patient admissions or reduced formal admissions to hospital.

It is unrealistic to expect people to travel far in order to attend an appointment. The therapist should therefore make appointments at a location that is easily accessible, such as a GP surgery. Secondary care service settings are to be avoided if at all possible, as these may be perceived as stigmatising. At times the client may be seen at their home, but this should be an offer not an imposition. The timing of the appointment needs to be agreed collaboratively; it may be necessary to offer appointments outside office hours.

Because the various indicators of risk do not yield a homogenous group with regard to symptom presentation, the therapist has to be aware of a wide range of cognitive models and draw upon these in order to deliver appropriate interventions. This makes this approach somewhat different from many of the interventions tested in CBT trials, which use manuals to very specifically define the symptom profile to be treated and the interventions to be utilised.

A CASE EXAMPLE: JOHN

A young man, John, presented to his GP, apparently experiencing delusional ideas. He believed that calamities such as accidents were going to happen to him, and also that he was able to cause unpleasant events to happen to other people, including an accident that happened to his friend. John thought that he was the Devil's son and was cursed. He also had ideas of reference, believing that articles in newspapers referred to him. He felt unable to discuss these experiences with his family and felt so frightened that people were attempting to harm him that he had stopped eating and was drinking only water for fear of being poisoned. When he was finally taken to see his GP, he was certain that he was going to be killed by a lethal injection. These ideas were extremely distressing to him. A relative at the time described an episode when he became so distressed while travelling on a bus that he had to get off a long way from his home. A shopkeeper, who obviously recognised John's distress and confusion, telephoned his relative who came to pick him up. These ideas were short-lived (approximately one week) and they resolved themselves spontaneously without the use of neuroleptic medication. The GP prescribed a course of antidepressant medication and referred John to the practice counsellor and also to a consultant psychiatrist.

The practice counsellor subsequently referred John to the local Department of Clinical Psychology and, after being assessed by one of the clinical psychologists, he was referred to our research team. He entered the study via the Brief Limited Intermittent Psychotic Symptoms (BLIPS) Group, as he had experienced frank psychotic symptoms that had resolved spontaneously after a short period of time.

At initial assessment, John's symptoms were measured using the Positive and Negative Syndromes Scale (PANSS; Kay, Fiszbein, & Opler, 1987). An attempt was also made to retrospectively assess John's symptoms at their worst, using the definitions contained in the PANSS positive symptoms subscale. His scores are shown in Fig. 12.2. As can be seen from the figure, there was limited evidence of psychotic ideation at the time of assessment, although John was very concerned about whether his BLIPS would recur and wanted to understand why this had occurred in the first place. Obviously, someone who has had experiences of this sort is then vulnerable to further symptoms. If they worry about this possibility they may become hypervigilant and this may increase the likelihood that this will happen. The aim of intervention with people in the BLIPS Group must therefore be to facilitate their escape from this vicious cycle.

Although John was experiencing minimal psychotic symptoms at the time of assessment, he was presenting as anxious, depressed, and emotionally and socially withdrawn—symptoms that have all been linked to the relapse prodrome (Birchwood et al., 1989). Social withdrawal has also been identified as a behavioural marker of the initial prodrome (Moller & Husby, 2000). There was also evidence of a loss of 50 points on his overall level of functioning as measured by the Global Assessment of Functioning (GAF; American Psychiatric Association, 1994), a simple 100-point measure of psychological, social, and occupational ability designed to be concordant with DSM-IV (American Psychiatric Association, 1994).

The client was randomised to treatment, which comprises psychological interventions, driven by the model previously presented. There were five therapy sessions required by John, the details of which are described below.

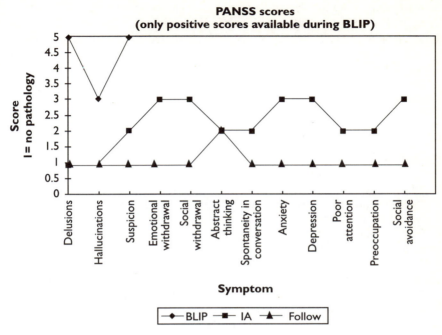

Figure 12.2 John's PANSS scores.

Session one

Before the beginning of the session, on the way to the interview room, John said that he did not feel much like talking and had very little to say. The process of engaging John was therefore difficult: it was necessary to socialise him to the cognitive model and explain the structure of therapy while also recognising that he had already been involved with a number of professionals. It is important to address patients' expectations of therapy during this initial phase. It transpired that John had anticipated his treatment would involve spending a great deal of time discussing his childhood, an expectation that he quickly abandoned. Emphasising the collaborative nature of therapy, that the focus of the treatment was in the here and now, and that the therapy would be problem-orientated, therefore facilitated the engagement process. The principal aim of the initial therapeutic assessment was to understand John's predominant concerns, which were about what had happened to him, his fear that it would happen again, and his anxiety in social situations. After assessing his recent history it was clear that he had been under significant amounts of stress because of a number of critical events: his father's problem drinking; the death of a best friend's father (who was also a problem drinker);

the ending of his relationship with a long-standing girlfriend; increased stress at work; and an attack by someone in a local pub who hit him with a bottle.

Quickly reviewing these incidents, it is hardly surprising that John was experiencing stress. This observation was presented back to him as a means of normalising his distress. The assault seemed to offer a clue about the origins of his paranoid beliefs. At the end of the session John was given a rationale for the intervention both verbally and in written form to take away, which is given in the panel.

BLIPS Group rationale

At some point in the recent past you will have experienced some odd thoughts, perceived things slightly different or maybe heard things such as noises or voices even when there was no one around. These things may have caused you some distress, or may even have led to people around you becoming concerned about you.

Around this time you may have been under more than usual amounts of stress for various reasons and this could have affected things like sleep, you might have started drinking more than usual, or even taking drugs. In combination, reduced sleep and increased stress can lead to people having "odd thoughts" which would be out of keeping with the way they generally think about things.

These strange experiences will have gone and you will possibly not want to talk about them much perhaps out of fear that they may return or because they were so upsetting that you just want to forget about them. It may be the case that these things never come back again and you will be fine. However, there is also a possibility that in the future if you are in a similar position with increased amounts of stress that you may react in a similar way.

What we feel, is that by tackling these difficulties rather than leaving them we can work to prevent any further difficulties in the future or certainly to minimise the potential of them happening in the future. The way we propose to do this is through a talking form of therapy which will look at the way you think about things and how these thoughts impact upon what you do and how you feel.

Session two

A tentative model of John's experiences was collaboratively discussed, and this was presented in the form of a longitudinal formulation, which is shown in Fig. 12.3. Time was also spent reviewing the influence of thoughts on

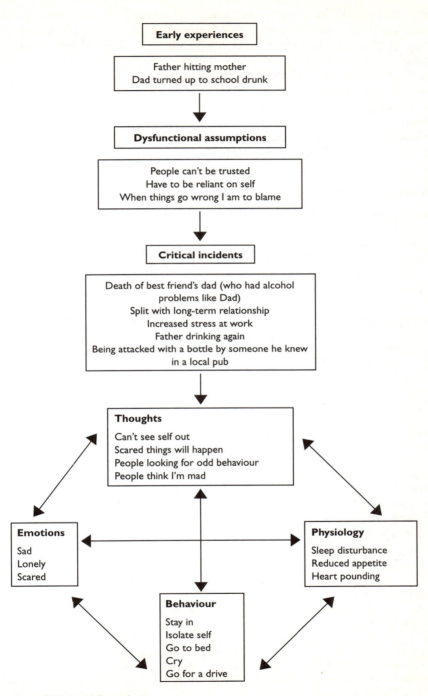

Figure 12.3 Initial formulation.

behaviours and emotions, taking the maintenance aspect of the formulation to illustrate how the process had continued. The remainder of the session was spent developing problem statements and choosing SMART (specific, measureable, achievable, realistic and time-limited) goals. This approach enables the patient and the therapist to agree targets that they can work towards over a relatively short period of time, ensuring that the patient has success experiences. Clearly defined goals also enable the patient to break down and define their problems rather than viewing them as a mass of over-whelming difficulties, increasing optimism. The resulting list of prioritised problems and goals is shown in Table 12.1.

Session three

During this session the main agenda item was to work on the first problem on the problem list—social anxiety and avoidance—as this was causing the most concern for John. The usual review of previous work was undertaken before-hand, and this revealed a recent incident that exemplified this difficulty.

John had been about to go shopping and was going to catch the train to a local shopping centre. However, while going for the train he met someone he knew who asked "how are things?": John became self-conscious, started to feel that people were watching him, and this made him scan the environment for other indicators of people watching him. He became introverted and unable to discuss anything with them, and subsequently returned home due to his feelings of fear and anxiety.

This incident was discussed in terms of the model. It was suggested that if John had had the opportunity to talk through his experiences with a

Table 12.1 John's prioritised problems and goals

Problem	Goal statement
One John was experiencing social anxiety that prevented him from going out and enjoying himself.	**One** For John to be able to go out at least once per week with friends who do not understand about his illness (such as his brother or friend) and be able to stay out for at least two hours without wanting to return home.
Two John wanted to prevent this from happening again.	**Two** We decided not to spend time on this at this point and recognised that this would be a hard goal to achieve and measure but was an understandable problem that he wanted to work on.

sympathetic person, he would have been able to reappraise the situation and consider alternative explanations of what was happening. John felt very unsure what he could say to people if they asked him how he was, so the therapist worked collaboratively with him to find a suitable form of words. Role-play was then utilised until he was comfortable with his chosen way of describing his experiences, and he was able to use it in a relaxed and comfortable manner. This discussion led to the joint development of a revision to the model of early psychosis presented to John, which took into account his particular history and experiences. This revised model is shown in Fig. 12.4.

The homework task agreed from this session was to go out and, if a similar situation arose, to try out John's statement about his experiences with an appropriate friend. Also, if John was approached by someone whom he felt comfortable talking to about his illness, then he should do so and monitor what they said. As John had not discussed his concerns with anyone from his social circle, this had prevented him from having access to normalising data. It was hypothesised that some of his friends may have had similar experiences, or if they had not, then they would nonetheless be supportive of him. The assumption we were testing was, therefore, "If I discuss it with people then they will think I am going mad".

Session four

At the homework review John found that he had only used the agreed form of words a couple of times, but that it had been available to him as a safety net had it been required. However, he had come across two other people in his

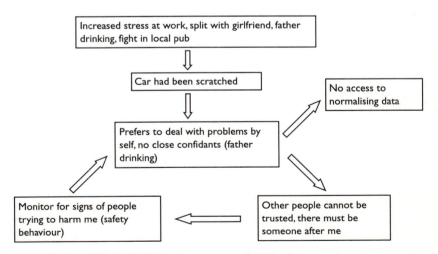

Figure 12.4 Idiosyncratic model of emergence of psychotic symptoms.

close circle of friends and had disclosed some of the things he had been experiencing, and this had turned out to be highly beneficial. Interestingly, both friends had experienced some form of psychotic symptoms. One person had experienced paranoia to the point where he had wanted to move away from the area, an apparent consequence of his use of illicit drugs. Also, a close relative reported seeing an hallucination one morning upon waking, which had appeared incredibly real and frightening. These two experiences served to normalise John's experiences and he felt significantly more relaxed as a consequence. In the homework review it also transpired that John had made significant progress towards his goal in relation to problem one, and was now socialising more, and with less distress and concern, than anticipated. He was able to stay out as long as he desired without his fears making him return home.

During this session the main agenda item was to focus on problem two, which involved reviewing signs and symptoms that had led to him becoming ill. The Early Signs Scale (Birchwood et al., 1989) was utilised as a way of structuring information and collecting data about what had happened. This served a useful purpose and we were able to develop a time frame for the prodrome being around 7–8 weeks. The homework from this session was for John to review the early signs and, at his request, for him rather than the therapist to consult with relatives and ascertain any further signs that should be included.

Session five

The main agenda item in this session was the development of an action plan, to include cognitive strategies, that John could employ, especially when he experienced increased stress and sleep disturbance, which seemed to be predictors of psychotic symptoms. It was important that John should have copies of the formulations we had developed regarding onset and development of problems, with strategies used in therapy to overcome them, and also details of the experiments we had undertaken. These were all to be reviewed in the event that he experienced difficulties in the future. Other non-cognitive strategies—for example contacting the GP—were included in the plan, with the intention that they could be used if early strategies failed and he entered the later stages of his relapse.

The agreement of this plan concluded the interventions. In five sessions he had made significant progress, to the point that he planned a trip away on holiday, was considering a change of career, and felt positive about the future. As John felt that his problems had been largely resolved as a consequence of the therapeutic intervention, no further sessions were planned. John agreed to be followed up at two monthly intervals by a research assistant. Details of his PANSS scores can be seen in Fig. 12.2. At two-month follow-up John was not experiencing any psychotic ideation, was not emotionally or socially withdrawn, and reported no symptoms of anxiety. John appeared quite comfortable talking to the assessor and reported going out with friends. He did report feeling a little fed up because of boredom but added that he could be easily cheered up. At four-month follow-up, John had changed his job and reported an active social life. At eight months all benefits had been maintained.

REFERENCES

American Psychiatric Association (1994). *Diagnostic and Statistical Manual of Mental Disorders (DSM)* (Fourth Edition). Washington DC: American Psychiatric Association Press.

Asarnow, J.R. (1988). Children at risk for schizophrenia: Converging lines of evidence. *Schizophrenia Bulletin, 14*, 613–631.

Beck, A.T. (1952). Successful outpatient psychotherapy of a chronic schizophrenic with a delusion based on borrowed guilt. *Psychiatry, 15*, 305–312.

Beck, A.T., & Rector, N. (2000). Cognitive therapy for schizophrenia: A new therapy for the new millennium. *American Journal of Psychotherapy, 54(3)*, 291–300.

Bentall, R.P., Kinderman, P., & Kaney, S. (1994). The self, attributional processes, and abnormal beliefs: Towards a model of persecutory delusions. *Behaviour Research and Therapy, 32*, 331–341.

Birchwood, M., & MacMillan, J.F. (1993). Early intervention in schizophrenia. *The Australian and New Zealand Journal of Psychiatry, 27*, 374–378.

Birchwood, M., Smith, J., Macmillan, F., Hogg, B., Prasad, R., Harvey, C., & Bering, S. (1989). Predicting relapse in schizophrenia: The development and implementation of an early signs monitoring system using patients and families as observers. *Psychological Medicine, 19*, 649–656.

Birchwood, M., Smith, J., Macmillan, F., & McGovern, D. (1998). Early intervention in psychotic relapse. In C. Brooker & J. Repper (Eds.), *Serious mental health problems in the community: Policy, practice, and research*. London: Bailliere Tindall.

Chadwick, P.D., & Lowe, C.F. (1990). Measurement and modification of delusional beliefs. *Journal of Consulting and Clinical Psychology, 58*, 225–232.

Chapman, L.J., Chapman, J.P., Kwapil, T.R., Eckblad, M., & Zinser, M.C. (1994). Putatively psychosis-prone subjects 10 years later. *Journal of Abnormal Psychology, 103(2)*, 171–183.

Drury, V., Birchwood, M., Cochrane, R., & Macmillan, F. (1996). Cognitive therapy and recovery from acute psychosis: A controlled trial—I Impact on Psychotic Symptoms. *British Journal of Psychiatry, 169*, 593–601.

Falloon, I.R.H. (1992). Early intervention for first episodes of schizophrenia: A preliminary exploration. *Psychiatry, 55*, 4–15.

Falloon, I.R.H., Kydd, R.R., Coverdale, J.H., & Laidlaw, T.M. (1996). Early detection and intervention for initial episodes of schizophrenia. *Schizophrenia Bulletin, 22(2)*, 271–282.

Gottesman, I.I. (1991). *Schizophrenia genesis: The origins of madness*. San Francisco: Freeman.

Gottesman, I.I., & Shields, J. (1982). *Schizophrenia: The epigenetic puzzle.* Cambridge: Cambridge University Press.

Gumley, A.I., & Power, K.G. (2000). Is targeting cognitive therapy during relapse in psychosis feasible? *Behavioural and Cognitive Psychotherapy, 28(2)*, 161–174.

Herz, M., & Melville, C. (1980). Relapse in schizophrenia. *American Journal of Psychiatry, 137*, 801–812.

Johnstone, E.C., Crow, T.J., Johnson, A., & Macmillan, J. (1986). The Northwick Park study of first episode schizophrenia, I: Presentations of the illness and problems relating to admission. *British Journal of Psychiatry, 148*, 115–120.

Kay, S.R., Fiszbein, A., & Opler, L.A. (1987). The Positive and Negative Syndrome Scale (PANSS) for schizophrenia. *Schizophrenia Bulletin, 13*, 261–276.

Kuipers, E., Garety, P., Fowler, D., Dunn, G., Bebbington, P., Freeman, D., & Hadley C. (1997). London-East Anglia randomised controlled trial of cognitive behavioural therapy for psychosis, I: Effects of the treatment phase. *British Journal of Psychiatry, 171*, 319–327.

Larsen, T.K., McGlashen, T.H., & Moe, L.C. (1996). First episode schizophrenia, I: Early course parameters. *Schizophrenia Bulletin, 22*, 241–256.

Linszen, D.H., Dingemans, P.M.A.J., Lenior, M.E., Scholte, W.F., Haan, L., & Goldstein, M.J. (1998). Early detection and intervention in schizophrenia. *International Clinical Psychopharmacology, 13(suppl. 3)*, 32–34.

Loebel, A.D., Lieberman, J.A., Alvir, J.M.J., Mayerhoff, D.I., Geisler, S.H., & Szymanski, S.R. (1992). Duration of psychosis and outcome in first episode schizophrenia. *American Journal of Psychiatry, 149*, 1183–1188.

McGlashen, T.H. (1996). Early detection and intervention in schizophrenia: Research. *Schizophrenia Bulletin, 22*: 327–345.

McGlashen, T.H., & Johannessen, J.O. (1996). Early detection and intervention with schizophrenia: rationale, *Schizophrenia Bulletin, 22*, 201–222.

McGrath, J., & Murray, R. (1995). Risk factors for schizophrenia: From conception to birth. In S.R. Hirsch & D.R. Weinberger (Eds), *Schizophrenia* (pp.187–205). Oxford: Blackwell Science.

Meehl, P.E. (1962). Schizotaxia, schizotypy and schizophrenia. *American Psychologist, 17*, 827–838.

Miller, T.J., & McGlashan, T.H. (2000). Early identification and intervention in psychotic illness. *American Journal of Psychiatry, 157(7)*, 1041–1050.

Moller, P., & Husby, R. (2000). The initial prodrome in schizoprenia: Searching for naturalistic core dimensions of experience and behaviour. *Schizophrenia Bulletin, 26(1)*, 217–232.

Morrison, A.P. (1998a). A cognitive analysis of the maintenance of auditory hallucinations: are voices to schizophrenia what bodily sensations are to panic? *Behavioural and Cognitive Psychotherapy, 26(4)*, 289–302.

Morrison, A.P. (1998b). Cognitive behaviour therapy for psychotic symptoms in schizophrenia. In N. Tarrier, A. Wells, & G. Haddock (Eds.), *Treating complex cases: The cognitive behavioural therapy approach* (pp.195–216). Chichester: Wiley.

Morrison, A.P. (2001). The interpretation of intrusions in psychosis: An integrative cognitive approach to hallucinations and delusions. *Behavioural and Cognitive Psychotherapy, 29*, 257–276.

Morrison, A.P., Haddock, G., & Tarrier, N. (1995). Intrusive thoughts and auditory hallucinations: A cognitive approach. *Behavioural and Cognitive Psychotherapy*, *23*, 265–280.

Mrazek, P.J., & Haggerty, R.J. (Eds.) (1994). *Reducing risks for mental disorders: Frontiers for preventative intervention research.* Washington, DC: National Academy Press.

Murray, R.M., & McGuffin, P. (1993). Genetic aspects of psychiatric disorders. In R.E. Kendell & A.K. Zealley (Eds.), *Companion to psychiatric studies* (pp. 227–261). Edinburgh: Churchill Livingstone.

Neuchterlein, K.H., & Dawson, M. (1984). A heuristic vulnerability stress model of schizophrenic episodes. *Schizophrenia Bulletin*, *10*, 300–312.

Olin, S.S., & Mednick, S.A. (1996). Risk factors of psychosis: identifying vulnerable populations premorbidly. *Schizophrenia Bulletin*, *22(2)*, 223–240.

Olin, S.S., Mednick, S.A., Cannon, T., Jacobsen, B., Parnas, J., Schulsinger, F., & Schulsinger, H. (1998). School teacher ratings predictive of psychiatric outcome 25 years later. *British Journal of Psychiatry*, *172(suppl. 33)*, 7–13.

Salkovskis, P.M. (1991). The importance of behaviour in the maintenance of anxiety and panic: A cognitive account. *Behavioural Psychotherapy*, *19*, 6–19.

Sensky, T., Turkington, D., Kingdon, D., Scott, J.L., Scott, J., Siddle, R., O'Carroll, M., & Barnes, T.R.E. (2000). A randomised controlled trial of cognitive behavioral therapy for persistent symptoms in schizophrenia resistant to medication. *Archives of General Psychiatry*, *57(2)*, 165–172.

Sham, P.C., Jones, P., Russell, A., Gilvarry, K., Bebbington, P., Lewis, S., Toone, B., & Murray, R. (1994). Age at onset, sex, and familial psychiatric morbidity in schizophrenia: Camberwell collaborative psychosis study. *British Journal of Psychiatry*, *165*, 466–473.

Sullivan, H.S. (1927). The onset of schizophrenia. Reprinted in *American Journal of Psychiatry*, *151(6)* (June 1994 Sesquicentennial Supplement), 135–139.

Tarrier, N., Yusupoff, L., Kinney, C., McCarthy, E., Gledhill, A., Haddock, G., & Morris, J. (1998). Randomised controlled trial of intensive cognitive behaviour therapy for patients with chronic schizophrenia. *British Medical Journal*, *317*, 303–307.

Watts, F.N., Powell, G.E., & Austin, S.V. (1973). The modification of abnormal beliefs. *Behaviour Journal of Medicine and Psychology*, *46*, 359–363.

Wyatt, R.J. (1995). Early intervention in schizophrenia: Can the course of the illness be altered? *Biological Psychiatry*, *38*, 1–3.

Yung, A., & McGorry, P.D. (1996). The prodromal phase of first episode psychosis: Past and current conceptualisations. *Schizophrenia Bulletin*, *22*, 353–370.

Yung, A., Phillips, L.J., McGorry, P.D., McFarlane, C.A., Francey, S., Harrigan, S., Patton, G.C., & Jackson, H.J. (1998). A step towards indicated prevention of schizophrenia. *British Journal of Psychiatry*, *172(suppl. 33)*, 14–20.

Zubin, J., & Spring, B. (1977). Vulnerability: A new view of schizophrenia. *Journal of Abnormal Psychology*, *86*, 103–126.

Chapter 13

Cognitive therapy for clients with bipolar disorder

Jan Scott

INTRODUCTION

The aims of therapy for bipolar disorder (BD) are to alleviate acute symptoms, restore psycho-social functioning, and prevent relapse and recurrence. The benefits of pharmacotherapy have dominated the literature on treatment. However, in day-to-day clinical settings, lithium prophylaxis protects only 25–50% of BD sufferers against further episodes (Dickson & Kendall, 1986) and the introduction of newer medications has not improved prognosis (Scott, 1995a). In the past two decades there has been a greater emphasis on stress diathesis models. This has led to the development of new aetiological theories of severe mental disorders that emphasise psychological aspects of vulnerability and risk and has also increased the acceptance of cognitive therapy (CT) as an adjunct to medication for individuals with treatment-resistant schizophrenia and severe and chronic depressive disorders (Scott & Wright, 1997). Research in BD has been limited, but as described later, there is evidence that CT may benefit this client group. This chapter explores current psychological models of BD. It comments on the clinical applicability of CT, and also reviews outcome research. Lastly, a case example is used to outline the basic structure of the intervention and highlight how CT may be used to address the problems typically faced by clients with BD.

THEORETICAL MODELS OF BIPOLAR DISORDER AND THE USE OF COGNITIVE THERAPY

Theoretical models: The story so far

At present, psychological theories of BD are relatively under-researched and there are few insights to aid our understanding and to explain how therapy achieves its effects (Lam & Wong, 1997; Scott, 2001a). However, it is possible to use an adaptation of Beck's original model of depression and mania to increase its utility in working with BD (Beck, 1996; Beck, Rush, Shaw, &

Emery, 1979; Healey & Williams, 1989; Scott, 1995b;). The description of this model should not be regarded as an empirical explanation of the aetiology of BD, but it provides a framework for understanding the psychopathology of this disorder and how cognitive and behavioural approaches may be targeted at specific symptoms and problems.

Beck's original cognitive model suggests that depressed mood states are accentuated by patterns of thinking that amplify mood shifts. For example, as people become depressed they become more negative in how they see themselves, their world, and their future (called the negative cognitive triad). Hence they tend to jump to negative conclusions, overgeneralise, see things in all-or-nothing terms, and personalise and self-blame to an excessive degree (cognitive distortions). Changes in behaviour, such as avoidance of social interaction may be a cause or a consequence of mood shifts and negative thinking. Cognitive vulnerability to depression is thought to arise as a consequence of dysfunctional underlying beliefs (e.g. "I'm unlovable"), which develop from early learning experiences and drive thinking and behaviour. It is hypothesised that these beliefs may be activated by life events that have specific meaning for that individual (e.g. rejection by a significant other).

Beck suggests that mania is a mirror image of depression and is characterised by a positive cognitive triad of self, world, and future, and positive cognitive distortions. The self is seen as extremely lovable and powerful with unlimited potential and attractiveness. The world is filled with wonderful possibilities, and experiences are viewed as overly positive. The future is seen as one of unlimited opportunity and promise. Hyperpositive thinking (stream of consciousness) is typified by cognitive distortions, as it is in depression, but in the opposite direction. For example, jumping to positive conclusions such as "I'm a winner; I can do anything"; underestimating risks such as "there's no danger"; minimising problems such as "nothing can go wrong"; and overvaluing immediate gratification such as "I will do this now". Thus, cognitive distortions reflected in thoughts provide biased confirmation of the positive cognitive triad of self, world, and future. Positive experiences are selectively attended to, and it is hypothesised that in this way underlying beliefs and self-schema that guide behaviour, thinking, and feeling are maintained and strengthened. It is hypothesised that dysfunctional beliefs are likely to involve high levels of social desirability (Scott, Stanton, Garland, & Ferrier, 2000; Winters & Neale, 1985). Examples of such underlying beliefs and self-schema include: "I'm special"; "Being manic helps me to overcome my shyness".

Beck's model of depression is well tested with reliable and valid questionnaires applied in research settings. However, given the ethical and practical difficulties of engaging manic patients in research, the model of mania is largely derivative, based on the careful observation of patients in a manic state. Interestingly, a recent study of BD patients demonstrated that, between episodes of illness, patients show similar patterns of cognitive vulnerability to individuals with unipolar depression. In comparison with healthy controls, BD patients had lower levels of self-esteem, higher levels of dysfunctional attitudes (particularly related to need for social approval and perfectionism), overgeneral memory, and poorer problem-solving skills (Scott et al., 2000). Scott et al. (2000) argue that whether or not these cognitive dysfunctions are a cause or a consequence of BD is not so important as the fact that the difficulties persist between episodes in patients who were adherent with prophylactic medication. Furthermore, the beliefs identified (e.g. "I'm different") are potentially dysfunctional when a positive or a negative valence is applied to them.

Although the above description has clinical validity, it fails to take into account the well-recognised biological aspects of vulnerability to BD. Beck (1996) concluded that a more complex model of cognitive processing (the Integrative Model) is needed to replace the original theory (now termed the Linear Schematic Processing Model) described above. A detailed discussion is beyond the scope of this chapter, but Beck's reformulation includes two main additions; the concepts of modes and charges, and additional refinements about precipitants of shifts in mood and thinking (see Fig. 13.1). Modes are an integrated network of sub-systems (cognitive, affective, motivational, and behavioural schemas) that can act in synchrony to produce goal-directed strategies. Charges (energy levels) explain activation of the modes, and account for shifts from quiescent states (normal) to activated states (abnormal). Importantly for the cognitive theory of BD, modes can be

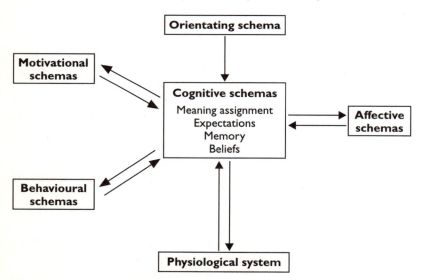

Figure 13.1 Beck's Integrative Model: Activation of the mode.

activated by external and internal events and, when activated, congruent memories are also activated. An orientating schema, described by Beck as a "kind of algorithm", sets the conditions necessary for activating the mode. It rapidly assigns a preliminary meaning to a situation and activation is spread across the network as the relevant mode is activated. In turn, this mode activates the schema. When a person is in a depressed or hypomanic/manic state, the orientating schema requires less evidence in order to make the "match".

The Integrative Model offers a more coherent explanation of the development of depression or hypomania. It also argues that belief in the meaning of negative thoughts leads to dysfunctional mood states. The goal of cognitive therapy is therefore to change dysfunctional interpretations as well as underlying dysfunctional beliefs (changes in construct accessibility). Beck writes that therapy for dysfunctional modes involves de-activation, modification, or neutralisation by the construction of an adaptive mode. This is achieved through interventions such as restructuring absolute and conditional rules (core schema) that shape interpretations, or by learning new skills, which can be applied in adverse circumstances and inhibit the action of dysfunctional beliefs.

This description represents an unproven but important theoretical model (Scott, 2001a). Two main problems exist. First, clinical data suggest that depressed and manic mental states cannot simply be regarded as polar opposites. For example, some of the most common symptoms of mania are dysphoria and irritability (Goodwin & Jamison, 1990). This undermines the notion that people with mania are happy and their thoughts predominantly positive. Secondly, although major life events are associated with the onset of affective episodes, there is no evidence that particular life events are associated more frequently with the onset of mania as compared with depression.

The clinical rationale for cognitive therapy

While research continues to explore integrative models of BD, clinicians should remember that there are some obvious and pragmatic reasons why CT may be beneficial to clients with the disorder. First, CT has all the hallmarks of an effective short-term psychotherapy. Secondly, the clinical picture can be formulated into an acceptable generic or specific CT model for all clients. Thirdly, the interventions can clearly target psycho-social functioning, comorbid disorders, and can ensure a sense of coherence between the clients' abstract and concrete experience of the disorder and the treatment strategies proposed (described as the cognitive representation of the disorder; Horne, 1997). The aspects are described in more detail in the following sub-sections.

An effective psychotherapy

Cognitive therapy shares the characteristics of a *clinically effective* short-term psychological intervention (Scott, 1995c) in that the therapy:

- is highly structured and based on a coherent model;
- provides the client with a clear rationale for the interventions made;
- promotes independent use of the skills learned;
- attributes change and progress to the individual's rather than the therapist's skilfulness; and
- enhances the individual's sense of self-efficacy.

The model is understandable

At a specific level, in order to understand BD and its impact on the individual, a conceptualisation that encompasses cognitive (thoughts, images, and beliefs), behavioural, affective, biological and environmental areas of the individual's life is required.

The generic approach described by Greenberger and Padesky (1996), with its clear acknowledgement of biology, is particularly useful in working with individuals with BD because it allows the therapist to emphasise a stress diathesis model that may also include neuroendocrine or other physical factors as precipitants of symptom shift (see Fig. 13.2). In order to use this approach in BD, the therapist should first ask the client to describe their own views about the causes of the disorder and their problems. Their aetiological theory is then incorporated within the framework of the model. Links between four aspects of the individual (cognitions, behaviour, mood, and biology), and the interaction between these and the environment (past and present events or experiences) are stressed. The therapist then explains that

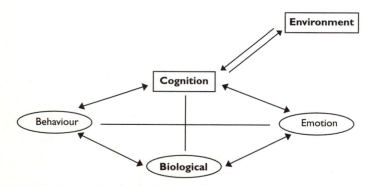

Figure 13.2 Basic conceptualisation of bipolar disorder. Source: Greenberger, D. and Padesky, C. (1996). *Mind over mood: A cognitive therapy treatment manual for clients.* New York: Guilford Press.

small changes in one of these five areas may lead to small changes in another area. This rationale is used to engage the client in CT through monitoring and linking changes in thoughts, behaviours, feelings, and the biological symptoms of BD. Many individuals will have been given a "biological" explanation of BD prior to coming to CT sessions. When the connections between the biological and other aspects of their experience are exposed, the client is readily able to understand the rationale for the use of CT (alone or in combination) without having to totally reject other causal models. This establishes the coherence within their cognitive representation of the disorder and allows an inroad into exploring attitudes towards, use of, and adherence with medication.

This approach is generally well received, particularly in the early stages of CT when the client is trying to make sense of the disorder and the proposed treatment. Virtually all aetiological "theories" can be incorporated in the model outlined, and the client gains confidence that the therapist is listening to their views about their problems and trying to help make sense of them. The therapist is not perceived as telling the client what they are experiencing nor dictating what they should do about it. However, during the course of CT, the therapist gradually moves the client on to a more sophisticated model of their disorder (see Fig. 13.3). The diagram presented here is a revision of the model proposed by Basco and Rush (1996). This formulation draws in all the symptoms and behaviours that the client experiences in a coherent way and, most importantly, it highlights the key role of change in sleep pattern. This symptom is often the strongest predictor of shift from euthymic to an abnormal mental state (Ehlers, Frank, & Kupfer, 1988). This formulation also allows the client to see the rationale for the specific interventions proposed for BD.

The model is adaptable to the individual

There are general and specific reasons for the use of CT that the therapist will wish to discuss with a client with BD. The general aims for employing this approach are to increase or enhance non-pharmacological coping skills, to enhance adherence to treatment, to help the individual recognise and manage psycho-social stressors, to teach CT strategies to deal with cognitive and behavioural problems, and to modify underlying maladaptive beliefs. Furthermore, Beck's model of CT may be used for clients with substance misuse problems, personality disorders, and psychotic disorders (Scott & Wright, 1997). It may be employed alone or in combination with medication, in an individual, couples, or family format, and in out or in-patient settings. This flexibility is important as clients with BD form a heterogeneous multi-problem group. Beck's approach (Beck et al., 1979) allows a consistent model to be applied to the whole spectrum of difficulties presented by such individuals, reducing the risk of confused messages about the treatment rationale.

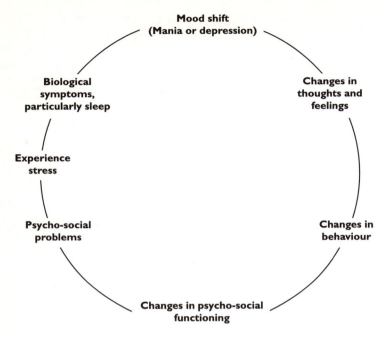

Figure 13.3 A more detailed conceptualisation of bipolar disorder. Adapted from Basco, M. and Rush, A. (1996). *Cognitive-behavioural treatment of manic-depressive disorder.* New York: Guilford Press.

The model is acceptable

The cognitive model offers the opportunity to help the client construct an accurate, coherent representation of the disorder, its likely impact, and the benefits of treatment. From the client's perspective, any coping strategy they choose to employ in dealing with their symptoms will be based on their ideas about five key issues:

- Identity: What is BD?
- Cause: What caused it?
- Time-line: How long will it last?
- Consequences: How will it/has it affected me?
- Cure: Can it be controlled or cured?

Although the content of the cognitive representations varies across different demographic and illness groups, its structure appears to remain constant (Skelton & Croyle, 1991). Adherence with CT and/or medication is most likely to occur if there is coherence between the patient's abstract ideas about the illness, their concrete experience of the symptoms, and the therapist's recommendations (Horne, 1997). Beliefs that modify the client's view of their disorder and its treatment may be unique to BD or the proposed treatment (e.g. medication does more harm than good), or may represent the general rules or assumptions that operate across the whole spectrum of the individual's life (e.g. "I must be in control"; "I must be perfect in everything I do"). Either way, classic cognitive behavioural approaches may be beneficial (Scott, 1999; 2001b).

DOES COGNITIVE THERAPY IMPROVE OUTCOME?

Encouraging anecdotal and single case reports on the use of CT in clients with BD have been published over the last 20 years (Chor, Mercier, & Halper, 1988; Scott, 1995b; Wright & Schrodt, 1992). There is also an emerging literature on the use of individual and group CT in small-scale open or randomised controlled trials (Bauer, & McBride, 1997; Cochran, 1984; Lam et al., 2000; Palmer, Williams, & Adams, 1995, 1998; Perry et al., 1999; Scott, Garland, & Moorhead, 2001).

The aim of Cochran's study was to apply cognitive therapy to enhance lithium adherence. It compared 28 patients randomly assigned to either six sessions of group CT or standard clinic care (Cochran, 1984). She reported enhanced lithium adherence in the therapy group where only 3 patients (21%) discontinued medication, compared with the standard clinic care group where 8 patients (57%) discontinued medication. There were fewer hospitalisations in the group receiving CT.

In Palmer et al.'s (1995) initial exploratory study, six clients with BD were offered CT in a group format. The focus of the programme was psycho-educational, recognising the process of change, strategies for coping, and interpersonal problems. Overall findings indicated that group therapy combined with mood stabilising medications was effective for some of the participants. Improvements were found in symptomatology and in overall social adjustment. All participants improved on one or more measures, although the pattern of change varied across individuals. Palmer et al.'s (1998) more recent study included a larger numbers of participants receiving group CT (=25) and a comparison group (=12) receiving treatment as usual only. The results showed that there was no difference in mood state between groups, but, in comparison with the control group, CT reduced non-specific symptomatology and increased social adjustment.

The "Life Goals" programme developed by Bauer and McBride (1997) is a structured, manual-based intervention that seeks to improve patients' management skills and their social and occupational functioning. Outcome data is not yet available, but a recent study analysed data on process goals and found that the manual could be used by therapists who were not greatly experienced with BD, and the programme was effective in terms of knowledge gained and goals achieved by patients (Bauer & McBride, 1997).

Perry et al. (1999) undertook the largest study so far (n=68), using cognitive and behavioural techniques to help people identify and manage early warning signs of relapse in a group of clients at high risk of further relapse of BD. The results demonstrated that, in comparison with the control group, the intervention group had significantly fewer manic relapses, significantly fewer days in hospital, higher levels of social functioning, and better work performance. However, the intervention did not have a significant impact on depression and the researchers suggested that more formal CT approaches might be important to produce significant changes in this area.

Scott, Garland, and Moorhead's pilot study of 42 subjects allowed examination of the benefits of 20 sessions of CT for BD and to develop a treatment manual for a large-scale multi-centre study. Patients were randomly allocated to CT in addition to treatment as usual or a waiting list control condition of treatment as usual for six months followed by CT plus treatment as usual. Preliminary results show protocol guided CT plus treatment as usual may benefit about 70% BD patients and is a highly acceptable treatment approach (90% of subjects endorsed this approach). The results also suggest that CT plus treatment as usual versus treatment as usual alone leads to fewer relapses (reduced from 42% to 18% per annum), significantly reduced symptom levels (for both depression and mania), and a 30% improvement in adherence to medication when CT is added to a waiting list condition of treatment as usual (Scott, Garland, & Moorhead, 2001). An outpatient CT study of BD of similar size (n=25) and design demonstrates comparable results with additional significant improvements in social adjustment (Lam, et al., 2000).

STRUCTURING COGNITIVE THERAPY

The case described later in this chapter highlights the adjustment problems that many clients with BD experience, and explores the use of CT in dealing with behavioural and cognitive symptoms of relapse in BD. Before introducing the case, some basic background information is given about the structure of the CT package. This will orientate novice therapists and provide an overview of the spectrum of techniques they may need to employ when working with people with BD (see the panel).

Early sessions are spent developing a formulation (see Fig. 13.3) and identifying the specific difficulties and consequences of the disorder that form key aspects of the individual's problem list. Defining problems under three broad headings—intrapersonal (e.g. low self-esteem), interpersonal (e.g. lack of social network; difficulties in relationships with family members) and basic problems (e.g. symptom frequency, severity, or course; early warning signs for

Typical cognitive therapy approaches to bipolar disorder	
General coping strategies	*Relapse prevention*

• **Knowledge**
 	
~ symptoms, effect on life-style
~ treatments and outcome
~ encouraging questions, providing information
 	
• **Self-regulation** (Ehlers et al., 1988): sleep, eating, exercise
 	
~ structured daily diary
 	
• **Self-monitoring**
 	
~ mood, thoughts, behaviours
~ changes in symptoms with events or treatment
 	
• **Adherence management**
 	
~ assume won't always adhere
~ explore fears, attitudes and thoughts
~ discuss advantages and disadvantages
~ what increases or decreases risks
	• **Identifying vulnerable periods**
	
	~ stressful events
	  (specific personal meaning)
	~ high-risk behaviours (alcohol, drug use)
	~ "Relapse signature": 2 symptoms recognised by >75% (avoid using mood, misattributed as health)
	
	3 components:
	  i. depression specific
	  ii. mania specific
	  iii. idiosyncratic
	
	• **Increase self-regulation and self-monitoring**
	
	• **Crisis management**
	
	~ hierarchy of coping: step by step
	~ no major decisions
	~ 48-hour delay
	~ third-party rule prior agreements for action with family and clinicians

relapse; difficulties coping with work; housing problems, etc.)—seems particularly helpful. Examples of key strategies include education about BD, facilitating adjustment, self-monitoring and self-regulation, enhancing medication adherence, and relapse prevention, and these are examined in the following sub-sections.

Education about BD

Verbal, written, and visual information are all useful in educating clients about BD. Clients deserve a frank description of the disorder, and the known facts about prognosis and the alternative treatment approaches. Again, getting clients to outline their baseline knowledge initially may allow important influences on their thinking to be identified and specific misunderstandings to be rectified. A number of leaflets, books, and videos have been produced (Manic Depression Fellowship, 1995; McKeon, 1992; Peet and Harvey,

1991), and these provide valuable material for early homework assignments and allow the opportunity to ask questions at later CT sessions. When setting such homework tasks it is useful to ensure the client is answering the key questions identified in the cognitive representation of illness (identity; cause; time-line; consequences; cure).

Facilitating adjustment

To some extent, adjustment problems such as anxiety about the future, fears about relationships, or concerns about what to say to people at work, will be partly resolved through provision of information and dealing with cognitive distortions relating to self-image, views of the world, and of the future. However, premorbid difficulties, such as the prevalence of abnormal personality traits and disorder (30–50%) should be borne in mind. Dysfunctional core beliefs will need modification and problem-solving skills may need to be developed to overcome adjustment problems and help reduce risk of relapse.

Partner or family attitudes towards the sufferer, the disorder, their beliefs about its causes, and knowledge about or attitudes towards treatment may influence clients' prognosis (Cochran & Gitlin, 1988; Scott, 1992). As such, supplementing individual CT with three to four family sessions may be desirable. When appropriate, partners or members of the family may be engaged as "co-therapists" outside the CT sessions (Scott, 1995b).

Self-monitoring and self-regulation

Many individuals with BD are keen to have as much control as they can over their emotional and behavioural fluctuations. They are quite prepared to record activity schedules and data on thoughts, feelings, and symptoms. In planning activity schedules, individuals are initially encouraged to include everything they wish to accomplish and then to determine the priorities and engage in the minimum required for effective functioning. Dysfunctional thought records (DTRs) may be used to explore evidence for mood lability and links between this and other symptoms of mania or depression, or DTRs may be used to examine individual reactions to BD and to treatment.

Daily mood graphs are used to identify fluctuations in quality and severity of mood shifts. Additional instructions can be agreed in advance and listed on the mood charts. For example, a client and therapist identified that if elation was rated at greater than 40%, increased self-monitoring would be undertaken; if elation ratings exceeded 60%, this would be a signal to seek professional help.

It has been reported previously that clients with BD benefit from maintaining regular patterns of sleep, physical activity, and eating (called the social rhythm metric; American Psychiatric Association, 1994). This should be encouraged, although not if it leads to too restrictive a lifestyle. Self-regulation does appear to increase stability in an individual's mental state and enhances their sense of self-efficacy (Scott, 1995b). Finally, many clients benefit from using affect regulation techniques as used more frequently for clients with personality dysfunction (Scott, Byers, & Turkington, 1993). Relaxation and "active" calming activities such as self-talk to slow down movements and speech, or suggestions to always sit down before getting into animated discussions (which reduces the frequency and magnitude of accessory body movements) may be useful.

Enhancing medication adherence

Given the prevalence of non-adherence, the therapist should assume that it might prove problematic to all individuals at some time. The critical factor in the successful management of medication adherence is creating an atmosphere where the client does not feel disapproved of and so is able to talk honestly about their concerns about drug treatments and their pattern of adherence. Discussion of the individual's cognitions about BD and fears about treatment and exploring practical and psychological barriers to adherence is a vital component of CT (Goodwin & Jamison, 1990; Rush, 1988).

At a practical level, highly complex treatment regimes make the risk of non-adherence greater, so simple schedules should be negotiated whenever possible (Goodwin & Jamison, 1990). Behavioural strategies such as "pairing" tablet taking with a routine daily activity may aid adherence (Rush, 1988; Wright & Thase, 1992). Noting situations where the risk of forgetting or omitting to take medication is high and developing behavioural prompts (e.g. a note stuck to a bathroom mirror) or exploring situation-specific negative automatic thoughts (e.g. "If I take the lithium before the weekly review, I'll be a zombie and make a fool of myself") may also identify barriers to adherence.

Two additional approaches can be used in this and other situations. First, a cost-benefit analysis table can be drawn up on the use of medication. Advantages and disadvantages for taking medication and advantages and disadvantages of not taking medication are assessed. Secondly, the option of seeking a "third-party opinion" from someone else whom the client trusts may also be useful (Newman & Beck, 1992).

Relapse prevention

Identifying personal factors that make an individual vulnerable to episodes of BD (e.g. underlying perfectionistic beliefs), or high-risk situations for relapse (e.g. work stress, or increased alcohol consumption) is a valuable intervention on its own and is a crucial aspect of CT for BD. Modifying underlying core beliefs is a key component of CT and the approaches employed in BD are the same as those used in other mental disorders (Padesky, 1994). If individuals cannot identify specific precipitants they may learn to recognise the signs and symptoms of relapse and identify what action they can take to control these.

Many events, although inevitable consequences of the lifecycle, signal a period of increased risk of relapse. Discovering the specific meaning of events previously associated with relapse (e.g. the breakdown of a relationship activating beliefs about being unlovable) may reduce the impact of similar experiences in the future. Strategies for anticipating events, and reviewing how to act or cope during and after such events can be developed (Scott, 1995b). Alternatively, identifying "high-risk behaviours" for relapse such as excess use of stimulants (alcohol or caffeine intake) or non-adherence, and trying to find alternative, safer activities can also be beneficial.

Retrospective examination of prodromal symptoms in previous episodes suggests that 85% of BD sufferers can identify at least two prodromal symptoms specific to depressive swings and 75% can identify two symptoms specific to hypomanic swings (Smith & Tarrier, 1992). These individual pro-dromal symptoms are termed the "relapse signature". For hypomania, physical prodroma such as sleep disturbance (Wehr, Sack, & Rosenthal, 1987) or other features related to activation level are better symptoms to monitor rather than affective state (Bauer et al., 1991). Elated mood is a less reliable discriminator because many clients may misattribute this to well-being rather than sickness (Smith & Tarrier, 1992). Having identified relapse symptoms on a flash card, sufferers (and their relatives) may engage in monitoring of early warning symptoms. In addition, a written hierarchy of coping responses can be developed in CT sessions. This might start with strategies such as increased attention to self-regulation of activities, cancelling meetings where important (or irreversible) decisions might be made, or setting an agreed spending limit. It may include "the 48-hour delay" rule where the client is discouraged from acting impulsively on a "good idea" immediately, but to weigh up the pros and cons and review their idea 2–3 days later (Newman & Beck, 1992). Further up the hierarchy, the point at which to change the medication regime is noted. Developing tactics to ensure that mental health service input is obtained even if the individuals' insight is fading (e.g. giving a trusted friend permission to institute contact with professionals), should also be included on the hierarchy. Prodromal periods for depression or mania may last for up to four weeks, allowing a significant period of time in which to make these interventions (Molner, Feeney, & Fava, 1988).

CASE STUDY: MARK'S STORY

Mark was a 37-year-old man who had experienced an episode of mania 4 months previously. He had a history of one previous episode of mania at the age of 35 years and of an episode of depression at the age of 30 years. He was referred for CT by a psychiatrist who was seeing him as an outpatient. Mark's pattern of adherence with medication was not clear, but two recent serum lithium levels had been below the therapeutic range despite increases in the prescribed dosage. Although Mark's current symptoms did not meet major depression criteria, he appeared sad and hopeless and his mood was quite labile.

Mark's progress after discharge had been erratic. He was not able to consistently attend his job as a company salesman, partly because of his fluctuating mental state with marked mood swings and partly because he avoided turning up after any interaction where he thought people did not approve of him. Rejection was a prominent theme at this time. Mark reported he met and then rather impulsively married his wife within six weeks in 1997 and moved to another city. However, the relationship had lasted only seven months before his wife left him. Mark was shocked, as he had not expected this. Having few friends in the area, he moved back to live with his sister and her husband, but then moved again when their second child was born, this time to live with his parents. His employer allowed him to transfer to a job of slightly lower status in a franchise near his parents' home. His manic episode began not long after this. Mark reported that his parents had been upset and initially angry at his disinhibited behaviour prior to hospitalisation, but had said virtually nothing about his illness since then.

There was a family history of bipolar affective disorders in two distant relatives and Mark's father had a history of recurrent unipolar depression. Mark's mother reportedly opposed medication for his father's depression and often stated that people with depression "should pull themselves together". His mother had not spoken about the other relatives and expressed relatively few opinions about Mark's manic episode. However, Mark perceived that his behaviour was constantly under scrutiny. His mother made negative comments on two or three occasions when Mark had gone out drinking with old school friends to a local pub. Mark reported that this perceived criticism and his own uncertainties about whether these "friends" really wanted him around or simply felt sorry for him and "let me tag along", had led him to stop socialising.

Mark's relationship with his father was better than that with his mother, but Mark's mother was critical of his father. Mark also recalled his mother comparing him unfavourably with his older siblings during his childhood. He reported that he had been born some years after his siblings (an eight-year gap). Mark believed that his parents had not really wanted a third child, he considered himself "the black sheep of the family", was a rather reluctant scholar, and never believed he was good enough. This pattern had been echoed at school where his sister had been a high achiever and a popular school sports captain. After university, she had set up a small business and was considered a "great success" by the family. His brother was also a very able scholar and was now married and working as an academic at an "Ivy League" university in the USA. Although Mark achieved moderately well at school and went on to college, he was easily drawn into minor trouble and he did not think the teachers approved of him. In retrospect, there was evidence from his late teens of mood swings, which he had largely "controlled" through the use of alcohol and recreational drugs such as Ecstasy.

The following sections briefly outline the issues covered over the course of therapy. Many of the techniques draw on our own work and that of others working in this area (Basco & Rush, 1996; Lam et al., 2000; Newman & Beck, 1992; Scott, 2001b; Wright & Thase, 1992).

Sessions 1–3: Engagement and socialisation

As with any individual presenting to CT, the initial sessions were used to socialise Mark into the model, to develop rapport with the therapist, and to identify a problem list. To understand the problems Mark was experiencing and to develop a preliminary conceptualisation, we used a model that links together five areas of the individual's life as described by Greenberger and Padesky (1996). As noted, this model (Fig. 13.2) is easier to grasp during the early sessions, but the client is gradually moved on to the more detailed conceptualisation (Fig. 13.3).

In the first session we identified the links between four aspects of Mark himself, namely his cognitions (including thoughts, images, beliefs), behaviour, mood, and biology, and the interaction between these and the fifth area, his environment (past and present events or experiences). This approach (see Fig. 13.2), with its clear acknowledgement of biology, was particularly useful as Mark had been told he was suffering from a disorder that may have a significant biological component. The therapist emphasised a stress diathesis model.

Mark was able to fit his own experiences to the model. For example, he noted that lack of energy (biological) was often linked with feeling down in his mood. He reported associated negative thoughts about himself ("I'm useless"; "People don't like failures"), and on those days he noted he would avoid going to work. Others in his environment, such as his supervisor at work, would express concern or criticise his behaviour and this led Mark to feel more depressed and anxious and to have further negative thoughts ("I'll lose my job"; "I'm lazy, I should try harder").

On other occasions, Mark reported feeling elated. He was very active, and his automatic thoughts were very positive ("I'm a very attractive and capable person"). He would go out with friends or stay up into the early hours of the morning watching videos or playing music from his collection of old LPs that he had stored at home. His mother would often criticise this behaviour and the atmosphere would become tense as Mark reacted to his mother's disapproval. Mark also noted that this often made him feel more depressed and to recall memories of his marriage and the onset of BD. He then experienced a cascade of negative thoughts ("I had everything and now I have nothing"; "I can't cope alone, I'll have to live with my parents forever"; "No-one will ever love me again, I'll be alone and never have a family of my own") associated with feelings of depression and hopelessness.

Using the model, the therapist then explained that small changes in one of these five areas may lead to small changes in another area (Greenberger & Padesky, 1996). This rationale was used to engage Mark in monitoring his thoughts, behaviours, feelings, and the biological symptoms of BD. In addition, this approach allowed an inroad into exploring the use of medication. The topic was introduced later in the assessment as Mark had already expressed negative views about his psychiatrist and the use of drugs. This tactic was well received and Mark gained confidence that the therapist was interested in a multi-modal approach. He also commented in his feedback at the end of the session that he finally felt that someone was listening to his views about his problems and trying to help him make sense of them, rather than telling him what he was experiencing and what he must do about it. Over two sessions, the following problem list was produced:

1 To gain knowledge and understanding of BD and its treatment, including the cognitive model and the role of CT.
2 To develop self-management strategies and stabilise social rhythms.
3 To decide on the advantages and disadvantages of taking medication and to identify problems in adhering with treatment.
4 To build up my self-esteem and confidence.
5 To develop my social network.
6 To improve my attendance and performance at work.
7 To become more independent by moving into my own accommodation.
8 To improve relationships with my family and help them understand my problems.
9 To identify what factors make me vulnerable to episodes of BD.
10 To identify high-risk situations for relapse and develop coping strategies.
11 To recognise the signs and symptoms of relapse and to identify what action I can take to control these.

This list was fairly comprehensive. It incorporated intrapersonal issues (low self-esteem) that could undermine progress, interpersonal problems (social network and family relationships), and basic problems relating to the client's employment and living situation. The list also included work on vulnerability factors, allowing underlying assumptions and beliefs to be explored, and relapse prevention. Between sessions, Mark agreed to review the list to help him and the therapist identify specific targets so they would both know when a problem had been adequately addressed. Mark also kept an activity schedule and began monitoring changes in mood and other symptoms. He read two articles on BD produced by the Manic Depression Fellowship, and found some other literature in his local library. The therapist also provided leaflets on lithium and other drug therapies.

Sessions 4 and 5: Education about BD, regulating activities, and enhancing adherence

The initial stage of CT progressed quite well. Mark was happier working with a more eclectic model and seemed to value the collaborative approach. Mark and the therapist also translated items on the problem list into specific treatment goals. For example, the initial target for problem one was to understand the cause, course, and prognosis of BD; the target with regard to medication adherence was to take more than 75% of the prescribed mood stabiliser, while the target for problem 7 was to have established himself in his own flat within 12 months. The therapist put a great deal of effort into active listening and summarising information and encouraged very frequent feedback from Mark on his thoughts and feelings about therapy, particularly any thoughts of rejection or breaks in his trust of the therapist.

Over a period of four weeks Mark became very knowledgeable about BD (developing his own cognitive representation and correcting misconceptions). Mark's cognitive representation acknowledged his familial vulnerability to develop BD, saw life stress as an important precipitant of episodes, but his view of the consequences of an episode were mixed. He still largely believed that the cure was in his own hands (trying harder would allow him to control his symptoms) and he remained somewhat sceptical about the benefits of medication. As he further understood BD, Mark decided to loan the educational leaflets to his mother and father, but he avoided the homework task to discuss BD with them. In imagining a discussion with them, Mark became anxious and had thoughts of being "defective and a failure". He was not confident he would be able to field questions they asked and was worried about how they would react. In the CT session, Mark and the therapist role-played the discussion he would try to have at home. This allowed specific cognitions relating to this scenario (particularly Mark's cognitions about his mother's negative appraisal of him) to be identified and evaluated in the session. Mark discovered that not only was his mother prejudiced about people with psychological problems (she regarded them as "inadequate"), Mark himself was prejudiced against people with mental disorder and this was undoubtedly contributing to his distress.

These thoughts were challenged through the use of a dysfunctional thoughts record (DTR) and through role-play. Role-play was also used to allow the therapist to model how to present information about BD. Mark then reviewed possible ways to explain BD that he thought would be acceptable to his father (a sufferer) and his mother (someone perceived as less sympathetic towards mental disorder). At the end of session four, Mark was not convinced by his alternative responses on the DTR and still had some anxieties about talking to his parents, and so the homework was renegotiated. He decided to explore information about creative and famous people with bipolar disorders and to gain a greater understanding of the issue of stigma. He also decided he would approach someone with whom he felt he had a greater degree of empathy and "practise" explaining his illness to that person. In the end, Mark chose to speak with his sister, as he perceived her to have shown greater understanding in the past, and to have been very supportive during his brief marriage and subsequent divorce.

Mark was keen to have as much control as he could over his emotional and behavioural fluctuations and had been quite rigorous in his collection of activity schedules and data on feelings and symptoms. He also kept automatic thought records, particularly regarding relationships with people at home and at work. Two particular issues emerged from these recordings. First, Mark showed less mood lability and was less likely to avoid work when he kept a regular pattern of sleep and activity. Mark now had evidence of this from his own homework assignments, that people with BD benefit from maintaining regular patterns such as sleep, physical activity, and eating (social rhythm metric; American Psychiatric Association, 1994). The therapist was able to reinforce Mark's discovery and help devise a regular timetable of activity, including things he enjoyed (such as weight training) as well as routine tasks such as getting to work on time. This pleased Mark and he reported this increased his sense of self-efficacy.

Mark also began to discuss his practical difficulties with regard to taking medication and admitted his adherence had been rather erratic over the past year. He had not felt able to discuss this previously because he thought the psychiatrist and general practitioner would disapprove of his non-adherence and he wanted to avoid criticism. His therapist helped him develop some simple strategies for overcoming "unintentional" non-adherence. Mark stuck a note by his alarm clock to remind him to take his medication in the morning and also kept a record of his adherence pattern.

In session five Mark identified that on the evening he went to play snooker straight from work he was at greater risk of not taking his second dose of lithium. On these occasions he would go with other people from the class to a local bar for a drink. In addition, if he was feeling happier and was not having thoughts of being rejected by others, he would be more likely to go out during weekends. This again appeared to reduce the likelihood of taking his late evening medication. Mark suggested he bring the time of his second dose of medication forward and monitor if this improved the situation. However, this data provided evidence of more "intentional" non-adherence indicating cognitive barriers to engaging with medication. Mark agreed it would be useful to keep a DTR relating to taking medication.

Sessions 6–8: Non-adherence and non-attendance

Mark was cheery at the next session. The discussions with his sister had gone well and he said he now felt ready to try to talk to his parents, and he set this as one of his homework tasks between sessions six and seven. Mark reported that the activity regulation and behavioural techniques for enhancing his adherence were beneficial. Although his DTR regarding medication in the two days prior to the session showed many negative thoughts such as "I'm a zombie", "I'm controlled by drugs", and "I'm inadequate, I should be able to cope without this crutch", he had only missed two evening doses of lithium in two weeks. The work on alternative responses to his DTR was put on the agenda, but most of session six was taken up with a discussion of lithium and the perceived benefits (e.g. symptom reduction and mood stabilisation) and barriers (e.g. side effects) of this treatment. However, Mark's view that "if I try harder I will succeed" was still rather fixed and the therapist realised she was struggling to retain the coherence between Mark's concrete and abstract experiences of BD and the rationale she was giving for the CT interventions. This difficulty emphasises the importance of proactively reviewing cognitive representations throughout treatment (as these do not remain static).

Mark reported that he was more tired, had gained weight despite his exercise programme, and he wondered if he was being lazy. He wished to determine if these problems could be overcome. The therapist and Mark explored this hypothesis, but came to the conclusion that his increased adherence may have increased the plasma level of the medication and that this might be having an affect on his weight and functioning. It was agreed that a serum lithium level would be checked to ensure it was within the therapeutic range and the therapist also suggested Mark ask the psychiatrist to review the dosage regime at the next outpatient session. Mark agreed to this and said he would try to look at the DTR himself before the next session. He reported at the end of the session feedback that he was happier, thought CT was helpful, and as he left the session he also commented on an upturn in his social life; he was dating "the woman of his dreams" whom he had just met at his fitness club.

The blood result showed Mark's serum lithium level to be at the upper limit of the therapeutic range and so the therapist made a note to put this on the agenda for discussion, with a possible goal of agreeing to a slight reduction in dosage regime to reduce side effects and maintain adherence.

Unfortunately, Mark failed to attend the next two scheduled sessions. The therapist wondered if the task of talking to his parents was too much for Mark, but this seemed an unlikely reason for non-attendance. Despite phone messages offering appointments, Mark did not contact the therapist until two weeks later, when he rang to say he would like to come for a final CT session. The therapist was surprised and decided to review the initial cognitive formulation to try to prepare for the session. Mark had described core beliefs about being different; when depressed (and even when euthymic) Mark regarded himself as not good enough and disliked (when he was hypomanic he saw himself as "special"). Mark often expected others to reject him when they got to know him. Mark also blamed himself for the onset of BD, stating that "if I had tried harder, this would not have happened".

Sessions 9–11: Re-engagement in CT

At session nine, all the factors noted above seemed relevant to what was happening. Mark told the therapist that he had found CT very helpful, the therapist had been "wonderful", but he now felt in control of his disorder and no longer needed to attend. He reported that he had seen the psychiatrist, but by then Mark had already halved the dose of lithium. A few days after the last session Mark stated that he had changed the dose because the side effects were a nuisance and he noted he actually felt better without it, particularly being more cheerful, less tired, and less sluggish in his thinking. Mark also felt he did not need medication because self-regulating his activity was clearly the best way forward. Mark and the psychiatrist had not been able to agree a compromise. Furthermore, he was going to marry the woman he had met at the fitness club and this would simultaneously resolve all his other problems—he would be able to leave his parents home (where things had been worse since his last session), and his new girlfriend also liked and wanted children.

As far as the therapist could establish, although Mark had prodromal symptoms of hypomania, this was not yet a full relapse. However, Mark only agreed to stay for the rest of the session with some considerable persuasion. This was done by the therapist getting Mark to agree to review the lists of symptoms Mark had compiled right at the beginning of CT. The lists identified the typical features of Mark's episodes of mania, mixed states, and depression. As Mark re-read the list he acknowledged that his present state may indictae that he was hypomanic. Together client and therapist gently challenged Mark's current beliefs that his improved mood state could be attributed to "well-being" and not BD, that all his improvements were a direct result of his own efforts, and that reducing the medication had no negative effects on his mental state. Initially, Mark thought there had been positive benefits from reducing his medication, as he felt better because he no longer suffered any side effects. As the session progressed Mark then revealed that he had only had three dates with his current girlfriend and he had not actually suggested marriage. However, Mark believed he was going to propose to her any day and if he did not he thought it was likely she would propose to him.

The therapist persisted with a gentle but steady line of Socratic questioning that helped Mark establish that his current positive state of mind might not be due to well-being, but might be an early sign of relapse. The therapist and Mark then reviewed Mark's symptoms as noted in his "relapse signature".

After examining the evidence together in considerable detail, he acknowledged that he had most of the symptoms listed and two of the three key symptoms of impending relapse (see the flashcard panel). The therapist explained that although Mark's self-regulation programme had undoubtedly been beneficial, non-adherence and stress might be contributing to his current presentation. The therapist also explained to Mark that although the side effects of lithium disappear early, often leading the individual to feel better in themselves, after a short delay BD symptoms may recur. The delayed onset of symptoms is not always associated with non-adherence in the client's mind (Rush, 1988). Mark only rated his belief in this explanation as 50%. However, he was prepared to delay proposing marriage to his girlfriend, as the evidence from his previous relationship demonstrated that getting married shortly after meeting someone may not be the best way to proceed. He also acknowledged "if it was really a good idea, it would still be a good idea in the future". Mark was not prepared to increase the dose of lithium. Mark wanted to prove to himself that if he tried hard he could control his symptoms, and asked if the therapist would support this or if the therapist was about to become "just another pill-pusher".

This presented a dilemma to the therapist. It was important to try to maintain collaboration within sessions and to re-engage Mark in therapy. However, he was at risk of a full relapse and the therapist was aware that this would have an extremely negative impact on Mark's view of himself, might

---

FLASHCARD FOR RELAPSE PREVENTION

My relapse signature is:

> Lack of sleep
> Poor concentration
> Excessive spending

When I start to go high it helps if I:

> Target my sleep pattern
> Cut out stimulants
> Actively calm myself
> Avoid major decisions
> Limit my spending

My specific technique is:

> 48-hour delay rule

The following individual may contact my doctor on my behalf:

> John Dobson, Tel. 0782 413243

damage the relationship with his new girlfriend and Mark's family, and his employers might not tolerate further disruption in his work attendance. Furthermore, Mark's relationship with his psychiatrist was currently strained. The therapist gave a clear message about the benefits of maintaining a therapeutic dose of medication and presented the reasons for this. Although Mark did not accept this view, the therapist and client eventually decided on an acceptable experiment as a compromise. Mark agreed to self-monitor a list of symptoms of hypomania and depression. The therapist negotiated with Mark that, if he continued on the lower dose of medication, they would increase the frequency of his CT sessions to twice weekly and have brief daily contact by telephone on the days between sessions. Mark agreed that if the self-monitoring demonstrated that he was beginning to relapse, he would resume a higher dose of medication. If the evidence was that his symptoms were under control, the frequency of sessions would gradually be reduced again over the following month and Mark could then make a decision as to whether to continue CT or not. This session lasted 90 minutes. At the end, Mark suggested he was prepared to undertake a trial of CT for a few more weeks and a further appointment was arranged for two days' time.

Mark attended sessions 10 and 11, and reported that his mental state had remained stable. He continued to attend work and maintained his agreement not to propose to his girlfriend. Mark reported some difficulties in his relationship with his mother, but he managed to avoid a major argument by agreeing to go to bed rather than stay up playing records one night. Session 11 also looked at Mark's ideas about trying harder. The therapist and client were able to conclude that although Mark was trying hard in his own right, if the concept of "trying harder" was reframed it could also include using medication, CT, and seeking out appropriate help and support from others. Overall, Mark concluded that his symptoms were reasonably stable and that he was maintaining some degree of self-control, but he accepted the rationale for close monitoring and frequent sessions. He also agreed to conduct a behavioural experiment in which he asked a close friend at work to help him with a project he was finding difficult to complete because of poor concentration.

Sessions 12 and 13: Introducing a third party

At the next session Mark was slightly disinhibited and, although he had not brought his self-monitoring record, he reported he had been out drinking till very late one night and had only gone to bed for three hours the next night. Since then his sleep pattern had been unpredictable and he had missed two days from work. Mark acknowledged that these features might be evidence of relapse and also that his own attempts to control his symptoms over the last few days, such as "dampening" his mood with alcohol, had not been successful. However, when the discussion turned to increasing medication, Mark was still reluctant to consider this option, despite Socratic questioning that reminded him of evidence of its benefit.

Two approaches were used to try to help Mark. First, a cost-benefit analysis was drawn up (see the panel) on the use of medication (Newman & Beck, 1992). Mark reluctantly acknowledged that this demonstrated more advantages and fewer disadvantages to taking medication. However, the therapist still sensed that the therapeutic collaboration was under threat, and Mark admitted he was less certain that the therapist was not trying to "hoodwink" him into this course of action.

Mark was offered the option of seeking a "third-party opinion" from someone else whom he trusted to get another view of his progress and current mental state, and to discuss medication. Mark decided that his sister was someone whose opinion he valued and a further session was arranged for that evening. This approach proved particularly helpful. When Mark's sister highlighted that he was not coping as well as previously, expressed her fears about relapse, and talked about how hard it had been during and after his hospitalisation, Mark appeared more able to believe that the therapist was working

---

COST-BENEFIT ANALYSIS OF TAKING MEDICATION

Advantages of taking medication

1. Treatment keeps me out of hospital
2. My family are less worried when I'm on medication
3. I know I'm doing everything I can to keep my illness under control

Advantages of not taking medication

1. I have less things to carry around and less things to remember
2. I'm in control of me, not the tablets

Disadvantages of taking medication

1. I hate blood tests
2. I've gained weight as a side effect
3. Medication can be toxic and you can get irreversible kidney damage from some drugs such as lithium

Disadvantages of not taking medication

1. There is a greater risk I'll have a relapse
2. I might have to go back into hospital and that might jeopardise my career
3. If my wife finds out she'll be upset
4. The doctor has expressed concern for my well-being if I don't use medication
5. Once, when depressed, I thought of killing myself—it was a frightening experience that I'd rather not have happen again

with him. Mark's sister had also rung the Manic Depression Fellowship tele-phone helpline to find out about lithium and alternative treatments. After this discussion, Mark agreed that refusing lithium and other major tranquillisers did not preclude a trial of a different tablet. He was started on carbamazepine (an alternative mood stabiliser) after being given information about its mode of action and a discussion of the side effects. Frequent CT appointments were maintained during this period to monitor progress and the change of treatment. With his sister's help, the therapist also negotiated with Mark that, if his symptoms deteriorated any further, he would attend the day hospital for at least two days per week.

Sessions 14–28: Vulnerability to relapse and coping strategies

Having narrowly avoided a relapse, Mark was initially disappointed with himself and pessimistic about his future. Relationships at home had con-tinued to be difficult, he was feeling anxious about work, and he had stopped dating his girlfriend. Mark said he did not feel he could face meeting his girlfriend because he felt embarrassed about a number of inappropriate comments he had made to her about their relationship and their future together. It took time for Mark to forgive himself for his recent behaviour. However, over several sessions, Mark concluded that he had not gone back to square one; he had neither been hospitalised nor experienced a full relapse. At work, he discussed his problems with his supervisor; at his own instigation a regular review session was set up at four-monthly intervals to monitor his coping. Mark identified that poor sleep pattern, excess alcohol intake, and getting into (or out of) relationships constituted vulnerable times for him. He also identified specific symptoms (besides elation) that might be early warning signs of relapse. Mark recorded important information about what strategies and behaviours were most effective when prodromal symptoms were present. These were further developed and a hierarchy of interventions was recorded by Mark and a copy given to his sister. The hierarchy began with increasing the frequency of, or re-instituting CT sessions. Later strat-egies included giving his sister permission to seek help on his behalf. Mark and his family attended CT for a joint session in which Mark took the lead in explaining more about BD and its treatment. This particularly helped Mark's mother understand the rationale for medication and CT, and Mark and his mother later attended two meetings held by a local support group for people with BD and their families.

Mark moved out of his parents' home about three months later. He also worked on modifying underlying core beliefs about being different (usually themes of being unlikeable and defective) using CT schema change methods (Padesky, 1994). In this case, it was only possible to modify rather than change the belief about being different. Although a review of Mark's life history revealed a balance in the evidence for and against "being different", Mark constantly drew on the fact that he had BD as evidence. However, he now saw the difference as due to symptoms of an illness rather than a comment on his personality. A great deal of input was offered to improve Mark's self-esteem. This drew on techniques described in detail by Fennell (1997), but particularly focused on the fragility of Mark's self-concept. People with BD often show great variablity in how they view themselves from day to day. The therapist and Mark established that in his case this variability seemed to stem from the fact that his self-esteem seemed to vary as a consequence of how he believed people were evaluating him at any time. Hence, if his supervisor at work frowned, Mark would jump to the conclusion that the supervisor was making a negative appraisal of Mark's performance. The approach initially targeted Mark's view of himself, trying to strengthen his ability to maintain a positive self-image in the face of any negative events or experiences. After some progress had been made, the therapist and Mark then tried to reduce Mark's vulnerability to shift to a negative view of himself by modifying his underlying belief that he needed to be approved of by everyone he met.

The final four CT sessions were spread out over several months. Between sessions, Mark was encouraged to use the CT techniques he had learned for self-management. He kept a personal log of how he coped with difficulties and monitored any fluctuations in symptoms. He also developed a more accurate picture of life events that did and life events that did not stress him. At 18-month follow-up he had had no further episodes of BD and his serum carbamazepine levels suggest sustained adherence with medication.

CONCLUSIONS

This chapter illustrates the potential use of CT for individuals with BD. Cognitive therapy appears to be an effective approach, but to develop a more coherent and empirical model, a greater understanding is required of individual and environmental vulnerability factors that may influence onset or outcome of episodes of BD. More research on commonly shared underlying beliefs in individuals at risk of BD, attitudes towards BD, and views about its treatment, will also aid our understanding of adjustment difficulties and psychological barriers to treatment adherence and good outcome.

On the evidence available, it appears that CT has specific characteristics that may benefit clients with BD. Its collaborative, educational style, the use of a step-by-step approach, and of guided discovery make it acceptable to individuals who wish to take an equal and active role in their therapy (Beck et al., 1979; Scott, 1995b). This is important because many individuals with BD resist and challenge a didactic approach to treatment (Miklowitz & Goldstein, 1990). Also, if the structure of CT sessions is maintained, clients may retain their focus on specific agenda items even when mildly elated or distractible (Scott, 1995b).

The model of CT for clients with BD may have similarities to the approach used with other severe disorders such as schizophrenia or in-patient depression (Scott & Wright, 1997). However, some modifications to recognised treatment packages may be useful. For example, Miklowitz and Goldstein (1990) noted that, in comparison with other client groups, individuals with BD are more overtly emotional and demanding during interactions with their family and significant others, while Scott (2001a) commented that clients with BD underestimate relationship difficulties. This suggests that, even if formal couples or family CT is not undertaken, enhancing the interpersonal focus of individual CT may be beneficial in the same way that it has proved helpful to clients with chronic depressive disorders (Markowitz, 1994; Scott et al., 1993). The CT approach also has to take into account that, between episodes, many individuals with BD function at a higher level than those with schizophrenia or chronic depression. As shifts in functioning level can occur quite rapidly, the therapist has to be prepared for significant variations in what can or cannot be tackled during a particular session. Groundwork must be done to reduce the risk of the client opting for premature discharge on the basis of overly optimistic subjective assessments of improvement. Miklowitz and Goldstein (1990) observed that clients with BD may interact in a more fast-paced, affective, and spontaneous manner than those with other severe mental health problems. Therapists need to be aware that these features may be signs of health or the prodroma of relapse. Also therapists need to avoid the temptation to "join the rush" and should take greater responsibility for establishing a clear structure and realistic pace for sessions. These caveats suggest that, for the time being, a formal course of CT for clients with BD should probably be undertaken by a CT therapist with a high level of expertise. However, other professionals may wish to use specific cognitive and behavioural techniques to improve medication adherence (Scott, 1999) or to reduce risk of manic relapse (Perry et al., 1999).

Finally, larger scale treatment intervention studies will be needed to establish the effectiveness of CT and to differentiate between the specific and non-specific benefits of therapy. Ultimately, it is important for clinicians and researchers to know not only if the use of CT is indicated, but also whether it helps the client with BD because it enhances medication adherence, changes cognitive representations of the disorder, leads to the development of compensatory skills or because it reduces vulnerability to relapse through schema change.

REFERENCES

American Psychiatric Association (1994). Practice guidelines for the treatment of patients with bipolar disorder. *American Journal of Psychiatry, 151 (suppl.)*, 1–36.

Basco, M., & Rush, A. (1996). *Cognitive-behavioural treatment of manic-depressive disorder*. New York: Guilford Press.

Bauer, M., Crits-Christoph, P., Ball, W., Dewees, E., McAllister, T., Alahi, P., Cacciola, J., & Whybrow, P. (1991). Independent assessment of manic and depressive symptoms by self-rating. *Archives of General Psychiatry, 48*, 807–812.

Bauer, M., & McBride, L. (1997). *Structured group psychotherapy for bipolar disorder: The Life Goals programme*. New York: Springer Publishing Company.

Beck, A.T. (1996). Beyond belief: A theory of modes, personality, and psychopathology. In P. Salkovskis (Ed.), *Frontiers of cognitive therapy*. New York: Guilford Press.

Beck, A.T., Rush, A.J., Shaw, B., & Emery, G. (1979). *Cognitive therapy of depression*. New York: John Wiley and Sons.

Chor, P., Mercier, M., & Halper, I. (1988). Use of cognitive therapy for treatment of a patient suffering from a bipolar affective disorder. *Journal of Cognitive Psychotherapy, 2*, 51–58.

Cochran, S. (1984). Preventing medical non-adherence in the outpatient treatment of bipolar affective disorder. *Journal of Consulting and Clinical Psychology, 52*, 873–878.

Cochran, S., & Gitlin, M. (1988). Attitudinal correlates of lithium adherence in bipolar affective disorders. *Journal of Nervous and Mental Diseases, 176*, 457–464.

Dickson, W., & Kendall, R. (1986). Does maintenance lithium therapy prevent recurrence of mania under ordinary clinical conditions? *Psychological Medicine, 16*, 521–530.

Ehlers, C., Frank, E., & Kupfer, D. (1988). Social zeitgebers and biological rhythms: A unified approach to understanding the aetiology of depression. *Archives of General Psychiatry, 45*, 948–952.

Fennell, M. (1997). Low self-esteem: A cognitive perspective. *Behavioural and Cognitive Psychotherapy, 25*, 1–26.

Goodwin, F., & Jamison, K. (1990). *Manic-depressive illness*. Oxford: Oxford University Press.

Greenberger, D., & Padesky, C. (1996). *Mind over mood: A cognitive therapy treatment manual for clients*. New York: Guilford Press.

Healey, D., & Williams, J.M.G. (1989). Moods, misattributions and mania: An interaction of biological and psychological factors in pathogenesis of mania. *Psychiatric Developments, 1*, 49–70.

Horne, R. (1997). Representations of medication and treatment: Advances in theory and measurement. In K. Petrie & J. Weinman (Eds.), *Perceptions of health and illness*. London: Harwood Academic Publishers.

Lam, D., Bright, J., Jones, S., Hayward, P., Shuck, N., Chisholm, D., & Sham, P. (2000). Cognitive therapy for bipolar disorders: A pilot study of relapse prevention. *Cognitive Therapy and Research, 24*, 503–520.

Lam, D., Jones, S., Hayward, P., & Bright, J. (1996). *Cognitive therapy for bipolar disorders*. Chichester: John Wiley.

Lam, D., & Wong, G. (1997). Prodromes, coping strategies, insight, and social functioning in bipolar affective disorders. *Psychological Medicine*, *27*, 1091–1100.

Manic Depression Fellowship (1995). *Inside out*. Twickenham, UK: MDF.

Markowitz, J. (1994). Psychotherapy of dysthymia. *American Journal of Psychiatry*, *151*, 114–121.

McKeon, P. (1992). *Coping with depression and elation*. London: Sheldon Press.

Miklowitz, D., & Goldstein, M. (1990). Behavioural family treatment for patients with bipolar affective disorder. *Behaviour Modification*, *14*, 457–489.

Molner, G., Feeney, M., & Fava, G. (1988). The duration and symptoms of bipolar prodromes. *American Journal of Psychiatry*, *145*, 1575–1578.

Newman, C., & Beck, A.T. (1992). *Cognitive therapy of rapid cycling bipolar affective disorder: A Treatment Manual*. Philadelphia: Center for Cognitive Therapy.

Padesky, C. (1994). Schema change processes in cognitive therapy. *Clinical Psychology and Psychotherapy*, *1*, 267–278.

Palmer, A., Williams, H., & Adams, M. (1995). Cognitive behaviour therapy in a group format for bipolar affective disorder. *Behavioural and Cognitive Psychotherapy*, *23*, 153–168.

Palmer, A., Williams, H., & Adams, M. (1998). The added benefits of group CBT for bipolar disorders: A comparison study with treatment as usual. Paper presented at the British Association of Behavioural and Cognitive Psychotherapists, Annual Meeting, Durham.

Peet, M., & Harvey, N. (1991). Lithium maintenance: 1. A standard education programme for patients. *British Journal of Psychiatry*, *158*, 197–200.

Perry, A., Tarrier, N., Morriss, R., McCarthy, E., & Limb, K. (1999). Randomised controlled trial of efficacy of teaching patients with bipolar disorder to identify early symptoms of relapse and obtain treatment. *British Medical Journal*, *318*, 149–153.

Rush, A. (1988). Cognitive approaches to adherence. In A. Frances & R. Hales (Eds.), *Review of psychiatry: Volume 8*. Washington, DC: APA Press.

Scott, J. (1992). Chronic depression: can cognitive therapy succeed when other treatments fail? *Behavioral Psychotherapy*, *20*, 25–34.

Scott, J. (1995a). Psychotherapy for bipolar disorder: An unmet need? *British Journal of Psychiatry*, *167*, 581–588.

Scott, J. (1995b). Cognitive therapy for clients with bipolar disorder: A case example. *Cognitive and Behavioural Practice*, *3*, 1–23.

Scott, J. (1995c). Editorial: Psychological treatments of depression. An update. *British Journal of Psychiatry*, *167*, 289–292.

Scott, J. (1999). Cognitive and behavioural approaches to medication adherence. *Advances in Psychiatric Treatment*, *5*, 338–347.

Scott, J. (2001a). Cognitive therapy as an adjunct to medication in bipolar disorders. *British Journal of Psychiatry supplement*, *178*, s164–168.

Scott, J. (2001b). *Overcoming mood swings: A self-help guide using cognitive and behavioural techniques*. London: Constable Robinson.

Scott, J., Byers, S., & Turkington, D. (1993). The chronic patient. In J. Wright, M. Thase, A.T. Beck, & J. Ludgate (Eds.), *Cognitive therapy with in-patients* (pp. 231–257). New York: Guilford Press.

Scott, J., Garland, A., & Moorhead, S. (2001). A pilot study of cognitive therapy in bipolar disorders. *Psychological Medicine*, *31*, 459–467.

Scott, J., Stanton, B., Garland, A., & Ferrier, N. (2000). Cognitive vulnerability to bipolar disorder. *Psychological Medicine*, *30*, 467–472.

Scott, J., & Wright, J. (1997). Cognitive therapy with severe and chronic mental disorders. In A. Frances & R. Hales (Eds.), *Review of Psychiatry: Volume 16* (pp. 153–201). Washington, DC: American Psychiatric Association Press.

Skelton, D., & Croyle, H. (1991). *Mental representation in health and illness*. New York: Springer Verlag.

Smith, J., & Tarrier, N. (1992). Prodromal symptoms in manic depressive psychosis. *Social Psychiatry and Psychiatric Epidemiology*, *27*, 245–248.

Wehr, T., Sack, D., & Rosenthal, N. (1987). Sleep reduction as a final common pathway in the genesis of mania. *American Journal of Psychiatry*, *144*, 201–203.

Winters, K., & Neale, J. (1985). Mania and low self-esteem. *Journal of Abnormal Psychology*, *94*, 282–290.

Wright, J., & Schrodt, R. (1992). Combined cognitive therapy and pharmacotherapy. In A. Freeman, K. Simon, L. Beutler, & H. Arowitz (Eds.), *Handbook of Cognitive Therapy* (pp. 124–161). New York: Plenum Press.

Wright, J., & Thase, M. (1992). Cognitive and biological therapies: A synthesis. *Psychiatric Annals*, *22*, 451–458.

Chapter 14

Cognitive behaviour therapy for patients with co-existing psychosis and substance use problems

Gillian Haddock, Christine Barrowclough, Jan Moring, Nicholas Tarrier, and Shôn Lewis

INTRODUCTION

Although a number of case series and randomised controlled trials have demonstrated that individual cognitive behaviour therapy (CBT) can produce clinically significant outcomes for patients with chronic psychosis (Kuipers et al., 1998; Tarrier et al., 1997, 1998), little attention has been paid to those patients who have co-existing problems of psychosis and substance use, despite reported estimates of the incidence of substance use problems being as high as 60% (Lehman & Dixon, 1995). Indeed, many researchers have either excluded those who have substance use problems from CBT studies, or, the needs of those included with substance use problems have been ignored. Furthermore, the efficacy of antipsychotic drugs in this population is, technically, unknown, because dual diagnosis is routinely an exclusion criterion from efficacy trials (Meuser & Lewis, in press). This may be partly related to the way services have been organised. Traditionally, services for people with mental health problems such as schizophrenia and those for substance use problems have been independent from each other and have tended to adopt differing treatment philosophies. For example, substance use services tend to emphasise that "recovery" is a possible outcome, whereas mental health services tend to view severe mental health problems within a rehabilitation framework, where the illness is viewed as having a long-term chronic course. Although these rationales make sense for the disorders that they are representing, when a patient presents with co-existing difficulties, clinicians are faced with a dilemma about which service will meet the needs of the client. In addition, generally, staff are not trained or experienced in the skills necessary to manage both disorders leading to patients receiving inadequate help for one aspect of their difficulties and staff feeling unskilled because they cannot provide the appropriate help for the patient.

If treatment of one disorder generalised to the other, then treatment in a single modality alone might be justified. However, evidence suggests that the needs of dual diagnosed patients are not met by services that are delivered separately. Dual diagnosis patients tend to fare worse than patients with severe mental health problems alone in terms of a range of outcomes. For example, higher and earlier relapse and readmission rates, they are more likely to present to accident and emergency services, and they tend to have higher levels of aggression and violence (Drake, Osher, & Wallach, 1989; Menezes et al., 1996), suggesting that the financial and service burden of dual diagnosis patients is high. In addition, anecdotal evidence suggests that mental health staff do not feel equipped to deal effectively with the complex needs of these patients and can sometimes feel unsympathetic to psychotic patients who engage in substance using behaviour despite receiving advice from services that it is unhelpful for their disorder.

There has been very little work to date in the UK evaluating the effectiveness of services for people with dual diagnoses of psychosis and substance use problems, although there have been a number of studies carried out in the USA. The available evidence is limited, although there are some indications that specialist integrated services are most helpful for dual diagnosis patients where the treatment for psychosis and substance use are delivered by mental health professionals skilled in the treatment of both psychosis and substance use problems (Drake et al., 1998; Ley et al., 1999). The rationale behind this is that the psychosis and substance use problems are not independent from each other and hence should be addressed simultaneously. In the UK, little evaluation of interventions has been undertaken: however, a recent randomised controlled trial carried out in Manchester demonstrated that an integrated cognitive behaviourally oriented service for patients with psychosis and drug and/or alcohol problems was effective in producing positive benefits on a number of outcomes (Haddock et al., 1999). The treatment was made up of interventions that research has shown to be most effective in treating the two disorders independently, and which were combined into an integrated treatment delivered by specialist therapists working in parallel with traditional services. The key elements of the treatment included motivational interviewing for substance use (Miller & Rollnick, 1991), individual cognitive behaviour therapy for psychosis (see Haddock et al., 1998), and family intervention (Barrowclough & Tarrier, 1992). The elements were not delivered in the traditional way usually adopted with each disorder alone, but were adapted for use with dually diagnosed patients. This chapter will describe the three aspects of treatment and how they were integrated, using illustrations from case examples.

MOTIVATIONAL INTERVIEWING

Motivational interviewing has been used effectively to enhance motivation to change substance use behaviour in non-psychotic populations (Bien, Miller, & Boroughs, 1993; Saunders, Wilkinson, & Phillips, 1995). It has been described fully in Miller and Rollnick (1991). Its application to substance use problems has been influenced by the stages of change model of Prochaska and DiClemente (1982), which has been described within substance use populations. Although this model has not been adequately validated with respect to psychotic patients, anecdotal evidence and clinical experience indicates that the approach has some validity in relation to psychotic patients with substance use problems. The model suggests that interventions should be linked to the patient's motivational stage. These stages are referred to as:

- pre-contemplation (i.e. substance use not perceived as a problem, no desire to change);
- contemplation (i.e. some awareness of problems associated with use, some indications that change is being considered);
- preparation/action (i.e. preparation and carrying out of change); and
- maintenance (i.e. maintaining and consolidating change, preventing relapse).

It is during the first two of these stages that motivational interviewing is particularly appropriate, as traditional interventions, such as direct advice to cease taking substances, may be at odds with the patient's view of their current substance use.

Motivational "type" interventions have been used with psychotic patients in relation to changing medication adherence (see Kemp et al., 1996), although they have not specifically been applied in relation to substance use problems. Motivational interviewing is described as therapy "style" rather than as an intervention in itself (Rollnick and Miller, 1995). It assumes that the responsibility for change in substance use behaviour lies with the patient and that change is only likely if the patient regards their substance use as problematic and identifies motivating factors towards change. As a result, motivational interviewing assumes that ambivalence about changing substance use is normal, not pathological, and that resolving this ambivalence is the key to change. This means that although the therapist has a clear aim to help the patient to confront any problems associated with their substance use, this aim is not made explicit and would not be brought up as an agenda item for a session by the therapist unless the patient wished to discuss it. This approach differs from traditional mental health approaches that have tended to adopt a psycho-educative perspective on substance use so that advice and discouragement to reduce or cease substance use is delivered. As a result, the motivational "style" clearly contrasts with traditional cognitive behavioural therapy. So if a patient expresses some doubts about whether or not to change substance use, the therapist would not focus on convincing the patient of the need to change, but would instead reflect back to the patient their ambivalence about change. The therapist avoids telling the client the advantages of, or need for change in substance use; instead the emphasis is focused on eliciting such statements from patients themselves. Reflective listening, summary statements, positive restructuring, and evocative questions can be utilised to elicit self-motivational statements. For example:

Patient: My family want me to stop using, but they don't realise how good the amphetamine makes me feel . . . I can reach another plane and communicate with the spirits when I'm using . . . and I don't want to lose that even though it gets me in a mess . . .

Therapist: It gets you in a mess . . . (*reflection*)

Patient: Yeh . . . last time I got picked up by the police . . . I'd nothing on, I don't know what had happened to my clothes . . . and then I ended up in hospital for weeks after . . .

Therapist: So . . . it sounds as though you enjoy using amphetamine because of how it makes you feel but sometimes things get in a mess and last time you ended up in hospital for some weeks . . . (*summary*)

Patient: Yeh . . . that was awful . . . I wouldn't want to go through that again . . . it gets me down when I think about it . . . (*self-motivational statement*)

Therapist: It sounds as though you've thought about things quite a bit, and not everyone would be prepared to do that . . . but then it's difficult to know what to do . . . on the one hand you enjoy using amphetamine, but on the other hand you say it gets you in a mess . . . (*restructuring/reflection*)

Patient: I know that my amphetamine use is going to do me in if I carry on for much longer . . .

Therapist: Does that bother you much?

Patient: Yes . . . I can't just ignore the problems . . . I ought to do something about my amphetamine use . . . (*self-motivational statement*)

The motivational interviewing style can be integrated with a CBT approach in order to increase patients' motivation to change their substance use behaviour while concurrently addressing issues relating to psychosis. In practice, this can be useful when first engaging with psychotic clients and can help in the establishment of an initial problem list. At this stage, the aim is for the patient to identify what they consider to be their key problems, which may or may not include drugs or alcohol. Indeed, many patients may not have considered their substance use as a problem because they had not noticed that they were consuming any more (or differently) from their peers. In addition, they may report positive benefits of drug or alcohol use that outweigh the disadvantages. For example, patients may report that drugs or alcohol can help them to cope better with their symptoms, or might help them to get along better when they are in social situations. As a result, careful exploration of any disadvantages is useful during early engagement sessions in order to assess the extent of any negative consequences of substance use. It is possible that there may be minimal negative consequences arising from substance use and therapy might then be focused on other problems that the patient identifies. However, in the Manchester trial, only patients who met DSM-IV criteria for substance abuse or dependence, and accordingly were experiencing problems associated with substance use, were included.

Assuming that substance use is problematic, the therapist utilises motivational interviewing skills of reflective listening, acceptance, and selective reinforcing of the patient's self-motivating statements during sessions. This will usually include responding to patient's expressions that substance use is problematic (e.g. "maybe I am drinking more than I should"), expressions of concern over substance use (e.g. "I sometimes wish I didn't spend quite so much on drugs"), expressions of desire or intention to change (e.g. "sometimes I think I should cut down on my drinking") and expressions of ability to change (e.g. "I can give up whenever I want"). The aim during initial sessions is to elicit change or motivational statements from the patient in relation to their substance use and engage the patient in developing a shared problem list. The initial list usually consists of the problems of severe mental illness such as distress about hallucinations and delusions or lack of motivation. At the same time the therapist will respond to disclosures about substance use with a view to helping the patient to suggest that this might be an area they would like to change. Once the patient identifies substance use as a problem and expresses a desire to change, then this can be part of the agenda in the usual way and assist the patient to achieve and maintain the change. However, the change process relating to substance use is lengthy and variable. The therapist should continue to adopt a motivational style to reinforce change, but also to monitor motivation, which may wax and wane throughout therapy.

Although the motivational interviewing style may be directed mainly towards substance use, discussion of other issues relating to psychosis may also be facilitated by the approach. For example, some patients have delusional ideas that make it difficult to put some important items on to an agenda, and it is not unusual for patients to have ambivalent feelings towards engaging with services or discussing the possibility of treatment or medication. Motivational approaches can be useful for addressing these issues. It may be useful in helping to resolve doubts or uncertainties about the origins of hallucinations or delusions where patients are struggling with whether something is externally generated or internally generated. As a result, initial agenda items such as "trying to stop MI5 from persecuting me" might be changed through motivational approaches into something that is more easily addressed—e.g. "trying to stop worrying about whether MI5 is after me".

INDIVIDUAL COGNITIVE BEHAVIOUR THERAPY (CBT)

The individual CBT that has been described for chronic psychotic patients (see Chadwick, Birchwood, & Trower, 1996; Fowler et al., 1995; Haddock & Tarrier, 1998; Kingdon & Turkington, 1994; Morrison, 1998) can be adapted for dual diagnosis patients and should include the following elements: therapy that is collaborative and based on a shared formulation, a focus on key cognitions, the application of guided discovery, the use of homework where appropriate, and the use of structure and agenda together with non-specific elements of empathy, understanding, and acceptance. The intervention process should cover: assessment, formulation, intervention, monitoring, and evaluation and keeping well/relapse prevention strategies. Agenda items during early sessions are most likely to include providing a rationale for CBT and engaging the patient in the approach, exploration of key problems and establishing an initial problem list. Leaflets explaining "what is CBT" can be useful at this stage to familiarise the patient to the approach. The emphasis during engagement is on communicating that the approach is collaborative and meant to help patients identify and resolve problems. If the patient has not acknowledged that substance use is a problem, this would not be identified on the problem list and the motivational interviewing approach described earlier should be adopted. The following problems are common to most patients with psychosis and are likely to come up with most patients at some time: problems regarding hallucinations, delusions, negative symptoms, social functioning, self-esteem, depression, anxiety, familial difficulties, medication and side effects, as well as financial and social problems. Although these areas are common for all psychotic patients, substance users may have pertinent problems relating to symptomatology that is masked or covered up by the substance use, financial problems relating to substance use, interpersonal and family difficulties related directly to disagreement regarding substance use, frequent and less predictable relapses, frequent hospitalisations, and problems relating to violence and aggression.

Once the patient is agreeable to exploring problems and initial problems have been identified, the therapist should negotiate a prioritised list that can be assessed in more detail. Sessions should be structured as follows:

1   Discussion of the previous week and how the patient has been in order to assess whether there are any issues that should be prioritised for the agenda and to assess the patient's mental state for continuing with the session.

2   A rationale for the session and establishment of a shared agenda. This will include a discussion of any homework and the implications of this, and specific items generated by the therapist and patient.

Cognitive behavioural assessment and formulation

Further assessment should be based around a thorough cognitive behavioural analysis of the problem, which ensures that issues relating to substance use are accounted for in the onset, occurrence, and maintenance of a symptom. Attention should be paid to how the symptom/problem presents currently and how the symptom has changed or developed over time. Important areas to cover are when the symptom first occurred, how this related to the onset of "illness" (if the patient describes his/her difficulties in this way), and the circumstances surrounding worsening or relapse of the symptom/problem. It is likely that this type of assessment will elicit some observations that substance use has occurred when there has been a worsening of the symptoms. These observations can be used within initial formulations to encourage discussion of issues relating to relapse and substance use. However, this should be carried out sensitively utilising a motivational interviewing style. In addition, attention should be paid to the patient's model of illness. It is not uncommon for substance use to be blamed for the maintenance or onset of their difficulties. Although, substance use may have played a part in this, this type of attribution can often lead to patients blaming all their "symptoms" on substance use and assuming that these would disappear if the substance use was reduced/ceased. Alternatively, a patient may attribute all his difficulties to external sources (such as aliens or a persecutory agent) or to illness. As a result, it is necessary for the therapist to explore models of illness as part of their assessment with a view to a collaborative working formulation being adopted by the patient as well as the therapist. This is also important when working with families (discussed later).

A working formulation should be the aim of the assessment. The complexity of the formulation that is shared between patient and therapist will depend on the nature of the patient's difficulties and on the patient's ability to discuss their symptoms in cognitive behavioural terms. It is usually advisable for the therapist to discuss and prepare a formulation with a supervisor before sharing this with a patient. The formulation should then be prepared in a form that can be easily proposed to the patient in simple and clear terms. It is much easier to build on a simple clear formulation than to start with something too complex, which interferes with the collaborative relationship between patient and therapist. The formulation should ideally be generated during a joint session with a patient, so that there is a shared "ownership" of the problem conceptualisation. The minimum aim at this point in terms of formulation is to describe the key problem/s in terms of their component thoughts, feelings, and behaviours in a way that reflects the experiences of the patient. The following brief case study illustrates how this can be done.

Jane: A case study

Jane had a 10-year history of psychosis. She took amphetamines and cannabis regularly and did not consider her drug use to be problematic. Her main symptom was a belief that there was a large, worldwide organisation that targeted her for persecution because of an incident when she owed money to her drug dealer. She experienced unpleasant thoughts being inserted into her mind and avoided going out because she was afraid that everyone could read her mind and hence be influenced by these unpleasant thoughts. She felt that taking drugs helped her to get out and about and helped her to cope with the unpleasant thoughts. She had had seven previous episodes where hospitalisation was necessary due to an increase in severity of her symptoms. During assessment, it became clear that there were links between how she felt, her thoughts, her drug use, and her symptoms. For example, she always experienced an increase in her worries about the persecutory organisation at the weekend. These times coincided with an increase in her drug taking over the previous couple of days. She received her financial benefits on Tuesdays and always spent the money on drugs. Her money was usually spent by Thursday resulting in her feeling down as she had no money left and upset that she would probably not be able to get any more until next benefit day. However, she knew that if she really hassled her mum that she would probably give her some money to tide her over. Her mum usually did give her some money but not before there were aggressive and sometimes violent rows between them. Jane was able to associate this pattern with the increase in her symptoms, and although she felt that the persecution was "real" she could acknowledge that she became more bothered by it when she was upset or distressed. She acknowledged that her lack of money, probable physiological reaction to drugs, and the familial difficulties all contributed to her feeling upset, and that if she were able to reduce the stress caused by these factors then she might be less bothered about the persecutory organisation.

This type of initial formulation can be used as a basis for deciding what interventions are necessary. In this case, they initially included continued motivational style to increase her motivation to change her substance use, strategies designed to increase her ability to manage her money, family intervention, and belief modification work to address her ideas of persecution. In addition, the understanding and conceptualisation of the case should continue because more information will be revealed over sessions that can be added to the formulation. For example, factors that have contributed to the onset of symptoms or illness and factors that contribute to relapse or hospitalisation may only become apparent later on in therapy. However, these areas are extremely important in understanding the wider context of a patient's symptoms and it is usually relevant to expand the formulation to include these areas to maximise and maintain change. The assessment and formulation of issues relating to family work in this case are described later in the chapter.

Individual CBT interventions

Once a shared understanding or agreement of factors that contribute to symptom or illness occurrence has been achieved, interventions are applied in the usual way (see Haddock & Slade, 1996). Delusions can be addressed using belief modification and reality-testing. Hallucinations can be treated using similar belief modification and reality-testing approaches, focusing, monitoring, and distraction. Negative symptoms can be modified using activity scheduling and goal setting. Other symptoms such as anxiety, depression, and low self-esteem can be addressed using traditional cognitive behavioural methods. Intervention relating to substance use will depend on the motivational stage of the patient, which will continue to be monitored throughout any intervention. However, the absence of motivation to change substance use does not prevent interventions for other symptoms from progressing. If the patient has expressed a desire to makes changes to substance use, then cognitive behavioural strategies will be adopted to assist with this. Assistance can be provided to help the individual to make change, and to maintain this once substance use behaviour is modified using relapse prevention strategies.

FAMILY INTERVENTION

Although some patients with psychosis and substance use problems may not reside with relatives, a substantial number will have regular contact with carers. Working with these carers is extremely important to assist mental health professionals to improve outcomes for patients, and for carers themselves to feel that their needs are met. It is well established that high expressed emotion households are associated with increased relapse risk for patients, and family interventions have demonstrated significant improvements in relapse rates for patients (Mari & Streiner, 1994). Given the dual problems for carers of coping with both mental illness and drug or alcohol misuse, indications from the Manchester schizophrenia and substance use study suggest that family interventions are very important for both dual diagnosis patients and their carers. The cognitive behaviourally oriented family intervention described by Barrowclough and Tarrier (1992) was adapted for use with substance using patients and their carers, modifications being to incorporate issues concerning substance use to each component of the intervention. The intervention sought to promote a family response that was consistent with the motivational interviewing style and the stages of change model: i.e. (i) responsibility for problems and their consequences needs to be left with the client and confrontation about substance use may create more resistance to change; and (ii) family help will be most effective when it matches the stage of change of the client. The stress reduction approach of the generic family intervention model and motivational enhancement approaches were in complete concordance, sharing a common framework about the kind of help that was likely to be most effective. For patients who are, at best, only at the contemplative stage of change, the intervention is directed at helping relatives to appreciate that attempts, on the one hand, to try and get/make someone change their substance use or, on the other hand, to buffer the consequences of the use would be counter-productive. Hence, the family is encouraged to embrace the deliberate strategy of doing nothing—not persuading, cajoling, or even encouraging clients to stop drinking or using drugs. This approach was promoted in the educational and subsequent interventions as an active and positive strategy of detachment, rather than a passive and negative way of behaving. It emphasised that the family need to leave it up to the client to make changes, but at the same time it is good to set boundaries and limits on the extent to which they will tolerate the substance use having adverse consequences on the family life. This includes not rescuing clients from the consequences of drug/alcohol use (for example, not bailing them out financially if they blow their money on drugs/alcohol; not covering up for their periods of drunkenness; and establishing reasonable house rules about acceptability of behaviour with age appropriate sanctions that the relative is willing to carry through if rules are broken). For patients who have identified the need for change and who have commenced active change, the emphasis on client responsibility would also endorse the relative supporting changes once they have happened, but not the relative attempting to initiate change.

The general approach to family intervention used in Manchester has been documented (Barrowclough & Tarrier, 1992). It begins with a detailed assessment of family problems and needs elicited from interviews, supplemented by questionnaires. Following from this assessment a collaborative problems and needs list is formulated that would typically include: (a) issues concerning the relatives' understanding of the illness; (b) relatives' distress; (c) coping difficulties; (d) dissatisfactions with particular aspects of the patient's behaviour; and (e) restrictions and hardships that the relative is suffering as a consequence of the illness. Additionally, family strengths would be highlighted using the problem list as a guide and the interventions to address the problems are then structured around three components: (1) education; (2) stress management and coping strategies; and (3) goal setting to promote patient and relative change. In the dual diagnosis study, using the motivational framework, problems associated with substance use were identified in the assessment phase, highlighted in the problem formulation, and addressed in each of the intervention components.

Common problems associated with the substance use identified in the education sessions were:

1   Relatives tending to blame patients for making their problems worse through substance misuse.

2   Underestimating the patient's symptomatology in relation to schizo-phrenia and tending to attribute all the problems to drugs or alcohol.

3   Relatives being reluctant to stand back and leave responsibility for change with clients, feeling that this would be tantamount to condoning substance use.

4   At the same time, making many sacrifices in terms of time and money in attempts to help the patient, but finding that these attempts did not resolve the problem.

The education sessions sought to acknowledge relatives' viewpoints, while beginning to work sensitively to offer alternative explanations and strategies where appropriate, thus setting the scene for bringing about family change in later stages of the intervention.

The stress management component of the intervention aimed to reduce intrafamilial stress in the household. It focused directly on the situations associated with stress. Cognitive behavioural assessment of these situations was carried out and collaborative ways of reducing stress were explored. The goal setting component in the family intervention aimed to improve the social functioning of the patient. Using the format of goal planning and seeing the whole family together, the aim was to teach the family a constructional approach to the problems of family members. This entails seeing problems as needs that might best be met through promoting positive behaviour change. An indirect aim was to reduce family stress by directing their attempts to assist the patient at methods that are constructional and have a high chance of success, hopefully replacing previous unsuccessful attempts that focused on trying to eradicate problem behaviours. In the context of the dual diag-nosis families, this emphasis was very important and helped to counter the feeling that, by suggesting they left responsibility for substance use with the patient, they were being asked to do nothing. It was presented as an opportunity to channel carers' efforts to help into plans that might promote positive client behaviours (rather than into fruitless arguments and frustrated attempts to control the substances). This component was closely linked to patient sessions and was a forum for addressing problem areas identified as common to both patients and relatives during the initial problem identifica-tion and formulation stage. Because of the emphasis on one-to-one client work in combination with the family intervention, attention was paid to the integration of patient alone, carer alone, and patient–carer sessions. This integration is illustrated in the following further discussion of Jane and her family.

Jane and her mother: A case study

Jane had been living with her mother (Ms M) throughout her illness. Ms M worked part-time in a supermarket. She used to work full-time but felt that if she was away from Jane, that Jane would get into "some sort of trouble" as a result of her drug using. In consequence, she tended to stay at home as much as possible for Jane, in case she got into difficulties and needed her mum to help. Ms M appreciated that Jane had a serious illness and thought that drugs had caused it. She thought that she was partly to blame as the illness emerged after she and her previous husband had divorced. She found Jane's drug use very upsetting and was constantly worried that Jane would hurt herself and that she would end up in hospital again. Jane's previous admissions had been preceded by suicide attempts that had been discovered by Ms M. She was extremely supportive of Jane, and helped her financially and with her day-to-day living. Ms M had few friends and did not go out very often, although she wished she could get out a bit more. Her main contacts were with Jane and her other daughter, Julie. Julie was married with two young children. She visited her mother often and relied heavily on her for child care. Julie thought Jane was a "waster" and took advantage of her mother. She felt that if Jane just tried harder and stopped taking drugs that everything would be OK. She was angry that her mother provided Jane with money for drugs and constantly reminded Jane of how she sponged from the family. However, Julie was fond of Jane and sometimes took her out with her friends. This had not happened recently because last time they went out Jane had a confrontation with Julie's friends whom she thought were talking about her behind her back.

It was clear that both Julie and her mum were very concerned about Jane and were keen to help in any way they could. As a result, both mum and Julie were assessed individually. Assessment revealed that Ms M had needs and/or required help in the following areas: knowledge about schizophrenia and the role of drugs in onset, maintenance and relapse, strategies to assist her to cope and manage relapse, strategies to help cope with Jane's drug use, strategies to help her cope with her worries and stress, and strategies to develop her own social functioning and independence. Some of these need areas were also common to Julie and to Jane. For example, all of the family had inaccurate views of factors that contribute to the onset and maintenance of schizophrenia. Areas of common need can be identified and intervention strategies can then be directed towards either the individual alone or towards the family together. The following are the initial problem lists that were agreed on for Jane and her family. As can be seen, initially, substance use was not listed as a problem for Jane, although the consequences of her substance use, in terms of symptom exacerbation and worries about relapse and finances are prominent.

- **Jane**

    1   Paranoia and worries about thought reading.
    2   Depression and low self-esteem.

3 Concerns regarding rows in the family.
4 Worry about future relapse.
5 Worry regarding finances.

- **Mum/Julie**

1 Problems in managing the consequences of Jane's drug use.
2 Stress associated with their worries and concerns over drugs, relapse.
3 Dissatisfaction with levels of own social functioning.

- **Shared problem list**

1 Inadequate up-to-date knowledge and information about cause, triggers, and maintenance factors in schizophrenia.
2 Inadequate up-to-date knowledge about the role of factors that worsen symptoms of schizophrenia (including drugs and alcohol).
3 Diagreements about money.
4 Disagreement about Jane's contributions to the housekeeping.

In relation to Jane and her family, 25 individual sessions were carried out with Jane addressing issues outlined above. In addition, five joint family sessions with Jane, her mum, and Julie took place to address areas of joint concern, seven sessions took place with mum alone, and three with Julie and mum together. Initial joint sessions were spent on discussing education about schizophrenia, its causes, treatment, outcome, etc. (see Barrowclough & Tarrier, 1992 for details of specific approaches). However, these joint sessions were followed up with mum and Julie alone in order to help them to make use of the knowledge acquired during education sessions. For example, Ms M's strategies to influence Jane's drug using did not appear to be working. As a result, therapy focused on helping her and Julie to try adopting a motivational style towards Jane in their interactions regarding drug use. Initially, Ms M and Julie thought that this approach would make things worse rather than better, as they believed that if they stopped encouraging her to stop taking drugs that she would do it even more. However, when it was suggested that this approach be accompanied by strategies to help the family to "manage" Jane's drug taking (e.g. an agreement to provide Jane with only set amounts of money, and a rule that drug taking only take place outside Ms M's house), the family felt able to attempt the approach. The intervention sought to promote a family response that was consistent with the stages of change model and the motivational interviewing style characterised by leaving responsibility for problems and their consequences with the client; recognising that confrontation about substance use may create more resistance to change; and realising that family help will be most effective when it matches the stage of change of the client. Hence, one of the issues targeted in the education sessions was the need for Jane to take sole responsibility for the drug use.

In the individual stress management component, Jane's mother was encouraged to appraise the advantages and disadvantages of spending as much time with Jane as possible, and through such a guided discovery process, helped to see that there were more cons than pros in maintaining this role. Part of this process involved the mother experimenting in leaving Jane alone some days and monitoring the consequences. This required some gentle challenging of Ms M's catastrophic beliefs about what might happen if her daughter were left to her own devices, alongside some help in problem solving how to distract herself from her own anxious thoughts. At the same time, she set limits with Jane about not taking drugs in the house, and about how much extra money her mother would provide her with. Although this caused some distress to both Jane and her mother at first, there was not a large change in Jane's drug taking behaviour and she did not get into trouble as her mother had predicted. In addition, her mother had spent the time away from Jane on meeting up with an old friend who had invited her to go away on holiday with her. She was considering taking her up on this. Jane was pleased her mother had gone out on her own and was pleased she wasn't continually "on her back". Jane had noticed that she was struggling financially without the extra money from her mother and was considering making changes to her drug use. Goal setting sessions involved Jane, her mother, and Julie, and focused on increasing Jane and Ms M's social functioning and on strategies to increase the finances available for housekeeping and for Jane to spend on herself. At this point, Jane expressed a desire to calculate the amount of money she spent on drugs and to limit this, so that she had some money left to give to her mum and to spend on things she wanted. For example, she was keen to have a holiday and to buy a bicycle and realised that she would not get them if she continued to spend her money on drugs. Julie volunteered to help her with this by taking her out more with friends who were not drug users. She also suggested that she and Jane save up to go away for the weekend together, albeit only if Jane did not take drugs while they were away. These goals were implemented and Jane's drug use decreased, resulting in a range of improvements in her own functioning and that of her mother. This was dovetailed with the individual intervention that continued to employ a motivational style when necessary and to work on her delusional beliefs. Her distress, preoccupation, and conviction in her persecutory ideas decreased during the intervention. These changes also coincided with an improvement in her mood and self-esteem.

CONCLUSIONS

The Manchester study of schizophrenia and substance use has demonstrated that positive outcomes can be obtained for people experiencing dual problems using an integrated treatment model. The benefits were not demonstrated for those patients in the trial who received treatment as usual. In fact, there was some indication that, over time, patients with dual problems deteriorated, demonstrating that specialist interventions are extremely important to improve outcomes for this group of patients. However, it is important that these type of specialist interventions are not delivered as isolated "add on" mental health services. Much effort was dedicated towards integrating the specialist approach into routine treatment during and at the end of the intervention in order that interventions that had been helpful could be continued (albeit on a less intensive level) and consolidated. This was found to be an important component of the intervention and was welcomed by patients and families. However, the majority of staff felt ill-equipped to follow-up specific motivational and cognitive behavioural interventions with these patients, indicating that there are important issues relating to staff support, training, and supervision that need to be addressed in this area.

REFERENCES

Barrowclough, C., & Tarrier, N. (1992). *Families of schizophrenic patients: Cognitive behavioural intervention*. London: Chapman and Hall.

Bien, T.H., Miller, W.R., & Boroughs, J.M. (1993). Motivational interviewing with alcohol outpatients. *Behavioural and Cognitive Psychotherapy*, *21*, 347–356.

Chadwick, P., Birchwood, M., & Trower, P. (1996). *Cognitive therapy for voices, delusions and paranoia*. Chichester: Wiley.

Drake, R.E., Mercer McFadden, C., Mueser, K.T., McHugo, G.J., & Bond, G.R. (1998). A review of integrated mental health and substance abuse treatment for patients with dual disorders. *Schizophrenia Bulletin*, *24*, 589–608.

Drake, R.E., Osher, F.C., & Wallach, M.A. (1989). Alcohol use and abuse in schizophrenia: A prospective community study. *Journal of Nervous and Mental Disease*, *177*, 408–414.

Fowler, D., Garety, P., & Kuipers, E. (1995). *Cognitive behaviour therapy for people with psychosis: A clinical handbook*. Chichester: Wiley.

Haddock, G., Barrowclough, C., Tarrier, N., Lewis, S., Moring, J., O'Brien, R., Schofield, N., McGovern, J., & Lowens, I. (1999). *CBT for psychosis and associated substance use problems*. Paper presented at the British Association of Behavioural and Cognitive Psychotherapies Annual Conference, University of Bristol.

Haddock, G., & Slade, P.D. (1996). *Cognitive behavioural interventions for psychotic disorders*. London: Routledge.

Haddock, G., & Tarrier, N. (1998). Assessment and formulation in the cognitive behavioural treatment of psychosis. In N. Tarrier, A. Wells, & G. Haddock (Eds.), *Treating complex cases: The cognitive behavioural approach* (pp. 155-175). Chichester: Wiley.

Haddock, G., Tarrier, N., Spaulding, W., Yusupoff, L., Kinney, C., & McCarthy, E. (1998). Individual cognitive behavioural interventions for hallucinations and delusions: A review. *Clinical Psychology Review*, *18*, 821–838.

Kemp, R., Hayward, P., Applethwaite, G., Everitt, B., & David, A. (1996). Compliance therapy in psychotic patients: Randomised controlled trial. *British Medical Journal, 312*, 345–349.

Kingdon, D., & Turkington, D. (1994). *Cognitive behavioural therapy of schizophrenia*. New York: Guilford Press.

Kuipers, E., Fowler, D., Garety, P., Chisholm, D., Freeman, G., Dunn, G., Bebbington, P., & Hadley, C. (1998). London-East Anglia randomised controlled trial of cognitive behavioural therapy for psychosis, III: Follow-up and economic evaluation at 18 months. *British Journal of Psychiatry, 173*, 61–68.

Kuipers, E., Garety, P., Fowler, D., Freeman, D., Dunn, G., Bebbington, P., Hadley, C., & Jones, S. (1997). The London-East Anglia randomised controlled trial of cognitive behaviour therapy for psychosis: Effects of the treatment phase. *British Journal of Psychiatry, 117*, 319–325.

Lehman, A.F., & Dixon, L.B. (1995). *Double jeopardy: Chronic mental illness and substance use disorders*. Chur, Switzerland: Harwood Academic Publishers.

Ley, A., Jeffery, D.P., McClaren, S., & Siegfried, N. (1999). Treatment programmes for people with both severe mental illness and substance misuse (Cochrane Review). In *The Cochrane Library, Issue 2*. Oxford: Update Software.

Mari, J.J., & Streiner, D.L. (1994). An overview of family interventions and relapse on schizophrenia: Meta-analysis of research findings. *Psychological Medicine, 24(3)*, 565–578.

Menezes, P.R., Johnson, S., Thornicroft, G., Marshall, J., Prosser, D., Bebbington, P., & Kuipers, E. (1996). Drug and alcohol problems among individuals with severe mental illnesses in South London. *British Journal of Psychiatry, 168*, 612–619.

Meuser, K.T., & Lewis, S.W. (in press). Treatment of substance misuse in schizophrenia. In P.F. Buckley & J. Waddington (Eds.), *Schizophrenia and mood disorders: The new drug therapies in clinical practice*. New York: Butterworth-Heinemann.

Miller, W.R., & Rollnick, S. (1991). *Motivational interviewing: Preparing people to change addictive behaviour*. New York: Guilford Press.

Morrison, A.P. (1998). Cognitive behaviour therapy for psychotic symptoms in schizophrenia. In N. Tarrier, A. Wells, & G. Haddock (Eds.), *Treating complex cases: The cognitive behavioural approach* (pp. 195–216). Chichester: Wiley.

Prochaska, J.O., & DiClemente, P.P. (1982). Transtheoretical therapy: Toward a more integrative model of change. *Psychotherapy: Theory, Research and Practice, 19*, 276–288.

Rollnick, S., & Miller, W.R. (1995). What is motivational interviewing? *Behavioural and Cognitive Psychotherapy, 23*, 325–334.

Saunders, B., Wilkinson, C., & Phillips, M. (1995). The impact of a brief motivational intervention with opiate users attending a methadone programme. *Addiction, 90*, 415–424.

Tarrier, N., Yusupoff, L., Kinney, C., McCarthy, E., Gledhill, A., Haddock, G., & Morris, J. (1998). A randomised controlled trial of intensive cognitive behaviour therapy for chronic schizophrenia. *British Medical Journal, 317*, 303–307.

Chapter 15

Enhancing appropriate adherence with neuroleptic medication

Two contrasting approaches

Fiona Randall, Pam Wood, Jennifer Day, Richard Bentall, Anne Rogers, and David Healy

INTRODUCTION

Research into psychotic patients' willingness to take neuroleptic medication has been dominated by quantitative studies carried out from a medical perspective, which have relied on the concept of "compliance". According to Haynes, Taylor, and Sackett (1979), compliance can be defined as: "The extent to which a person's behaviour in terms of taking medications, following diets, or executing lifestyle changes, coincides with medical or health advice". However, the concept of compliance has been criticised because it appears to be paternalistic and suggests an unequal relationship between the patient and the prescriber. It assumes that a decision to refuse medication is always irrational and health-damaging. This presumption has been compounded in professionals' views of people with mental health problems, who are often dismissed as "lacking in insight" if they doubt the value of medical treatment.

Later studies substituted the term "adherence" in an attempt to acknowledge the presumed autonomy of the patient, although it is questionable whether this amounts to much more than a terminological advance. More recently the term "concordance" has been proposed, which acknowledges that patients' and prescribers' views may differ and promotes negotiation and collaboration (Royal Pharmaceutical Society of Great Britain, 1997). In this negotiation, it is emphasised that the health professional should respect the views of patients, even if they differ from their own, and work with this to form an alliance. Within this framework adherence with medication may be more likely to occur. Although this approach is consistent with research findings in a range of health settings that emphasise health beliefs and autonomy, there is little research evidence of strategies that improve concordance.

It is difficult to measure adherence accurately. However, reported adherence rates in people with a diagnosis of schizophrenia average out at about 50% (Kampman & Lehtinen, 1999; Kane, 1985). Although it is sometimes assumed that mental health patients are particularly reluctant to follow medical advice, this rate is similar to that found in studies of other long-term conditions such as hypertension (Ley, 1992). Unfortunately, the consequences of non-adherence with neuroleptic medication can be dramatic. Non-adherence is associated with increased rates of involuntary detention, longer hospital admissions, and slower recovery from psychotic symptoms (McEvoy, Howe, & Hogarty, 1984). It has been described as the single most important cause of relapse and readmission to hospital (Pool & Elder, 1986). Indeed, relapse rates have been shown to be up to five times higher in people who choose not to take medication compared with people who adhere to neuro-leptic regimens (Robinson et al., 1999). This leads to significant costs to individuals, their families, and health service providers.

In any review of the research on interventions designed to improve adherence in people with a diagnosis of schizophrenia, it is important to acknowledge that this should only be a goal when patients are prescribed appropriate treatment. Ideally, a treatment should be prescribed at a safe dosage, be effective, and have minimal side effects. In the treatment of schizo-phrenia this ideal can be difficult to achieve. Some 20% to 30% of people with a diagnosis of schizophrenia fail to respond to neuroleptic medication and a further proportion only respond partially (Conley & Buchanan, 1997). The side effects of neuroleptic medication are diverse, distressing and, very rarely, fatal (Bentall et al., 1996). Although the new atypical antipsychotics are an improvement on conventional neuroleptics, they are still associated with a significant risk of side effects, which include excess weight gain, sexual dys-function, and—in the case of clozapine—agranulocytosis, a potentially fatal blood disorder. Actual prescribing practices vary widely and treatment that departs from the evidence base is often observed. This may consist of pre-scribing above maximum recommended doses, polyprescribing, and the main-tenance of patients on high doses of medication when they have failed to show any clinical response. Kissling (1994) has suggested that inadequate prescrib-ing is a cause of unnecessarily high relapse rates in schizophrenia patients. We therefore recommend that strategies to improve adherence should only be implemented where there is evidence that the prescribed medication is within prescribing guidelines, is effective and has minimum side effects.

A number of psycho-social interventions have been designed to enhance adherence with neuroleptic medication. Educational approaches tend to improve knowledge about medication but not adherence rates (Boczkowski, Zeichner, & Desanto, 1985; Macpherson, Jerrom, & Hughes, 1996). However, Kelly and Scott (1990) found that educating patients and their families about schizophrenia, about treatment, and about communicating with health pro-fessionals significantly improved adherence.

Other researchers have developed interventions that place more emphasis on improving relationships between patients and mental health professionals. Eckman and Liberman (1990) developed a short training scheme for profes-sionals to enable them to teach adherence-related skills to patients. This included teaching skills in four areas: (a) obtaining information about medication, (b) administering medication and evaluating its benefits, (c) identifying medication side effects, and (d) negotiating with health professionals. Patients' adherence (assessed by psychiatrists and caregivers) increased significantly after training.

Corrigan, Liberman, and Engel (1990) used strategies to enhance collaboration between the patient and the prescriber in order to negotiate treatment regimens, and this also resulted in significant improvements in adherence. More recently, Kemp et al. (1996) carried out a randomised controlled trial of compliance therapy, a new intervention based on motivational interviewing and cognitive approaches to psychotic symptoms. This intervention resulted in significant improvements in insight, attitudes to treatment, and observer-rated compliance, and these were maintained at 18-month follow-up (Kemp et al., 1998).

In this chapter we describe two interventions designed to improve adherence in people with a diagnosis of schizophrenia or schizoaffective disorder, which are currently being evaluated in a large randomised controlled trial. The trial is taking place in the north-west of England and north Wales and is funded by the Medical Research Council. It has three arms: a treatment as usual control group, a compliance intervention group, and a novel alliance intervention group. The compliance intervention consists of providing information about medication, its indications, and potential side effects, destigmatising mental illness and medication-taking, and behavioural strategies to help patients remember when to take their drugs. The philosophy behind this approach is similar to that of some of the earlier educational interventions—the patient is given strong advice that they should take their medical treatment as prescribed. The alliance intervention, which is similar to Kemp et al.'s motivational interviewing approach, builds on our previous research that has focused on clients' experiences of medication (Rogers et al., 1998). It includes self-monitoring of symptoms and side effects experienced by individuals, exploring ideas and beliefs about mental health problems and medication, and learning how to negotiate with mental health professionals by means of role-play. The philosophy behind this approach is that the patient should be regarded as a rational consumer, and should be encouraged to evaluate the value of medication for him or herself. It is assumed that this will usually result in "appropriate adherence"; that is, enhanced adherence if and only if the medication is having overall positive effects.

One aim of the trial was to determine whether these quite simple yet different approaches have differential outcomes in terms of attitudes towards medication, adherence to treatment, and avoidance of relapse. However, because the interventions were part of a trial, they were constrained by manuals that determined their content. Of necessity, this prevented the therapists from responding as flexibly to the participants' needs as would be desirable in routine clinical practice.

CASE STUDY 1: COMPLIANCE INTERVENTION

History and initial assessment

NP was a 16-year-old woman living with her mother; her father and brother left the family home at about the same time as the intervention began. She had recently started attending college. NP began hearing voices when she was 15 and subsequently spent 2 months in a Young Persons Unit, which was her first contact with psychiatric services. Afterwards, she returned home but stopped taking her medication. As a consequence she became overactive and psychotic again and, soon after, she was hospitalised. It was at this point that she was recruited to the project. Although she was initially diagnosed as hypomanic, her psychiatrist reclassified her as suffering from schizoaffective disorder according to ICD-10 criteria, a diagnosis that was concordant with our initial assessment of her. Her medication at the time of this assessment was risperidone 6mg and benperidol 250mg daily.

Prior to the intervention NP was given a baseline battery of tests administered by DC, including the Positive and Negative Syndrome Scale (PANSS; Kay, Fiszbein, & Opler, 1987). During this assessment, NP talked openly about hearing unpleasant voices, having "odd thoughts" about killing people, and "dreaming" (seeing visions of people) while she was still awake. She said she had smelt dog faeces in her home although no dog had ever been in the house. She said that she also believed that the radio was communicating with her. NP confided to the assessor that her brother had raped her on several occasions and there was also some suspicion, by the staff on the ward, that she had been sexually abused by her father. Her fears about being raped again caused her to feel panic at night and sadness during the day.

NP presented as a softly spoken, friendly, and intelligent young woman. She described herself as loud and hyperactive. She compared herself negatively with other people because of her problems and also because of her excess weight. She believed she had a psychiatric problem and that she needed medication to calm her down. NP did not feel ready to be discharged from hospital as she felt her parents did not want her to go home.

Intervention

The intervention was carried out by PW. NP was keen to participate in the intervention and was generally talkative. However, on occasions she became quiet, which she attributed to feeling tired as a result of her medication.

The intervention took seven sessions, the content of which was determined by the manual prepared for the trial. Some of these took place in NP's home after she had been discharged from hospital. Most were much shorter than conventional cognitive behaviour therapy (CBT) sessions, reflecting their simpler and more structured format.

Session 1: Orientation

NP was informed that the overall aims of the intervention were (i) to help her understand the nature and purpose of her medication; (ii) to help her find better ways of taking her medication; and (iii) to help her cope with any side effects that she might be experiencing. In order to help her begin to think about some of these issues, NP was asked to describe herself when feeling both psychologically well and unwell, and to say what sort of things she believed influenced her mental health. During this task, she described her "ill" self as depressed, lacking in confidence, tense, anxious, and suffering from unpleasant thoughts and hallucinations. In contrast, she described her "well" self as calm, stable, happy and normal. She believed that stress at home, or from her peer group and society made her feel ill, whereas positive events in her life, such as making friends, made her feel well. When asked what she could do to achieve a feeling of well-being, NP readily offered that medication could help her. She said that initially she had been unable to accept that she was unwell but, as her problems had persisted, she had been forced to accept that there was something wrong with her. (In this respect, she differed from many other patients seen in the project, who sometimes completely denied that they had psychiatric difficulties. In such cases, we began by asking the participant to discuss how other people appear when mentally well and when ill. Diagnoses given by doctors were often mentioned by participants at this point. However, this issue did not arise in the case of NP.)

The rest of the session was educational, and much more didactic. As part of a normalising strategy, it was explained that mental illness existed on a continuum with normal functioning, and NP was told about famous people who had suffered from psychiatric problems. She was then given a brief and fairly conventional description of the symptoms of schizophrenia and schizoaffective disorder. The session concluded with a discussion of the benefits and costs associated with being in hospital. As NP accepted her need for hospitalisation, this presented no difficulty. However, with patients who believe that their hospitalisation is unnecessary, we have found it useful to discuss how their problems are viewed by the medical staff, and to suggest to them that the ward is an environment in which they can receive support through a difficult period.

Session 2: Prevention of relapse

This session took place in NP's home as her doctor had decided to discharge her from hospital. Its aim was to discuss the medication she had been prescribed. After being asked to briefly recall the content of the previous session, NP was asked to list her medication and dosage. It was clear she knew the names of her medication but not dosages, so these were explained to her. The rest of the session consisted of education about the nature of the medication.

If participants were keen to discuss their medication history or side effects at this stage, it has been our practice to reassure them that these issues will be returned to in later sessions.

The following important points were introduced and discussed. In order to introduce the idea that the medication has a preventative function, the therapist made a list in two columns, one column for short-term medications (e.g. antibiotics for throat infections, aspirin for toothache) and one for long-term medications (e.g. for heart disease, diabetes, schizophrenia, depression). NP was asked to consider the differences between the two types of treatment and, in order to reinforce the concept of prophylactic treatment, an analogy was made between psychosis and diabetes. NP was easily able to come up with examples of illnesses requiring long-term medication and found the diabetes analogy helpful. Other participants have required considerable prompting at this point.

This led naturally to a discussion of the consequences of suddenly stopping medication against medical advice. It was explained that relapses could occur many months after discontinuing in this way. NP conceded that her admission to hospital had been a consequence of her decision to stop taking her medication. She had experienced difficulty sleeping while taking it and had found the regimen inconvenient. She had often forgotten doses and had then consciously stopped altogether in the hope she would be able to sleep better. On becoming increasingly agitated over the following week, she had run away from home with a friend. The therapist used this information to reinforce the idea that patients do not always know when they are becoming ill.

Finally, the therapist discussed the time course of neuroleptic treatment, explaining that patients who resumed taking their medication sometimes had to wait some weeks before experiencing benefits. At the end of the session, NP was asked to summarise the main points that had been covered, which she was able to do.

Session 3: Information about neuroleptics

In the first part of this session, more detailed information about neuroleptic medication was offered to NP. She was given a standard United Kingdom Psychiatric Pharmacy Group leaflet on neuroleptics and was asked to study it with the therapist. The leaflet covers what neuroleptics are for (the names: antipsychotic and tranquilliser are also highlighted), who is prescribed them, and problems and contraindications (e.g. kidney problems, other medications, pregnancy). The non-addictive nature of neuroleptics and their interaction with alcohol are also discussed in the leaflet. NP stated that her current side effects were drowsiness, increased appetite and weight gain, feeling dizzy, and aching muscles. The therapist stressed that doctors try to choose medications with few side effects but that this can be difficult.

NP was told the difference between the approved and proprietary names of her medication, using an analogy with baked beans, which are marketed with many different brand names. The effects of decreasing and increasing doses without her doctor's advice were also discussed to emphasise the importance of following her prescription. It was explained that, if she forgot a dose but remembered within two hours, she should take it; otherwise she should wait until the next scheduled dose.

Session 4: Individual costs and benefits of medication

After being asked to recall the contents of the previous session, NP was asked to list the benefits and costs of her drug treatment. She said that she felt the medication made her feel more relaxed and calm and stopped her from hearing voices. In her opinion, these benefits outweighed the side effects. NP was told about research findings indicating that people who continue to take their neuroleptic medication are much less likely to be readmitted to hospital than those who do not continue.

NP listed the costs of medication as feeling drowsy, aching muscles, putting on weight so that she was not able to fit into some of her clothes, less frequent periods, and feeling dizzy when standing up quickly. She was also experiencing some urine leakage, which she was discussing with her GP. We have found that many participants experience relief on discovering that a puzzling symptom is probably a side effect.

It was stressed that people respond differently to neuroleptic medication, both in terms of benefits and side effects. NP was informed that it was therefore important that she tell the doctor about any positive and negative effects so that her progress on her medication could be assessed. The most bothersome side effect NP experienced was weight gain and the therapist discussed two possible explanations for this: carbohydrate craving and decreased metabolism. NP had started going to an aerobics class with her mother and had also started to cut out fatty foods. She was hopeful this was working as she noted that she was not continuing to put on weight. She had already discussed her infrequent periods with her CPN and was not concerned about this. It also transpired that NP had agreed with her doctor that her evening dose, previously taken at 8pm, could now be taken at 10pm so that she could stay out later in the evenings.

Sessions 5 and 6: Reasons for not taking medication and positive coping statements

NP and the therapist discussed reasons why she does not take her medication and how this problem could be overcome using positive coping statements. A very basic CBT approach was used and practical solutions were discussed in the following session.

NP was asked to think of a time when she had forgotten to take her medication and to discuss the circumstances surrounding this. She said she only occasionally forgot her medication in the morning if she was tired and overslept but that, as her mother usually reminded her, this was not really much of a problem. She felt that she had got into a routine with taking her medication. In the case of patients who report greater difficulties, we work on possible solutions using a problem-solving approach. Possible solutions might include asking a family member to remind them, starting a tick-off calendar, keeping the medication next to the kettle, and so on. Attention is also paid to participants' attitudes towards forgetting.

The same approach was used on occasions when NP had not taken her medication because of side effects or feelings of embarrassment. She discussed her experience of recently stopping her medication and recalled how quickly she had deteriorated to the point of needing hospitalisation. The therapist referred back to previous sessions in which NP had weighed up the costs and benefits of taking medication and she used these examples to frame positive coping statements to take her medication.

Session 7: Discussion of practical solutions to taking medications and review of past sessions

It was agreed that this would be the last session. NP was asked if she had any concerns or doubts about taking her medication.

Various practical options were discussed in relation to problems voiced in the previous session. A plan of action was agreed upon to help NP continue taking her medication. She decided to take a pillbox with her to enable her to take her medication when away from home. Pillboxes, which are available from pharmacists, have separate compartments for each dose and can be pre-loaded, so that it becomes obvious when a dose has been missed. Many medications, such as the contraceptive pill, are now dispensed in blister packs that have this function. However, NP reported that her main strategy for continuing the medication would be to recall its positive effects. Any negative thoughts about the treatment would be counterbalanced with positive statements about the medication as discussed previously. NP was able to give a good review of the past sessions.

Outcome

We obtained both qualitative and quantitative outcome data for NP. Her PANSS scores pre-intervention were 18 on the positive scale, 12 on the negative scale, and 36 on the general psychopathology scale. At 6-month follow-up her scores were 13, 13, and 18 respectively. Her scores on Hogan et al.'s (1981) Drug Attitude Scale (a measure of subjective attitude towards neuroleptics ranging from negative -30 to positive $+30$) were $+16$ at pre-intervention and +26 for all subsequent assessments. We assessed knowledge about neuroleptic medication using a scale developed specifically for the study. On this she scored one pre-intervention and four at both post-intervention and six months, and this reduced to three at one-year follow-up. Specific knowledge about her own medication was scored two at pre-intervention, increased to four at post-intervention and, encouragingly, six for both six-month and one-year follow up. These scores indicate a marked increase in her understanding of her drug treatment.

A qualitative interview was carried out by an independent assessor at the one-year follow-up point. NP stated that the sessions "gave me assurance like that I didn't really need to worry about the illness and there is help out there". About taking her medication she said, "I wanted to take it more because . . . I'd been told" [about the medication]. It transpired that NP had asked to speak to a pharmacist about a new medication she had been prescribed as she wanted to know more about it before agreeing to take it.

CASE STUDY 2: ALLIANCE INTERVENTION

History and initial assessment

BC was a 46-year-old man who lived alone in a bedsit and who had experienced visual hallucinations for many years. A brother and sister lived close by him and he was particularly close to his brother. There was a family history of mental illness. His mother and an uncle had both received psychiatric treatment at some point in their lives.

BC's visual hallucinations had consisted of coloured orbs of blue and gold, which he had accepted as part of his life until his admission to hospital. It was only when he started to see a black orb, and to hear voices blaspheming him and calling him a homosexual, that he became disturbed and had sought psychiatric help. At his first assessment BC presented as a pleasant and cooperative person who was keen to embark on the intervention.

It became apparent that BC had been taking stelazine for many years, which had been prescribed by his GP. However, it also became apparent in the sessions that he was unaware of its true function and believed that he had been taking an antidepressant "to help me cope with my nerves". At the time the intervention commenced, he was in receipt of olanzapine 10mg and paroxetine 20mg daily.

Session 1: Orientation

FR was the therapist. At the beginning of the first session, the aims of the intervention were described in much the same terms used with participants assigned to the compliance condition. BC was then asked to tell the therapist how he came to be in hospital. We have found that this is a useful way of establishing rapport, and introducing the idea that there are many different ways of construing psychiatric disorders. This idea is an important feature of the alliance intervention, because it provides a framework within which patients can choose the account of their difficulties that they find personally most helpful, while at the same time accepting that others (for example, mental health professionals) hold different and equally valid accounts.

BC's account was similar to that given to the independent assessor, and emphasised his distress on hearing voices. Other patients have used this opportunity to describe traumas that led up to hospitalisation, or to reflect on the trauma of being hospitalised. However, BC believed that hospital was the best place to be at that point in time, as he felt safer. Unlike some patients, he did not have any particular complaints about the hospital or his treatment.

Session 2: Keeping track of progress

One important theme of the alliance intervention is encouraging patients to evaluate their treatment for themselves. To do this, participants are asked to keep a personally tailored 15-item Self-Assessment Questionnaire (SAQ: see the panel). Three distressing symptoms are elicited, together with three frequently experienced side effects. These items are then written into the questionnaire and participants are asked to rate them for severity and distress on simple 11-point scales, daily, or at least as often as possible.

It can sometimes be difficult to negotiate items to be included in the SAQ. We have found that this is particularly the case for patients suffering from severe negative symptoms, who may experience difficulty describing what is troubling them. Ideally, the items should be generated by the patient but, in such cases, it may be necessary to suggest possible examples. In the case of

---

Self-Assessment Questionnaire

0–10 point scale (not at all–a great deal)

Unusual experiences or feelings

Distress

Side effects

Attitudes to medication
* medication help
* distress caused by side effects
* problems caused by mental illness

BC, it became apparent that he believed his main problem to be tension and anxiety, which he felt most severely when visiting his local town centre. Alongside this symptom, BC decided to monitor his increasing panic attacks and the extent to which he saw the coloured orbs.

Lack of concentration, memory problems, and dizziness were the most distressing symptoms that BC could attribute to his medication. The therapist discussed the possibility that some of these could be due to the mental health problems he was experiencing. It seemed likely that the dizziness could be related to his panic attacks.

As a consequence of these discussions, BC began to think more clearly about the nature of his difficulties. When asked to summarise them he was able to do so with ease. He clearly understood the rationale behind self-monitoring. He thought the concept was worthwhile and a potentially useful tool in future negotiations with health professionals about his medication.

BC completed his SAQ and reviewed changes in his symptoms at the beginning of all subsequent sessions (see Figs. 15.1 and 15.2).

Session 3: Exploring ideas about mental health

The main aim of the session was to allow the patient to formulate his own model of his mental health problems drawing on different accounts that he had discovered or encountered. He was asked to recall any explanations

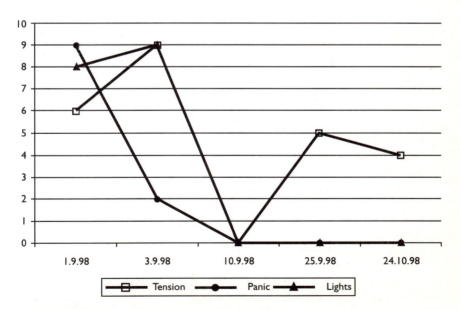

Figure 15.1 Distress caused by BC's unusual experiences.

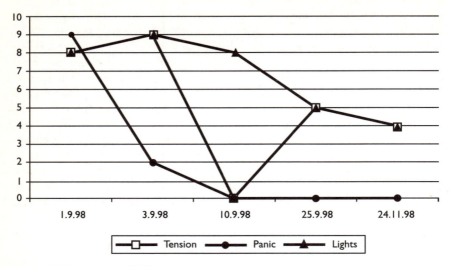

Figure 15.2 Frequency of BC's unusual experiences.

of his symptoms that he had either entertained himself or recalled hearing discussed by someone else. He was able to come up with a number of examples:

- According to BC's psychiatrist, the flashing lights were associated with epilepsy or schizophrenia and the voices were symptoms of schizophrenia. For this reason, BC had been given neuroleptic medication. BC thought it possible that he did actually suffer from a mental illness as his psychiatrist asserted; he was convinced on this point.
- Some years ago BC went to a spiritual medium. According to his account, other people in the room at the time had claimed to see the coloured orbs. In this context, these lights were seen as spiritually significant and related to "people on the other side" who were deceased. BC found this account quite frightening.
- BC's brother had always told him that he would be better off not taking the medication. He did not believe in medication and argued that BC relied on it too much. His brother did not offer suggestions about alternative treatment and seemed to believe that BC should just "get on with it".
- BC's own view was that he did suffer from a mental health problem causing him to feel anxious, fearful of others, and, at times, depressed. However, he also believed that he was more vulnerable to stress than other people and that there could be a genetic link between himself and those in his family who suffered from similar problems. This view was

complicated by BC's spiritual convictions, which were quite strong, and which led him to conclude that his visual hallucinations were quite separate and not due to mental health problems.

In the past BC has practised homeopathy, taken vitamins, and exercised to help himself in an attempt to achieve mental stability. He felt that this had not prevented his admission to hospital but he had maintained these practices anyway. The session concluded with a discussion about stigmatisation. BC felt that some people had given him the "cold shoulder" because of his spiritual beliefs but he chose to ignore them. He was able to summarise the session well and agreed with the suggestion that there are many different models of mental health problems. He filled in his SAQ form for the day and the reduction in panic attacks and apparently paradoxical increase in the distress these cause him was discussed. BC said that this was because he had not visited town during the week because of his fear of having a panic attack.

Sessions 4 and 5: Medication history

This session dealt with BC's questions about medication and involved taking a brief history of his medication taking. BC was first prescribed stelazine 6mg by his GP after he first experienced the visual hallucinations, 18 years prior to the intervention. He has been taking it until his recent hospitalisation, whereupon his medication had been changed to olanzapine and paroxetine. BC described an ideal medication as one that "makes me well, mentally sound, calms me down, and relaxes me". He felt that olanzapine helped "a little bit". BC's worst experience while taking medication had occurred when he had been withdrawn from stelazine, which made him feel "extremely uncomfortable and stressed up". The best thing the medication had done for him was "cure me to a basic extent and has made life more tolerable".

BC was able to summarise adequately the session and afterwards filled in his SAQ form.

Sessions 5, 6, and 7: Communicating with professionals

Latter sessions focused on the importance of communicating with professionals and informing them of both positive and negative effects of medication. The aim of these sessions was to empower the patient to act as a rational consumer, asserting his right to adequate treatment. Many patients find this a quite difficult concept to grasp, as they have been indoctrinated over many years not to question medical judgements. It is therefore important to explain to patients their right to adequate treatment, while at the same time emphasising the virtues of polite and clear communications with professionals.

BC felt that he was already quite proficient at this. As a consequence, role-plays of interviews with psychiatrists were not required. Instead, during these brief sessions, BC was encouraged to decide what he hoped to achieve at forthcoming meetings with his psychiatrist (what questions he wanted to ask, what information he wished to convey about how his treatment was progressing). During following sessions, BC's account of his meetings with his psychiatrist were evaluated against these goals. BC successfully communicated to the consultant that he felt his medication was at too low a dose to be very effective. As a consequence, his medication dose was increased on two separate occasions.

These elements of the alliance intervention were much more problematic in the case of patients who had difficult relationships with their psychiatrists, especially when a reduction in medication dose was required. A limitation of the alliance intervention is that no control is exerted over the behaviour of the prescriber. Although we have occasionally worked with patients who have had their carefully thought out requests rebuffed by unsympathetic medical staff, this has fortunately only occurred exceptionally. More often we have found that the prescriber's helpful response to the patient's change in attitude has encouraged a sense of increased self-efficacy in the latter. In some cases this has been accompanied by substantial improvements in the patient's sense of optimism, accompanied by a shift in mood towards the positive.

On the last visit BC said that he did not suffer from the panic attacks any more. Although he continued to see hallucinatory lights these did not appear to distress him any more. He was about to be discharged from hospital and had decided to live with his brother for company.

Outcome

BC's PANSS scores pre-intervention were 15 on the positive scale, 20 on the negative scale, and 38 on the general psychopathology scale. Post-intervention his scores were 18, 12, and 31, and at 6-month follow-up they were 17, 17 and 31 respectively. These changes were not clinically significant; indeed positive symptoms increased during this period. What did change was BC's distress as a consequence of these symptoms, which was markedly reduced at follow-up.

The main effect of the intervention was to encourage more positive attitudes towards neuroleptic medication. BC's DAI scores were zero at pre-intervention, indicating almost an indifference to the drugs. They were +18 post-intervention and +26 at 6-month follow-up. Although BC's knowledge about medication was not targeted by the intervention, this substantially increased, mainly because he felt enabled to seek advice and information from his keyworker and others. BC's general knowledge about neuroleptic medication was two pre-intervention, four at post-intervention, and three at 6-month follow-up. Specific knowledge about his own medication was three pre-intervention, which increased to six both post-intervention and at six-month follow-up.

DISCUSSION

We have described two highly structured and relatively simple interventions that we are evaluating in an ongoing clinical trial. Because of the nature of the trial, these interventions are highly constrained, limiting opportunities for the therapists to explore problems other than adherence to neuroleptic medication. This meant, for example, that the therapist was unable to discuss NP's experience of abusive sexual relationships with her. Clearly, this kind of limitation would be undesirable in the routine clinical practice of experienced cognitive behaviour therapists. However, this limitation must be offset against the advantage of having available interventions that can be carried out by moderately experienced clinicians who lack specific training in cognitive behavioural techniques. Given the number of patients who are in receipt of neuroleptics, it is unrealistic to expect that trained therapists will be available to address adherence issues in any but a tiny minority of patients.

In describing the interventions, we have chosen case studies that were relatively unproblematic. Our experience is that the majority of patients can be helped in much the same way as NP and BC. However, not all can. In extreme cases, patients may flatly deny that they have a psychiatric difficulty, assert that they are attending hospital because of a general medical condition, or remain mute. Sometimes by proceeding slowly and patiently it is possible to make some progress with such patients, but often it is not.

We have characterised our two interventions as deriving from very different philosophies. This raises questions about which intervention is "best". At present we have no firm data that addresses this issue, so the following points are necessarily subjective and provisional. Our experience is that the alliance intervention is more helpful than the compliance intervention with patients who have a negative or rejecting attitude towards medical care. The compliance intervention, on the other hand, seems particularly suited to patients who have a positive attitude towards their treatment, but who have not been provided with adequate information about its benefits and side effects. (Perhaps the most shocking discovery we have made in our work to date is that by far the majority of patients we have encountered have not received systematic instruction about the nature or effects of their medication.)

Of course, the two interventions are not as different as they might seem at first. During the alliance intervention, patients often request specific information about their drugs, in which case we have provided them with exactly the same information received by the compliance group. We have also encouraged alliance patients to seek information about their treatment elsewhere— from their doctor, from ward staff, from libraries, or even from the Internet. It is possible to think of a spectrum of interventions, ranging from "pure" compliance therapy at one end to "pure" alliance therapy at the other. A competent clinician should be able to pitch an intervention at any point along this spectrum according to the needs of the patient.

REFERENCES

Bentall, R.P., Day, J., Rogers, A., Healy, D., & Stevenson, R.C. (1996). Side effects of neuroleptic medication: Assessment and impact on outcome of psychotic disorders. In M. Moscarelli, A. Rupp, & N. Sartorius (Eds.), *Handbook of mental health economics and health policy, volume I: Schizophrenia* (pp.133–148). London: John Wiley & Sons Ltd.

Boczkowski, J.A., Zeichner, A., & Desanto, N. (1985). Neuroleptic compliance among chronic schizophrenic outpatients. *Journal of Consulting and Clinical Psychology, 53*, 666–671.

Conley, R.R., & Buchanan, R.W. (1997). Evaluation of treatment-resistant schizophrenia. *Schizophrenia Bulletin, 23*, 663–674.

Corrigan, P.W., Liberman, R.P., & Engel, J.D. (1990). From non-compliance to collaboration in the treatment of schizophrenia. *Hospital and Community Psychiatry, 41*, 1203–1211.

Eckman, T.A., & Liberman, R.P. (1990). A large-scale field test of a medication management skills training programme for people with schizophrenia. *Psychosocial Rehabilitation Journal, 13*, 31–35.

Haynes, R.B., Taylor, D.W., & Sackett, D.L. (1979). *Compliance in health care.* Baltimore, MD: Johns Hopkins University Press.

Hogan, T.P., Awad, A.G., & Eastwood, R. (1983). A self-report scale predictive of drug compliance in schizophrenics: Reliability and discriminative validity. *Psychological Medicine, 13*, 177–183.

Kampman, O., & Lehtinen, K. (1999). Compliance in psychoses. *Acta Psychiatrica Scandinavica, 100*, 167–175.

Kane, J.M. (1985). Compliance issues in outpatient treatment. *Journal of Clinical Psychopharmacology, 5*, 22S–27S.

Kay, S.R., Fiszbein, A., & Opler, L.A. (1987). The Positive and Negative Syndrome Scale (PANSS) for schizophrenia. *Schizophrenia Bulletin, 13*, 261–276.

Kelly, G.R., & Scott, J.E. (1990). Medication compliance and health education among chronic outpatients with mental disorders. *Medical Care, 28*, 1181–1197.

Kemp, R., Hayward, P., Applewhaite, G., et al. (1996). Compliance therapy in psychotic patients: Randomised controlled trial. *British Medical Journal, 312*, 345–349.

Kemp, R., Kirov, G., Everitt, B., Hayward, P., & David, A. (1998). Randomised controlled trial of compliance therapy. *British Journal of Psychiatry, 172*, 413–419.

Kissling, W. (1994). Compliance, quality assurance, and standards for relapse prevention in schizophrenia. *Acta Psychiatrica Scandinavica, 89*, 16–24.

Ley, P. (Ed.) (1992). The problem of patients' non-compliance. In *Communicating with patients: Improving communication, satisfaction, and compliance.* London: Chapman & Hall.

Macpherson, R., Jerrom, B., & Hughes, A. (1996). A controlled study of education about drug treatment in schizophrenia. *British Journal of Psychiatry, 168*, 709–717.

McEvoy, J.P, Howe, A.C., & Hogarty, G.E. (1984). Differences in the nature of relapse and subsequent in-patient course between medication compliant and non-compliant schizophrenic patients. *Journal of Nervous and Mental Disease, 172*, 412–416.

Pool, V.E., & Elder, S.T. (1986). A selected review of the literature and an empirical analysis of drug treatment compliance by schizophrenic patients. *International Review of Applied Psychology, 35*, 547–576.

Robinson, D. et al. (1999). Predictors of relapse following response from a first episode of schizophrenia or schizoaffective disorder. *Archives of General Psychiatry, 56*, 241–247.

Rogers, A., Day, J., Williams, B., Randall, F., Wood, P., Healy, D., & Bentall, R.P. (1998). The meaning and management of neuroleptic medication: A study of patients with a diagnosis of schizophrenia. *Social Science and Medicine, 47*, 1313–1323.

Royal Pharmaceutical Society of Great Britain (1997). *From compliance to concordance: Towards shared goals in medicine taking*. London: RPSGB.

Index

Note: page numbers in *italics* refer to figures, page numbers in **bold** refer to tables and information presented in boxes.

ABC framework 109, 112, **113**, 120–1, 123, 187

Adams, M. 243

adapted automatic thoughts diary 27–8, **29–30**

adapted pie chart records 27, 28, **31–3**

adherence: antimanic drugs 242–3, 247, 253, 254, 255, 256, 257–9; cognitive therapy 242–3, 254–5; neuroleptic medication 40, 67, 281–95

agendas, sessional 21

alcohol abuse 266, 268

alternative explanations 17, 92, 153; in attributional therapy 206–7, 209–10, 214; development tools for 28; in multi-factor theory 179–80, 185–6, 187–8, 192; and the onset of psychosis 223–4; salience of 192

ambivalence 267–9

amphetamines 53, 56, 202, 207, 208–9, 268

analysis-to-protocol 85

anger 193

Antecedent and Coping Interview (ACI) 87–90

AnTI 38, 39, **55**

antimanic drugs, adherence 242–3, 247, 253, 254, 255, 256, 257–9

anxiety: catastrophic misinterpretations 148, 154, 156–66, 167–70; and information processing biases 25, 26–7, *26*, *27*, 28; and paranoid delusions 173, 176–8, 181, 182, 184, 192

anxiety psychosis 69

appraisal, patient's: of auditory hallucinations 109, 110, 133; and coping ability 79, 80, 86; of paranoid delusions 178, 179

arbitrary inference 61, 65, 174, 199

assessment: Antecedent and Coping Interview 87–90; of antecedent stimuli/context 88–9; of auditory hallucinations 38–40, 87–8, 113–15, 136, 202–5, **203–4**; of catastrophic misinterpretations of anxiety 154–6; of emotional reactions 88; of general functioning 39; of paranoid delusions 38–40, 87, 117, 155, 202–5, **203–4**, 226, *227*; pretherapy 21–2; of psycho-social features 83; of psychological features 83; of social features 83; in social rank theory 113–15, 117; of substance abuse 271; of suitability for treatment 42; of the therapeutic relationship 44–5, *see also specific rating systems*

attention: narrowing 91, 96–7; selective 141–2, 166; self-focused 133–4, 141–2; switching 91

attributional biases 66–7, 202–5, **204**, 271; externalising 197, 199, 205; personalising 198, 199, 205, 206

attributional therapy 197–214, *198*; attribution measures **204**, 205; case report 200–14; qualitative analysis of attributional change 205–8; search strategies 198–200, 205, 206, 214; termination strategies 198–200, 205, 206, 214

auditory hallucinations 46, 49, 113–15, *116*; activating events 109, 112, **113**,

123, 139; assessment 38–40, 87–8,
113–15, 136, 202–5, **203–4**; and
attention 141–2; attributional
approach to 200–14, **203–4**;
benevolent 111; cognitive approach to
108, 125, 135–44, **138**, *143*, *145*; and
cognitive biases 132–3; cognitive
models of 132–5; command type 108,
109, 110, 121–6; compliance with 109,
110–11, 123, 125; consequences of 109,
112, **113**; coping strategies 94, 95–6,
97; as defence mechanism 133;
definition 132; emotional reactions to
88; and entrapment 108, 109, 110, 111;
malevolent 111; and medication
adherence 284, 289; as misattribution
of an internal source to an external
source 132–3, 134; modulators 139;
analogy with panic disorder 148;
patient's appraisal of 109, 110, 133;
patient's beliefs about 109, 112, **113**,
142; patient's interpretations of 62–3,
133, 134, 138–40, **141**; patient's
relationship to 108, 109, 110, 111–12,
114, 126; power of 109, 110–12, 114,
123; social rank approach to 108–16,
121–6, **127–9**; and subordination 109,
110, 111–12, 123, 124–6
Auditory Hallucinations Rating Scale
(AHRS) 202
Austin, S.V. 154
automatic thoughts diary, adapted 27–8,
29–30
autonomy 5, 11, 281, 283
avoidance behaviours 177, 187
awareness training 92

Baker, A. 134
Baker, G. 133
Barrowclough, Christine 265–80
Basco, M. 241
Bauer, M. 243–4
Bebbington, P. 66, 134
Beck, Aaron T. 3–14, 15–18, 19, 20, 37,
46, 82, 144, 223, 236–9
Beck Anxiety Inventory 181, 189, *191*
Beck Depression Inventory (BDI) 38, 39,
55, 181, 189, *191*
Beckett, R. 134
behavioural modification 79–80
behavioural responses, and psychotic
symptoms 82

behavioural tests 28, 34–6, **35**, 50–2, 94,
137, 153, 161–3, 165
belief–congruent behaviour 82
beliefs: adaptation 60; core 165–6;
correction 20; in mania 237;
modification 72, 73, 93–4, 150, 153–4;
normal 61; regarding psychotic
symptoms 80, 109, 112, **113**, 142,
165–6; self 17, *see also* delusions
Beliefs About Voices Questionnaire
(BAVO) 113–14
Benn, Andy 197–216
Benson, J.E. 198
Bentall, Richard P. 66, 92, 132–3, 175,
178, 197–8, 200, 219–35, 281–95
Berrios, G. 61
biological aetiology: bipolar disorder
240, *240*, 241; schizophrenia 149, 150,
152, 219
bipolar disorder 135, 140, 236–61;
adjustment facilitation 246; case
report 248–60; clinical rationale for
cognitive therapy 239–43;
formulations for *242*, 244–8, 250,
251–2; generic approach 240–1, *240*;
outcome measures 243–4; patient
education 245–6, 252, 260; relapse
prevention **245**, 247–8, 255–60, **257**;
self-monitoring/self-regulation 246–7,
248, 253, 257; structuring CT for
244–8, **245**; theoretical models 236–43,
238, *240*, *242*, 250, 251
Birchwood, Max 37, 63, 82, 108–31, 133,
134–5, 178
Bjorkman, T. 135
Blackburn, I.M. 43
booster sessions 166, 192
borrowed guilt 3, 7, 10, 12–13, 16, 17
Brabban, Alison 59–75
brainstorming 158
Brief Limited Intermittent Psychotic
Symptoms (BLIPS) Group 226,
228
bucket–filling analogy 71, *71*

California Psychotherapeutic Alliance
Scale (CALPAS) 44–5
carbamazepine 259
care in the community 41
carers, formal 104
catastrophic misinterpretation 148, 154,
156–66, 167–70

causal attributions *see* attributional biases; attributional therapy
Chadwick, P.D. 37, 63, 82, 133, 134–5, 150, 153–4, 174, 178
charges 238–9
Chisholm, D. 134
Clark, D.M. 170
Cochran, S. 243
cognitions, basis of 19–20
cognitive biases: attributional 66–7, 197–9, 202–6, **204**, 271; patient's understanding of 65; and psychotic symptoms 61, 66–7, 82, 132–3, *see also* reasoning biases
cognitive dissonance 60, 61–2
cognitive model 20, 46, 79; and auditory hallucinations 132–5; Beck's Integrative Model 238–9, *238*; Beck's original model 236–8, 241; generic 15; and the onset of psychosis 223–5, *224*, 231; and panic disorder 148–9, 154, 170; and schizophrenia 82; simple 65, *70*, 72
cognitive responses, and psychotic symptoms 82
cognitive therapy model 37
cognitive triad: negative 237; positive 237
collaboration 20, 167
compliance: auditory hallucinations 109, 110–11, 123, 125; medication 281
compulsive behaviour 4, 39–41, 46
conclusions, jumping to 61, 65, 174, 199
concordance 281
conditional assumption formation 46–8
confirmation bias 174
conspiracy, fears of 22–3, 25–35, 136–8
containment 67
context, and psychotic symptoms 88–9
controlling behaviour 5, 11
coping strategies 79–104; acquisition period 98; assessment of psychotic symptoms 87–90; attention narrowing 91, 96–7; attention switching 91; awareness training 92; behaviour experiments 94; belief modification 93–4; for bipolar disorder **245**, 259–60; case report 95–8; de-arousing techniques 92, 97; definition 86; efficacy 84–6; enhancement 94–5; increased activity levels 93, 96–7; internal dialogue 91–2; intervention 90–5, 96–8, 100, *101*; methods 91–4;

model of psychotic illness 82; modified self-statements 91–2; reattribution 92, 97; reality-testing 94, 97; relapse prevention 84, 98–104, *99*, *101*; and self-esteem 99–102, *101*; social engagement/disengagement 93; training 90–4
Coping Strategy Enhancement (CSE) 84–6
core beliefs 165–6
Corrigan, P.W. 283
cost–benefit analysis, medication use 258, **258**, 287
counselling, supportive 84, 85, 104
critical incidents 48, 112
Crow, T.J. 220
cultural issues 133, *see also* ethnic minorities

DAI 294
data gathering bias 174
Davidson, K.M. 43
Day, Jennifer 281–95
de-arousing techniques 92, 97
defence mechanisms: auditory hallucinations as 133; delusions as 66–7, 69–70, 72, 175
defining cognitive therapy 19, 37
delusional memories 69, 73
delusional mood 61
delusions: in anxiety psychosis 67–72; and belief modification 150, 153–4; catastrophic misinterpretations of anxiety 148, 154, 156–66, 167–70; and cognitive biases 61; defensive function 66–7, 69–70, 72; definition 62; efficacy of cognitive treatment 85, 135; formation 61; grandiose 121; and meaning 61–2; modification v confrontation 72, 73; reality-testing 38, 48, 50–2, 56, *56*; of reference 174–5; as unique entity 61, *see also* paranoid delusions
Delusions Rating Scale (DRS) *see* Psychotic Symptom Rating Scale
depression: and auditory hallucinations 110; Beck's model of 236–9; in bipolar disorder 248, 249, 250–1; cognitive vulnerability to 237; and paranoid delusions 178–9, 181, 182–3, 187, 192, *see also* bipolar disorder
developmental formulations 28–36, *34*

diagnosis, problematic nature in
    schizophrenia 63
dichotomous thinking 65
DiClemente, P.P. 267
"disaster averting" behaviours 39–40, 41,
    46
disfigurement, delusions of 116–21
dissonant states 60
dominance 108, 115, 124
downward arrow technique 160, 164
drop out rates 85
Drug Attitude Scale 288–9
drugs: abuse 24, 28, 142, 202, 207, 208–9,
    265–79, *see also* medication;
    medication adherence
DSM–IV 132
Dudley, R.E.J. 174
Dunn, G. 134
Dunn, Hazel 37–58
duration of untreated psychosis (DUP)
    220
dysfunctional thought records (DTRs)
    138, 139, 160, 246, 252, 253

early experiences, link with psychotic
    symptoms 5–8, 11, 15, 23–4, 28, *34*, 46,
    66, 68–9, 115, 122, 181
Early Signs Scale 232
early warning signs 54, **54**, 55, 248, 255–6
Eckman, J.A. 282–3
education: regarding bipolar disorder
    245–6, 252, 260; regarding cognitive
    therapy 20; regarding medication 282,
    283, 286–7; regarding substance abuse
    274–5
efficacy, cognitive therapy 84–6, 134–5
Emery, G. 19, 37
emotions: emphasis on in cognitive
    therapy 20; and psychotic symptoms
    88, 173, 176–9, 192, 193
engagement 43–4, 86, 118, 167, 225–6,
    250–2
Engel, J.D. 283
entrapment 108, 109, 110, 111, 126
escape behaviours 177
Escher, A.D.M.A.C. 62–3
ethnic minorities 116–26
"experiential approach" 20
externalising bias 197, 199, 205

family dynamics: in a case of bipolar
    disorder 246, 249–50, 252–3, 259; in a

case of catastrophic misinterpretation
    of anxiety 157–8; power relationships
    112, 115, 122, 123, 124–5, 126
family intervention 104, 266, 273–8
father–daughter relationship 68
father–son relationship: in a case of
    bipolar disorder 249, 252–3; in a case
    of chronic schizophrenia 4–5, 7–13,
    15–17
Fennell, M. 104, 260
Ferrier, N. 238
five systems model 157, 161–2
flashcards **257**
forms: adapted automatic thoughts diary
    27–8, **29–30**; adapted pie chart records
    27, 28, **31–3**; behavioural experiment
    type **35**; standard 27
formulations 46–54, *47*, 56, *56*, 173; in
    attributional therapy 208–9, 213; for
    auditory hallucinations 96–8, 115,
    138–43, **138**, *143*, 144; for bipolar
    disorder *242*, 244–8, 250, 251–2; for
    catastrophic misinterpretation of
    anxiety 157, 161, 164, 166–70, *168*,
    168–9; coping strategy type 96–8;
    definition 62; for delusional beliefs
    69–73, *70–1*, 96–8, 115, *116*, 120–1,
    120, 136–8, 174, 179, 182–6, *183*,
    192–3, 208–9; longitudinal 167–70,
    169, 228–30, *229*; in multi-factorial
    therapy 174, 179, 182–4, *183*, 185–6,
    192–3; in preventive treatment 228–30,
    229; schema level 65–6; sharing with
    patients 63–4; in a simple cognitive
    model 65, *70*, 72; in social rank theory
    115, *116*, 120–1, *120*; in a stress
    vulnerability model 64–5, 71; for
    substance abuse 271; symptom level
    167, *168*, *see also* interventions
Fowler, D. 134
Fowler, F. 65–6
Francey, S. 222
Freeman, Daniel 134, 173–96
French, Paul 219–35
Frith, C.D. 133–4, 174–5
fundamental attribution error 199

gains, therapeutic 56–7
Garety, Philippa A. 61, 65–6, 134, 173–96
Garland, A. 238, 244
general functioning, assessment 39–40
generic approach 15, 240–1, *240*

genetic vulnerability, to schizophrenia 149, 150, 152, 219
Gilbert, D.T. 198–9
Gilbert, Paul 108–31
Giuliano, T.A. 198
Global Assessment of Functioning (GAF) 226
goals 20; lists 22–3, 48–9, 136, 185, 230, **231**, 252; reasons for focusing on 48; route to achievement 48; setting 274, 275, 278
"going out", difficulties with 22, 23
Goldstein, M. 261
Greenberger, D. 240, 250
group identity 119–21, *120*
guilt 3, 7, 10, 12–13, 16, 17, 40

Haddock, Gillian 92, 133, 134, 220, 265–80
Hadley, C. 134
Hafna, R.J. 72
Haggerty, R.J. 221
hallucinations 85, 273; visual 114, 121, 289, 292–3, *see also* auditory hallucinations
Hansson, L. 135
Harrigan, S. 222
Harrow, M. 62
Harwood, S. 134
Havers, S. 133
Haynes, R.B. 281
Healy, David 281–95
Heilbrum, A.R. 133
Hemsley, D.R. 61
high–risk individuals: identification of 221–2; preventive therapy for 219–33
Hogan, T.P. 288
homework 21; for auditory hallucinations 138, 206; for bipolar disorder 246, 252–3; for catastrophic misinterpretation of anxiety 157, 159, 160, 161; for delusional beliefs 51–2, 187, 231–2; for improving self-esteem 102
homoerotic impulses 4, 9, 11
Honig, A. 62–3
"hot thoughts" 160
Hovland, C. 44
humiliation 110, 126
Husby, R. 225
hyperpositive thinking 237
hypervigilance 133, 142, 161, 226

hypothesis preservation 60, 82

ICD-10 284
idealisation 5
ideas, overvalued 73
identification 9, 11, 12–13, 16, 17
identity 119–21, *120*
imagery techniques 17
imagination 16, 19
incest 284
increased activity levels 93, 96–7
individualised approach 241; substance abuse/psychosis dual diagnosis 266, 270–3; treatment of schizophrenia 151–3, 167, *168*, 170–1
information processing biases 26–7, *26*, *27*, 176–7, 182–3
insight 11, 13
Institute of Psychiatry 66
Integrative Model 238–9, *238*
"intellectual approach" 20
internal dialogue 91–2
Internal, Personal and Situational Attributions Questionnaire (IPSAQ) **204**, 205
interpretative biases 25–7, 28, *see also* reinterpretation
interventions 25–8, 42–57, 115, 124–5; in attributional therapy 209–12, 213; for bipolar disorder 250–60; for catastrophic misinterpretation of anxiety 155–70, **156**, *168–9*; coping strategy type 90–5, 96–8, 100, *101*; for delusions of disfigurement 118–21, *120*; for medication adherence 283, 284–8, 289–94, 295; multi-factorial 173–4, 184–8, 192, 193; preventive 222–3, 227–32; in social rank theory 115, 118–21, *120*, 124–5; for substance abuse/psychosis dual diagnosis 266, 273; theoretical background 149–50, *see also* formulations
interviews: Antecedent and Coping Interview 87–90; motivational for substance abuse 266–9; structured 17

Jackson, H.J. 222
Janis, I. 44
Jaspers, K. 61
John, C.H. 174
Johnson, A. 220
Johnstone, E.C. 220

Junginger, J. 110

Kaney, S. 66, 197, 220, 223
Kanfer, F.H. 79–80, 92
Karoly, P. 79–80, 92
Kelley, H.H. 44
Kelly, G.R. 282
Kemp, R. 283
Kinderman, Peter 197–216, 220, 223
Kingdon, D.G. 63, 133, 154, 167
Kinney, C.F. 86
Kissling, W. 282
Knight, Alice 219–35
Kuipers, E. 65–6, 66, 134

Lampl, H. 12
latent content 11, 12
"laughing bouts" 50
learning 59–60, 90
Lewis, Shôn 265–80
Liberman, R.P. 282–3
life skills training 150
life stresses: critical incidents 48, 112;
    link with schema and psychotic
    symptoms 59–73; and relapse
    prevention 98; and schizophrenia 149,
    150, 152, 219, see also early experience
Limb, K. 244
lithium 236, 243, 253, 254, 255, 256, 259
Lowe, C.F. 150, 153–4

McBride, L. 243–4
McCarthy, E. 244
McFarlane, C.A. 222
McGorry, P.D. 222
Macmillan, J. 220
McNulty, S.E. 198
Manchester trial 104
mania 236–9, 248–9, 250, see also bipolar
    disorder
Marks, I. 92
Meaden, Alan 108–31
meaning: and delusions 61–2; search for
    59–73
Medical Research Council 283
medication: in bipolar disorder 236,
    242–3, 247, 253, 254, 255, 256, 257–9;
    compliance 281; concordance 281;
    preventive treatment 222, see also
    medication adherence
medication adherence 40, 67, 281–95;
    alliance intervention 283, 289–94, 295;

appropriate dosages 282; in bipolar
    disorder 242–3, 247, 253, 254, 255,
    256, 257–9; case reports 284–95;
    compliance intervention 283, 284–9,
    295; consequences of non–adherence
    282; coping strategies for 287–8;
    cost–benefit analysis 258, **258**, 287;
    education 282, 283, 286–7; outcomes
    288–9, 294; patient's evaluation of the
    impact of 53; self–monitoring 290–1,
    291, *292*; and side effects 282, 287
Meehl, Paul 219
memories, delusional 69, 73
mental health professional–patient
    relations: medication adherence 282–3,
    293–4, *see also* therapeutic relationship
metacognitive processes 28, 178
Miklowitz, D. 261
Miller, W.R. 267
Milton, F. 72
"mind–reading" 50–2
misinterpretations: correction 37, 50–2,
    56, *56*, *see also* catastrophic
    misinterpretations
modes 238–9
Moller, P. 225
mood: delusional 26–7, *26*, *27*, 61; low
    132; thought connection 65, 72
Moorhead, S. 244
Moring, Jan 265–80
Morrison, Anthony P. 132–47, 219–35
Morriss, R. 244
mother–daughter relationship 68, 275–6,
    277–8
mother–son relationship: in a case of
    bipolar disorder 249, 250–1, 252–3,
    259; in a case of chronic schizophrenia
    5, 11; in a case of paranoia 23
motivation 44
motivational interviews 266–9
Mrazek, P.J. 221
multi–factorial approach 173–93; case
    report 180–91, 192–3; contemporary
    theories on persecutory delusions
    174–6; theoretical ideas from neurosis
    176–9; therapeutic approach 179–80

narcolepsy 53
negative symptoms 85
neuroleptic medication: adherence 40,
    67, 281–95; atypical 222; preventive
    222

neurosis: parallels with psychosis 173–4, 176–9, 193, *see also specific neuroses*
neutralising behaviours 39–40, 41, 46
"noise in the night" illustration 187–8
Noordhoorn, E.O. 62–3
normalisation 51, 52, 65, 186, 206
Northwick Park study 220
"not knowing" 60
Nuechterlein, K.H. 79
number of patients needed to treat (NNT) 85

obsessional thoughts 4, 8–9
obsessive-compulsive disorder 40–1, 46
olanzapine 222, 289, 293
onset of psychotic illness: impact 99–100; model of 223–5, *224*, 231
operant conditioning principles 150
outcome measures 55, **55**, 144, *145*, 151–2, 189–91, *189–91*; attributional therapy for paranoia and hallucinations 212–13; bipolar disorder 243–4; medication adherence 288–9, 294; preventive treatment *227*, 232–3; in social rank theory 120–1, 126
Over, D.E. 174
overvalued ideas 73

Padesky, C. 240, 250
Palmer, A. 243
panic disorder, cognitive model 148–9, 154, 170
paranoid delusions: and anxiety 173, 176–8, 181, 182, 184, 192; assessment 38–40, 87, 117, 155, 202–5, **203–4**, 226, *227*; attributional approach to 197–8, *198*, 200–14, **203–4**; behavioural tests for 52; and borrowed guilt 3, 7, 10, 12–13, 16, 17; case reports 3–4, 6–13, 15–17, 19, 21–36, 39–40, 45–6, 49, 52, 95–8, 121, 123, 125, 136–8, **138**, 154–70, 180–93; catastrophic misinterpretation of anxiety 154–70; and cognitive biases 174; contemporary theories of 174–6; coping strategies for 95–6, 97–8, 100–2, *101*; as defence mechanisms 175; and depression 178–9, 181, 182–3, 187, 192; of disfigurement 116–21; dynamic processes of 11, 12; and emotional processes 173, 176–9, 192, 193; formation 175, 179, 185–6, 193;

goal lists for 49; imagery 11; jealousy/betrayal theme 114, 115, *116*; latent content 11, 12; maintenance 175, 179, 182, *183*, 185–6, 187–8, 193; multi-factorial perspective 173–93; patient's appraisal of 178, 179; patient's interpretation/relationship with 179; preventive treatment 226; and reasoning biases 174, 183–4, 187–8, 193; and social rank theory 114, 115, 116–21, *116*, 125; and substance abuse 272, 273; and theory of mind 174–5
Parkinsonism, post–encephalitic 4–5
patient contributions 56–7
patient motivation 44
patient understanding 21, 27–8, 62, 64, 185–6, 242–3, *see also* insight
Patton, G.C. 222
Patwa, V.K. 72
perception 60
"peripheral questioning" 154
Perry, A. 244
Persaud, R. 92
person level approach *see* individualised approach
personal resources *see* coping strategies; self-efficacy
personalising bias 198, 199, 205, 206
persuasive communication 44
Phillips, L.J. 222
physical health, preoccupation with 46, 49–50
physiological sensation, catastrophic misinterpretation of 148, 154, 156–66, 167–70
pie chart records, adapted 27, 28, **31–3**
Positive and Negative Syndrome Scale (PANSS) 21, 38, **55**, 135, **135**, 155, 202, **203**, 213, 226, *227*, 232, 284, 288, 294
positive symptoms *see* auditory hallucinations; delusions; hallucinations; paranoid delusions
Post-Traumatic Stress Disorder (PTSD) 99
Powell, G.E. 154
power relationships: in families 112, 115, 122, 123, 124–5, 126; with voices 109, 110–12, 114, 123
Power Scale 114, 123, **128–9**
Present State Examination 87
preventive treatment 219–33; case

reports 225–33; engagement 225–6; identifying high-risk individuals 220–2; indicated 221; interventions 222–3, 227–32; onset of psychosis 223–5, *224*; primary 221; secondary 220–1; selective 221; universal 221; value of 220–1, *see also* relapse prevention
principles of cognitive therapy 20–1
probabilistic reasoning 61
problem lists 45–6, 136, 143; for bipolar disorder 244–5, 251, 252; for substance abuse/psychosis dual diagnosis 269, 274, 276–7
problem-solving format 21, 22–3, 84, 98
Prochaska, J.O. 267
prodromal symptoms 98, 220, 222, 226, 248, 255–6, 259
progress, therapeutic 42–57
PSE–10 188
psycho-social features: assessment 83, *see also* life stresses
psychological features, assessment 83
psychological reactance 153, 154
psychotherapy 3–13, 15–18
Psychotic Symptom Rating Scale (PSYRATS) 38, **55**, 87, 135, **135**, 138, *138*, *145*, 155, 156, 166, **166**, 202, **203**, 213
psychotic symptoms 85; antecedent stimuli 88–9, 96, 100, *101*; assessment 38–9, 87–90; behavioural responses 82; cognitive responses 82; consequences of 81–2, *81*, 89; context 88–9; coping strategies 80, 84, 90; emotions accompanying 88; feedback loops *81*, 82, 100; induction 162–3; link with life events and schema 59–73; models of 37, 80–3, *81*; nature and variation 87–8; and psycho-social stress 152; re-emergence 98; vulnerabilities to 80, *81*, *see also* negative symptoms; positive symptoms
punishment 12–13, 16

racial identity 119–20
Randall, Fiona 281–95
Rattenbury, F. 62
Raune, D. 66
reattribution 92, 97
reality, misconstructions of 19, *see also* delusions; paranoid delusions

reality-testing 20, 38, 48, 50–2, 56, *56*, 94, 97, 153, 187; failure 16, 17, *see also* behavioural tests
reasoning biases 174, 183–4, 187–8, 193, 197–9, *see also* cognitive biases
record keeping, patient's: for bipolar disorder 246, 252, 253; for medication adherence 290–1; for paranoid delusions 186–7, *see also* dysfunctional thought records
referral 22, 38, 226
reinterpretation 27–8, 38
relapse prevention: for auditory hallucinations 144; for bipolar disorder **245**, 247–8, 255–60, **257**; coping strategies for 84, 98–104; and life stresses 98; and medication adherence 282, 285–6; patient identification of early warning signs 53–4, 55; and self-esteem 99–104, *99*, *101*; and symptom re-emergence 98, *see also* preventive treatment
relapse signature 248, 255–6
Renton, Julia 19–36
repression 5
risperidone 40, 182, 284
ritualised behaviours 39–40, 41, 46
Rogers, Anne 281–95
role–plays 18, 252
Rollnick, S. 267
Romme, M.A.J. 62–3
routine care 84–6
Rush, A. 19, 37, 241
Rush, A.J. 19, 37

Sackett, D.L. 281
safety behaviours 163–4, 177–8, 187, 193
Safran, J.D. 42
Salkovskis, P.M. 177
Saslow, G. 79
schema theory 16–17, 59–73, 112; compensatory schema 61–2, 65–6, 69; core maladaptive schema 65–6, 69; schema activation 69; schema as basis of cognitions 20; schema formation 46–8; schema modification 166; schematic vulnerability 67, 73; self-schemas 16–17, 99–102, *99*, *101*, 103–4, 237; therapeutic formulations 65–6
schizoaffective disorder 283, 284
schizophrenia 37, 41, 149–52; aetiology

149, 150, 152, 219–20; auditory hallucinations 132, 133; case reports 3–13, 15–18, 59, 95–8, 148, 155–70; chronic 3–13, 15–18; coping strategies 80, 84, 91, 92, 93, 95–8; de-arousing techniques 92; engagement 86; family intervention 104; individualised treatment of 151–4, 167, *168*, 170–1; medication adherence 281, 282, 283; misconstructions of reality 19; models of 80, *81*, 82–3, 149–50; outcome data 151–2; preventive treatment 221; problematic nature of the diagnosis 63, 148, 151–2, 170; and self-esteem 99; and self-referent beliefs 115; and substance abuse 276, 278–9; theory of mind 174–5; variability in presentation 151
schizotaxia 219
Scott, J.E. 282
Scott, Jan 236–64
search strategies 198–200, 205, 206, 214
Segal, Z.V. 42
selective abstraction 65
selective attention 141–2, 166
Self-Assessment Questionnaire (SAQ) 290–1, **290**
self-efficacy 79
self-esteem: and attributional biases 202–5, **204**; in bipolar disorder 260; and compensatory schema 69; delusional maintenance 66–7, 72; improvement 102–4; loss 126; low 99–104, *99*, 178–9, 181, 182; measures of 202–5, **204**
self-focused attention 133–4, 141–2
self-harm 117, 118, 121, 122, *see also* suicide
self-image 15–18
self-monitoring: bipolar disorder 246, 248, 257; drug adherence 290–1, *291*, *292*; and the onset of psychosis 224, *see also* dysfunctional thought records; record keeping, patient's
self-referent beliefs 115
self-regulation 79–104, 246–7, 253
self-schemas: in mania 237; negative 99–102, *99*, *101*, 103–4; poorly defined 16–17
self-statements, modified 91–2
self-worth 132
"selling" the cognitive model 44

sessional agendas 21
Shaw, B.F. 19, 37
sibling relationships 68
side effects 40, 53
Slade, P.D. 92, 133
social anxiety and avoidance 23, 93, 132, 230–1
Social Cognitive Behavioural Therapy 104
Social Comparison Rating Scale **127**
social evaluative beliefs 119–21
social features, assessment 83
Social Functioning Scale 39
Social Rank Scale 123
social rank theory 108–26, **127–9**; ABC framework 109, 112, **113**, 120–1, 123, 187; case reports 113–26, *116*, *120*; model 110–13
social skills training 150
socialisation 44, 250–2
Socrates trial 167, 200, 201, 202, 212
Socratic method (guided discovery) 21, 255, 258
Spring, B. 64, 80
Stanton, B. 238
stelazine 289, 293
Stoll, F. 62
Strauss, J.S. 61
stress diathesis models 179, 236, 240, 250
stress management, familial 274, 275, 278
stress vulnerability model 64–5, 71, 79–80, 149–50, 176, 182, 219, 223–4
structured nature of cognitive therapy 21
Subjective Units of Distress (SUDs) scales 187
subordination 109, 110, 111–12, 123, 124–6
substance abuse 24, 28, 142, 202, 207–9, 265–79; assessment 271; case reports 272, 275–8; family intervention 266, 273–8; formulations 271; individualised CT 266, 270–3; motivational interviews for 266–9; patient ambivalence regarding 267–9
suicide 19, 22, 25, 36, 39, 122
Suitability for Short-Term Cognitive Therapy Rating Scale 42
suitability for treatment 42
Svensson, B. 135
symptoms *see* psychotic symptoms

Tarrier, Nicholas 79–107, 133, 134, 135, 220, 244, 265–80
Taylor, D.W. 281
termination strategies 198–200, 205, 206, 214
theory of mind 174–5, 198
therapeutic gains 56–7
therapeutic relationship 11; assessment 44–5; building 184–5; containment 67; emphasis of 21, 38, 42–5; engagement 43–4; patient's concerns about 41; sharing formulations 64
therapists: fallibility 73; playing down the role of 56–7; qualities of 43, 44; "selling" the cognitive model 44
thioridazine 40
third-party involvement 258–9
thought–mood connection 65, 72
time limited nature of cognitive therapy 21
Trower, Peter 37, 108–31, 178
Turkington, Douglas 59–75, 133, 154

Ugarteburu, I. 134
understanding: patient 21, 27–8, 62, 64, 185–6, 242–3, *see also* insight

violent behaviour, towards others 109, 111, 121, 122, 123
visual hallucinations 114, 121, 289, 292–3
vocational training 118–19
voices *see* auditory hallucinations

Walford, Lara 219–35
Watt, F.N. 154
Williams, H. 243
Williams, Steven 148–72
Wood, Pam 281–95
worrying 192–3

Young, A.W. 174
Yung, A. 222
Yusupoff, L. 134

Zubin, J. 64, 80